A SURVIVAL GUIDE TO
CHILDREN'S NURSING

Titles in this series:

*This book is dedicated, with honour, respect and devotion,
to our supportive and loving parents and family.*

For Elsevier
Content Strategist: Mairi McCubbin
Content Development Specialist: Sheila Black
Project Manager: Sruthi Viswam
Designer: Miles Hitchen
Illustration Manager: Jennifer Rose

A SURVIVAL GUIDE TO
CHILDREN'S NURSING

Sharon Edwards MSc DipN(Lon) PGCEA RGN

Senior Lecturer, Faculty of Society and Health, Buckinghamshire New University, Uxbridge, UK

Imelda Coyne BSc(HONS) MA PhD DipN RSCN RGN RNT FEANS

Professor in Children's Nursing, School of Nursing and Midwifery, Trinity College Dublin, Ireland

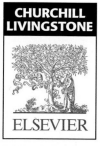

CHURCHILL
LIVINGSTONE

ELSEVIER

Edinburgh London New York Oxford Philadelphia St Louis Sydney Toronto 2013

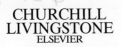
ISBN 978-0-7020-4227-0

British Library Cataloguing in Publication Data
A catalogue record for this book is available from the British Library

Library of Congress Cataloging in Publication Data
A catalog record for this book is available from the Library of Congress

Notices
Knowledge and best practice in this field are constantly changing. As new research and experience broaden our understanding, changes in research methods, professional practices, or medical treatment may become necessary.

Practitioners and researchers must always rely on their own experience and knowledge in evaluating and using any information, methods, compounds, or experiments described herein. In using such information or methods they should be mindful of their own safety and the safety of others, including parties for whom they have a professional responsibility.

With respect to any drug or pharmaceutical products identified, readers are advised to check the most current information provided (i) on procedures featured or (ii) by the manufacturer of each product to be administered, to verify the recommended dose or formula, the method and duration of administration, and contraindications. It is the responsibility of practitioners, relying on their own experience and knowledge of their patients, to make diagnoses, to determine dosages and the best treatment for each individual patient, and to take all appropriate safety precautions.

To the fullest extent of the law, neither the Publisher nor the authors, contributors, or editors, assume any liability for any injury and/or damage to persons or property as a matter of products liability, negligence or otherwise, or from any use or operation of any methods, products, instructions, or ideas contained in the material herein.

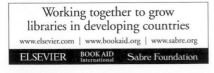
Printed in China

Contents

Contents

Preface

The ability to provide good evidence-based care for children of all ages in hospitals and in the community is what children's nurses, both pre- and post-qualification, seek to achieve. This does not profess to be the sole book of choice within children's nursing but to act in a supportive and informative way to the novice children's nurse practitioner, and to provoke further reading of current literature within the speciality. The book is a compact, pocket-sized companion that we hope will come to be regarded by its users as a friend that children's nurses can refer to while working.

The aim of this book is to provide an insight into children's nursing and highlight the important physiological, psychological and social areas, alongside legal issues, and ethical and moral dilemmas that children's nurses may face on a daily basis. It also aims to be a survival guide and constant companion during those first early days in practice as a student and provide answers to some of the many questions you will continue to ask well beyond your qualification and early years as a staff nurse in children's nursing. As children's nursing involves many different disciplines, the book is aimed not only at student nurses and qualified nurses undertaking relevant specialist courses/modules but also at student and qualified operating department practitioners, paramedics, physiotherapists, medical students, radiographers and occupational therapists. The objective is that, as team players in the decision-making process within children's nursing, they will develop a better working environment.

The book is divided into six sections covering aspects of care and management related to children's nursing today. You will find information on caring for children from birth to 16 years of age, emergency care of a child, assessment of children, haemodynamic monitoring, diagnostic procedures, children's nursing interventions, and common conditions related to medical and surgical conditions using a systems approach. In addition, the book includes mental ill health in children (a new and expanding area in children's nursing), psychological and ethical care, including areas related to professional practice, palliative care and drugs. The factual information provided will assist in your provision of holistic care, to improve your patient care and to enable you to do more than just 'survive' in children's wards today. Question boxes have been inserted throughout the book to stimulate further thought, reflection and discussion. You will find at the back of the book a reference list to support the book and some relevant web pages/sites that might further inform and develop your understanding of the practice of caring for children.

Children's wards may be noisy, busy, emotionally charged, daunting and containing complex technology, but for those of us who have spent a number of years in caring for children it is usually a welcoming, friendly and supportive environment. It is this picture we want to put across in our book. We wish to help open the doors to the very special area of expertise that is children's nursing. We hope that this small book will inspire you to spend time improving your knowledge and understanding, so that you can provide warm and sensitive care to children and families, using your competencies and evidence-based interventions.

Uxbridge and Dublin, 2012

Sharon Edwards
Imelda Coyne

Section 1

General principles of children's nursing

1.1 Introduction

Children's wards are dedicated to the management of children with acute or chronic illness, injuries or complications. They are specially staffed and equipped for the prevention of complications or the reduction of their severity.

For some, children's nursing may be a daunting prospect. You may have queries and concerns prior to going to a children's ward. This book aims to answer some of the questions you may have. Remember, even though you may not know it, there are skills you already have that you can apply to children's nursing. Experience and skills acquired in other areas of life will equip you and prepare you for your children's nursing experience.

What to expect

What is expected of the role of the children's nurse?

- Work as part of the multidisciplinary team
- Provide psychological and physiological care to children that is individualized and holistic
- Be an advocate for the child and parents
- Provide support for the families' needs
- Care for relatives of the child and significant others
- Display appropriate and effective communication skills
- Take part in ethical and moral decision making
- Prioritize care

- Assist with and undertake research-based care
- Accept changing practices and innovations
- Gain an awareness of self-development
- Support and educate less-qualified colleagues
- Record observations/document care
- Attend to all invasive lines
- Administer medications.

The multidisciplinary team (MDT)

Medical staff

- Includes clinical directors of paediatrics or medical/surgical directorates. Specialist doctors may be involved in the management of the paediatric environment. Some paediatric areas are staffed by individual specialists from other disciplines such as anaesthesia or medicine.

Physiotherapist

- Assists with children's respiratory functions, e.g. breathing pattern and depth to prevent complications
- Preserves existing motor skills, restores mobility, and considers the role of all limbs whether strong or weak
- Works towards reducing stiffness, contractions and spasticity
- Re-educates motor function, co-ordination and balance.

Occupational therapist

- Restores children's ability to perform daily activities. This may involve relearning skills (e.g. feeding or dressing) and adapting objects that the child can use.
- Evaluates children's perceptual and cognitive functions
- Assesses the need for modifications in a child's home.

Speech and language therapist

- Assesses children's swallowing and gag ability
- Provides specialized speech therapy, communication advice and aids to assist with speech.

Dietician

- Ascertains nutritional and fluid requirements
- Gives advice regarding enteral or parenteral feeding requirements and regimes.

Social worker

- Discusses long-term or short-term care options with a child and their family
- Supports families and the child by assisting with social issues, e.g. financial support at home
- Can provide carers and home adjustments.

Play specialist

- Is essential in the provision of play therapy
- Prepares children for procedures and events.

Other staff:

- Secretarial support
- Porters
- Technicians for servicing equipment
- Chaplains, priests or relevant officials of all religions
- Clinical pharmacists
- School teachers.

Children are different

Children are in a state of constant development, both physically and psychosocially. Children are not 'mini adults', as was previously thought many years ago. They have their own special requirements that must be met in specific ways. Their ability to cope with hospitalization is influenced by their age, developmental stage and previous experiences. This is what makes their needs different from those of adults.

Development aspects of a child (Piaget theory of development)

Generally, children are viewed as one group that think the same way. However, children's cognitive development (the ability to reason, think and understand) alters with age. Thus the child's views and experiences of illness and hospitalization will be affected by his/her stage of cognitive development. It can be hard to know how much a child can understand and how to communicate with children of varying ages. This is where Jean Piaget's (1896–1980) theory of development can be a useful guide. Knowledge of this four-staged theory will help you to understand how children interpret illness.

The four stages of this theory are:

1. Sensorimotor (birth to 2 years)
2. Preoperational (2–6 years)
3. Concrete operational (6–11 years)
4. Formal operational (11 years plus).

The stages of development and how they influence a child's beliefs and understanding are outlined below:

Sensorimotor (birth to 2 years)

Learning is mainly through the senses and physical activity. Babies are born with a large collection of reflexes (physical responses triggered involuntarily by a specific stimulus) (Bee and Boyd 2009). They use sucking, grasping and hearing to make sense of their surroundings. Babies are sensitive to sound and can link familiar objects with sound, for example mother with her voice. The child is strongly attached to familiar caregivers and will display upset when separated from them.

The toddler period (18–24 months) can be difficult for some children. They can have a temperament profile of high activity, intensity of emotion and low adaptability. It can be frustrating for this age group when they are unable to communicate their needs. From 2 years onwards, language acquisition is a key development.

Preoperational stage: 2–6 years

Phenomenism is the most developmentally immature explanation of illness at this stage. The child is unable to explain illness (e.g. How do people get colds? From the sun or the wind. How does the sun give you a cold? It just does that's all. God does it in the sky).

Contagion is a more mature concept of the prelogical stage. The cause of illness is seen to be located in objects or people who are in proximity to the child, but not necessarily touching them (e.g. How do people get colds? When somebody comes near you. How? I don't know, by magic I think).

In the preoperational stage, children's concerns are:

- Separation anxiety, leading to feelings of insecurity, abandonment, anxiety, loneliness

- Inaccurate understanding of the body can lead to fears of mutilation

- Changes in rituals, routines, and an unfamiliar environment can cause a child to feel insecure

- Inability to reason beyond the present and immediate environment so explanations have to be related to the here and now

- Illness may be seen as punishment so child needs demonstrations of love and affection to reassure him/her about this.

Concrete operational stage: 6–11 years

This stage is where differentiation of self from others occurs. A child is less egocentric and can apply thinking and reasoning to real objects and events. They can be confused about location of internal organs. Illness concepts are defined as contamination and internalization.

Contamination means that a child can distinguish between cause and effect in illness (e.g. If somebody has got a rash and you touch them you get it; if you go outside in the cold without a coat, the cold touches your body and goes all over it).

Internalization is a more mature understanding of the fact that illness may be located within the body but have an external cause (e.g. you breathe in cold air and get a cough; if someone with a cold kisses you, the germs go in your mouth and make you ill).

In the concrete operational stage, children's concerns are:

- Fear of loss of motor skills
- Worry about separation from school and peers
- Mutilation fantasies
- Increased concerns related to modesty and privacy
- Imposed passivity may be seen as punishment.

Formal operational stage: 11 years plus

Child can understand and explain illness in complex terms. They are able to reason logically, think in abstract terms, and systematically explore problems. Illness concepts may be physiological and psychological (e.g. worry and stress can cause ulcers and heart disease and it is possible to get in a state and worry yourself sick).

In the formal operational stage, children's concerns are:

- Altered body image due to puberty
- Lack of privacy
- Separation from peers, school and family
- Frustration with being dependent on others for help
- Threats of helplessness, and strong desire for mastery
- Dislike of being excluded, so will want to be involved in discussions about care and treatment decisions
- Prone to construe beyond their knowledge so may assume headaches to be a brain tumour.

Be aware that children's understanding can vary considerably depending on their life experiences. These ages are approximate to each stage as some children mature quicker and are more capable of processing information than others. Hence, this is a flexible guide that will help you provide developmentally appropriate care and reduce the negative effects of hospitalization for the child.

Reflection

Reflection is a way in which professionals pay attention to significant aspects of an experience they had in order to make sense of it within the context of their work. One can reflect during an action or after an experience has taken place (Schon 1983). Continuing professional development is essential in nursing and reflection facilitates this (Palmer et al 1994). By reflecting on and taking action to resolve the contradictions that occur in their practice, children's nurses can self-evaluate and come to know themselves. Consequently, they learn to become increasingly effective in their chosen field and they develop unique nursing knowledge.

This advocates the use of some sort of guide to ensure this happens and there are many cognitive models of reflection available, for example Boud et al (1985), Gibbs reflective cycle (1988) (see Fig. 1.1) and Johns model of structured reflection (1995) (see Table 1.1).

Boud et al (1985) Returning to the situation

What

- is the purpose of returning to the situation?
- exactly occurred in your own words?

- did other people do?
- do you see as key aspects of the situation?

So what

- were you feeling at the time?
- are your feelings now?
- were the effects of what you did or did not do?
- what 'good' emerged from this situation?
- were your experiences in comparison with your colleagues?
- are the main reasons for feeling differently from your colleagues?

Now what

- are the implications for your colleagues or the clients?
- needs to happen to alter the situation?

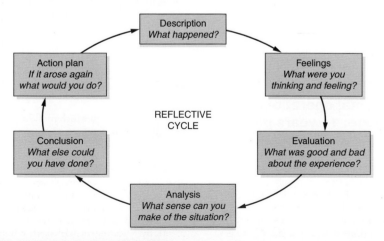

Fig. 1.1 The Reflective Cycle (Gibbs 1988)

Table 1.1 Johns' model of structured reflection (10th edition)	
Write a description of the experience	
Cue questions	
Aesthetics	What was I trying to achieve? Why did I respond as I did? What were the consequences of that for: the patient? others? myself? How was this person feeling? (Or these persons?) How did I know this?
Personal	How did I feel in this situation? What internal factors were influencing me?
Ethics	How did I feel in this situation? What factors made me act in incongruent ways?
Empirics	What knowledge did or should have informed me?
Reflexivity	How does this connect with previous experiences? Could I handle this better in similar situations? What would be the consequences of alternative actions for: the patient? others? myself? How do I now feel about this experience? Can I support myself and others better as a consequence? Has this changed my ways of knowing?

- are you going to do about the situation?
- happens if you decide not to alter anything?
- might you do differently if faced with a similar situation again?
- are the best ways of getting further information about the situation should it arise again?

Critical thinking

Critical thinking involves the development of cognitive processes such as higher-level thinking and reasoning. It encourages the individual to become open-minded, consider alternative perspectives, and respect the right of others to hold different opinions

7

(Clarke & Holt 2001). Critical thinking can be used when situations or problems arise whereby there is no definitive answer. Children's nurses need to be equipped and ready to find solutions, make decisions, and solve unique and complex problems within their clinical environment. As a children's nurse you will have to contend with tensions, prioritize care and deal with difficult technical terms when trying to get your view across. Critical thinking can facilitate your expression or articulate to others the sensitivity, complexity of making decisions in practice (Edwards 2007). To think critically, one needs to be inquisitive, curious, enthusiastic, willing to seek the truth and courageous about asking questions to obtain the best action for patients. Table 1.2 shows the phases involved in the critical thinking process.

Table 1.2 Main areas to consider as part of critical thinking

Phase 1		
1.	Interpretation and organization of the information	Descriptions of the situation or problem
		Logically assemble the information in the mind or on paper
		Use a concept or mind map starting with a broad concept with linking words that are interrelated and connected.
		If possible attempt to apply a systematic, organized and diligent approach to the situation (disorganized and abstract is also satisfactory at this time)
2.	Hidden assumptions	What are these?
		Values, attitudes and beliefs held by all those involved, are they opposite to your own beliefs or interests
		Consider positive and negative judgements that might be included
		Try to be open minded
3.	Nursing knowledge involved (both objective and subjective)	Look for the evidence: theoretical/research
		The ethical principles involved
		Knowledge from past experiences (personal or professional)
		Practical knowledge/skills
		What are your gut feelings about this – use your intuition
4.	Break down the situation/ information into parts	Is there a relationship between the parts?
		How does one effect the other?
		Analysis – examination of the ideas/arguments and possible courses of action.

Table 1.2 Main areas to consider as part of critical thinking—cont'd

5.	Consider all of the options	Include other people's views/perspectives
		Continual questioning of the issues involved
		Consideration of all of the possibilities
		Flexibility – view the situation in many different ways with a variety of ideas.
		Be inquisitive, curious, courageous about asking questions to obtain all of the information
6.	Are there any conflicting issues	What are they?
		Nurse–patient
		Professional–ethical
		Nurse–nurse/doctor–nurse/other HCP–nurse
		Air the concerns with each other
		Team-working, communication, negotiation skills to resolve conflicts
7.	Consider all of the options, again, synthesizing of ideas	Try to make sense of the muddle that is formulating in your mind or on paper
		Put them in some type of order with the preferred solution and consider the consequences of one decision over another
		Delete the ones that no longer apply or there are no resources, can never happen
		What is the best way forward and why?
8.	A decision has to be made	A decision/solution/conclusion has to be reached
		Self confidence and trusting own reasoning when making decisions / solving problems
Phase 2		
9.	Defending the decision	A reason why that decision was made
		How the decision was reached
		Has to be explained how the decision was arrived at
		Justification has to be given
10.	Accountability and responsibility for the decision made	Taking / accepting responsibility for the decision that has been made
		Being accountable legally, ethically and professionally

(Continued)

Table 1.2 Main areas to consider as part of critical thinking—cont'd		
11.	Evaluation of the process	Critical reflection/reflective practice
		Self-regulation/changing practices in the light of new insight and knowledge
		Correcting oneself if found to be wrong
		Learning from the situation/process/action plan for future learning needs
		Personal learning and continuing professional development (CPD)
12.	Creativity and innovation	Implementation of the decision/solution
		Implementing change, doing things in a different way, being creative and innovative (may go back to the start)
		Changing, refining or developing new policies/procedures
		Moving practice forward, doing things differently due to knowledge gained

Infection control issues

Patients who are admitted to a children's ward are immunologically vulnerable and invariably have a reduced immune response. This may be due to the individual child's general condition, their inability to take nutrition, or fasting practices in hospital. It might be due to prescribed treatments or drug therapies such as antibiotics, non-steroidal anti-inflammatory drugs (NSAIDs), antacids, chemotherapy and steroids. The children's nurse must be vigilant in relation to infection control practices to prevent the child from obtaining a hospital-acquired infection. Listed below are a number of areas that children's nurses need to be aware of so they can address a child's potential reduced immune response.

Broad-spectrum antibiotics

- These antibiotics do not only destroy the invading bacteria, but also devastate the normal flora present in the gastrointestinal tract (GIT) and can lead to diarrhoea.

- Broad-spectrum antibiotics destroy resident flora living in the mucous membranes of the mouth and vagina, allowing pathogens (commonly *Candida albicans*, which causes thrush) to colonize, leading to fungal infections.

NSAIDs

These are prescribed to relieve pain. This group of drugs works by reducing the release of prostaglandin during the inflammatory response. Prostaglandin has a number of roles in the body:

- Sends messages to the brain and pain may be felt
- Simulates the inflammatory response, which leads to swelling, putting pressure on localized nerve endings, resulting in pain, redness and heat
- Stimulates the clotting cascade, so any interference with its release can induce bleeding of the nose, vagina, or bleeding from wounds, etc.
- Controls renal blood flow and if prostaglandin is reduced then glomerular filtration rate (GFR) will be reduced leading to sodium and water retention
- NSAIDs are acidic and increase the acidity of the stomach and so can lead to the formation of ulcers; strict adherence to administering these drugs after meal times is essential (Galbraith et al 2008)
- It is essential that children taking NSAIDs should not take other protein-bound anticoagulants (such as aspirin) as these displace highly protein-bound drugs from proteins, leading to more free anticoagulants in the bloodstream
- These drugs reduce the inflammatory response and as such healing mechanism may also be delayed.

Antacids

- Antacids are drugs that neutralize acidity of the gastric juice
- Can give rise to an increase in production of bacteria living in the stomach, small and large intestine, which can lead to diarrhoea.

Administration of chemotherapy and radiotherapy

- Administration of chemotherapy and radiotherapy can depress the bone marrow
- Bone marrow produces neutrophils and monocytes, which mature to become macrophages
- Administration of chemotherapy and radiotherapy can lead to increased risk of patients becoming neutropenic, which leads to an increased risk of septicaemia.

Steroids

- Steroid hormones are synthesized by the adrenal cortex, and cortisol is a naturally occurring hormone
- Corticosteroids are anti-inflammatory and suppress the immune response, which affects healing; this can lead to susceptibility to infection and impaired wound healing
- Patient may be exposed to bacteria, which would not normally breach innate immune defences (Galbraith et al 2008).

Reduced nutritional intake

Adequate nutritional intake (e.g. glucose, fats, protein, vitamins and minerals) is required to produce the cells and molecules of innate immunity. If nutrients are not available, new molecules and cells cannot be produced, reducing the body's innate defence's protection against infection. The nutritional requirements for wound healing (see Section 2) include an adequate protein intake. Proteins supply the amino acids necessary for repair and regeneration of tissues, and produce many of the proteins involved in the immune responses. There are hospital practices that exacerbate bad nutrition and hence affect the child's immune response:

- Preoperative patients only need to be fasted for 4–6 hours.

- Postoperative feeding should be initiated immediately; leaving fasting until the return of bowel sounds is traditional, ritualistic and unnecessary.

- The prescription of 5% dextrose solution to maintain nutrition only promotes malnutrition as one litre of 5% dextrose solution contains approximately 800 kcal.

Note: All healthcare professionals and families can reduce the risk of transmission of hospital-acquired infection in children by following infection control practices, as outlined in Table 1.3.

Care planning and documentation

In paediatrics, the care is always discussed and planned with the primary carer as they know the child best and are usually very involved in the delivery of the care together with the nurses. The care needs to be planned and negotiated so that everyone is clear and happy with each others' roles and contribution. This always needs to be documented.

Key points to remember about nursing documentation:

- Should contain all the relevant information needed to care for the child

- Should be a structured plan based on a holistic assessment of the child's and family's needs

- Should be discussed and planned with both the child and primary carer(s)

- Should reflect primary carer's preferred contribution to the child's care

- Should be personalized to each child

- Should be written clearly and legibly with black pen

- Should be updated, reviewed and evaluated regularly to ensure relevancy.

Nursing models

Care plans are normally structured around an organizing framework, called a nursing model such as the Partnership Model. Some paediatric units prefer the philosophy of family-centred care. This is where the care is planned around the whole family, not just the individual child/person, and in which all the family members are recognized as care recipients.

Nursing process

Nursing models should include all four steps of the nursing process: assessment, planning, implementation and evaluation. These four steps will help to identify the child's needs and write a care plan to meet those needs.

Table 1.3 Infection control practices

Type	Reasons	Practice
The use of a single room	This is generally used to protect staff and other patients in the ward area (isolation) or to simply protect the patient due to immunosuppression (protective isolation)	Protective clothing is not generally required, visitors do not go from patient to patient and are not in contact with other patients Visitors do not handle infectious material Wash hands before and after the visitor leave the room is all that is necessary
Hand-washing	This is responsible for a large proportion of cross infection, and is the most important method of preventing the spread of infection (Finn 1997)	Thorough hand washing before attending a patient ensures the majority of micro-organisms acquired transiently from other patients are removed An awareness of micro-organisms demonstrates the importance of thoroughly washing and drying hands
Protective clothing	The transmission of micro-organisms on staff clothing is possible, but unlikely It is more likely to arise on the front Contaminated uniforms with body fluids increases the microbial load, plastic aprons provide adequate protection as they are impermeable	Plastic aprons under cloth gowns if there is a risk of spillage Disposable gloves for any activity Discarded after use and wash hands If no contact occurs with other patients, infection is unlikely to spread if the nurse leaves the room
Masks and eye protection	Recommended for infections that are spread by respiratory droplets They do not work when wet, as damp masks do not filter micro-organisms effectively	Not necessary for most procedures Are important to protect health care workers and should be worn for any activity where there is a risk of body fluid splashing into the face

(Continued)

Table 1.3 Infection control practices—cont'd

Type	Reasons	Practice
	Efficiency diminishes when worn for long periods	
	Easily contaminated by the hands during repositioning or removal, and as such are unreliable against airborne infections, especially viral (ICNA 1984)	
Waste material	If contaminated with blood or body fluids should be discarded in a yellow waste bag, in the patient's room	All body fluids should be safely discarded directly into a bedpan washer or macerator
	The outer surface of waste bags does not become significantly contaminated, no reason to enclose the waste in a second bag	
Equipment	Beds, curtains, bedclothes, toys, bedpans, sphygmomanometers	If it is known that microorganisms can contain spores and able to survive when food is scarce, hot water or special chemicals may be required to cleaning
	The majority of micro-organisms are not able to survive in the absence of moisture, warmth and nutrients, then as long as the equipment and other surface areas are kept clean and dry, the potential for the multiplication of bacteria will be removed	

Assessment

The first step in the development of a care plan is the thorough assessment of the child's physical, psychological and social needs, along with the family's needs. You need to:

- Explain to the child the purpose of the assessment and seek their agreement

- Undertake a comprehensive assessment using a child- and family-centred approach
- Obtain information directly from the child as much as possible to demonstrate respect for their knowledge and experience

- If assessing a non-verbal child or infant, seek the relevant information from the parents or primary carer
- Identify the physical, psychological, social, developmental, cultural, spiritual and sexual needs of the child
- Assess and record baseline observations and report anything out of normal range
- Ask the child and carer if they have any questions or concerns and address those concerns
- Provide information about the process and prepare child and carer for what to expect
- Obtain informed consent for any interventions or investigations planned.

Planning

This includes setting goals/outcomes and identifying specific interventions to fulfil these goals and expected outcomes. These need to be documented clearly and legibly.

- From the assessment identify the short-, medium- and long-term needs of the child.
- Take account of how child or young person would like to be involved in the delivery of their care.
- Take account of parents', carers' and family members' views of the child's care needs and how they would like to contribute to their child's care.
- Then set the goals/outcomes and identify specific interventions to fulfil these goals and expected outcomes.
- Negotiate and agree the care plan with the child and primary carer, taking account of all relevant information.

- Agree roles and responsibilities with those involved in caring for the child.
- Explain the care plans to the child and family and clarify any information that is unclear.
- Care plans should be individualized to each child and family situation.
- Document and record all relevant information and communication during the care planning process.

Implementation

This involves carrying out the interventions planned and recording the child's response to the interventions.

- Prioritize the interventions required and carry out the interventions according to the care plan.
- Ensure care is delivered consistently to meet the goals/outcomes.
- Work with MDT to meet the identified healthcare needs.
- Work in partnership with parents and primary carers to deliver the care required.
- Record and monitor child's response to the interventions.
- Keep child and carer informed on the progress and outcomes of interventions and investigations.
- Be flexible in the delivery of interventions that are non-urgent.

Evaluation

This involves reviewing how the interventions have worked, and determining any changes which need to be made to the care plan.

- Ensure that any changes made are negotiated and agreed with the child and carer.

- Monitor the quality of the care plans to ensure delivery of evidence-based care.
- Evaluate the quality of care delivered.
- Ensure that care is individualized and uses a child and family centred approach.

Essential skills for preregistration students

The Nursing and Midwifery Council (2007) have identified essential skills suitable for pre-registration students necessary for entry to the branch programme and for entry to the register. The skills are listed under five key areas:

1. Care, compassion and communication
2. Organizational aspects of care
3. Infection prevention and control
4. Nutrition and fluid management
5. Medicine management.

The new standards for preregistration nursing education introduced in 2010 will replace the existing *Standards of proficiency for preregistration nursing education* (NMC 2004).

Government directives in children's nursing

Many organizations have developed core principles to promote better standards of hospital care for children and their families and to safeguard children's rights. The National Services Framework (NSF) (Department of Health 2003)

have set standards for children in hospital to ensure that:

- hospital services meet the needs of children, young people and their parents, and
- they provide effective and safe care, through appropriately trained and skilled staff working in suitable, child-friendly, and safe environments.

It would be useful to read the documents that fully outline these standards which can be located on the website www.nhs.uk/NHSEngland/NSF/Pages/Children.aspx.

More recently, a common core set of knowledge and skills for all people who work with children has been identified (Children's Workforce Development Council 2010) and these link closely with the NSF standards. The common core has been divided into six key areas which sets out the basic knowledge and skills that everyone who works with children are expected to have.

Core set of knowledge and skills

1. Effective communication and engagement with children, young people and families.
2. Child and young person development.
3. Safeguarding and promoting the welfare of children.
4. Supporting transitions.
5. Multi-agency working.
6. Sharing information.

The Department of Health and Department for Children, Schools and Families have produced a long-term strategy to improve health outcomes for all children (Department of Health & Department for Education and

Skills 2009). The *Healthy Lives, Brighter Futures: Strategy* builds on the *National Service Framework for Children, Young people and Maternity Services* and the *Every Child Matters* reforms to improve the quality and consistency of services provided for children and families.

Voluntary organizations

In Europe the EACH organization (European Association for Children in Hospital) promotes the welfare of all children, before, during and after a hospital stay. EACH is made up of 19 associations from Europe, which promote the care of hospitalized children through the EACH charter. The EACH Charter contains a list of 10 rights for all children in hospital (www.each-for-sick-children.org/each-charter). These are listed in Table 1.4.

For further information on promoting the needs of all sick children and young people within the healthcare system in the British Isles, access:

Action for Sick Children, UK (www.actionforsickchildren.org/news.asp)
Action for Sick Children, Scotland (http://www.ascscotland.org.uk/)
Children in Hospital Ireland (CHI) (http://www.childreninhospital.ie/).

Table 1.4 The 10 rights of children in hospital	
Article 1	Children shall be admitted to hospital only if the care they require cannot be equally well provided at home or on a day basis
Article 2	Children in hospital shall have the right to have their parents or parent substitute with them at all times
Article 3	Accommodation should be offered to all parents and they should be helped and encouraged to stay
	Parents should not need to incur additional costs or suffer loss of income
	In order to share in the care of their child, parents should be kept informed about ward routine and their active participation encouraged
Article 4	Children and parents shall have the right to be informed in a manner appropriate to age and understanding
	Steps should be taken to mitigate physical and emotional stress
Article 5	Children and parents have the right to informed participation in all decisions involving their health care
	Every child shall be protected from unnecessary medical treatment and investigation

(Continued)

Table 1.4 The 10 rights of children in hospital—cont'd	
Article 6	Children shall be cared for together with children who have the same developmental needs and shall not be admitted to adult wards
	There should be no age restrictions for visitors to children in hospital
Article 7	Children shall have full opportunity for play, recreation and education suited to their age and condition and shall be in an environment designed, furnished, staffed and equipped to meet their needs
Article 8	Children shall be cared for by staff whose training and skills enable them to respond to the physical, emotional and developmental needs of children and families
Article 9	Continuity of care should be ensured by the team caring for children
Article 10	Children shall be treated with tact and understanding and their privacy shall be respected at all times

1.2 Emergency care of a child

Cardiac/respiratory arrest/CPR/BLS/ILS, DC shock

Cardiopulmonary resuscitation (CPR)

Many calls in practice are peri-arrests, which have implications for survival and soon will take over from cardiac arrest calls. Children's nurses are now encouraged to call when children have two or more of the criteria outlined in Table 1.5.

■ Early recognition
  – Most cardiac arrests are predictable; early warning signs are:
    • A drop in blood pressure and reduced oxygen saturation
    • Chest pain
    • Disorientation/confusion/unresponsive
    • Changes in breathing
    • Feeling unwell/faint/dizzy
    • Feeling sick/blurred vision
    • Pale/sweating/cold and clammy
    • Blue/cyanosed
    • Changes in baseline observations.
  – When these signs occur a precardiac arrest call can be given.
■ The reasons why children arrest are listed in Table 1.6.
■ Early assessment is often considered in relation to three areas:
  – D – Danger: consider the danger to the self and the patient/environment is safe
  – R – Response: talking to/shaking patient/touching patient; do not shake too hard tap the shoulder.
  – S – Shout for help: loudly and clearly, this is an emergency so be assertive:
    • get the trolley
    • make a call 2222

Table 1.5 Medical emergency team calling criteria

Acute change in:	Physiology:
Airway	Threatened
Breathing	All respiratory arrests Respiratory rate <5/min Respiratory rate >36/min
Circulation	All cardiac arrests Pulse rate <40 beats/min Pulse rate >140 beats/min Systolic blood pressure <90 mmHg
Neurology	Sudden decrease in level of consciousness Decrease in GCS of >2 points Repeated or prolonged seizures
Other	Any patient causing concern who does not fit the above criteria

Table 1.6 Reasons why children arrest

Airway problems	Cardiac problems	
	Primary	Secondary
Central nervous system	Coronary syndrome	Asphyxia
Blood	Dysthymias	Hypoxaemia
Vomit	Increased blood	Blood loss
Foreign body	pressure	Hypothermia
Trauma	Heart disease	Septic shock
Infection	Valve disease	
Inflammation	Drugs	
Laryngospasm	Hereditary	
Bronchospasm	Electrolytes	
Inhalation/burns	Acid–base changes	
Drugs (suppression)	Electrocution	
Pain (breathing inadequately)		
Pneumothorax/haemothorax		
Chronic obstructive pulmonary disease		
Pulmonary embolism		
Adult respiratory distress syndrome		

- check information about where you are on the ward, room, etc.
- crash trolley needed.

Life support

- A = airway, open airway – look for signs of life
  - patient response
  - open airway
  - check for signs of life
  - pulse check
  - this should take no more than 10 seconds.
- B = Breathing
  - check normal breathing
  - look, listen and feel
  - pattern and depth
  - chest movements are equal on both sides.
- C = Circulation
  - Chest compressions in the centre of the chest 30:2
  - older child palm of two hands linked together (as for adult)
  - younger child use palm of one hand only
  - baby or young child two fingers of dominant hand
  - 4–5 cm depth (varies dependent on child's age, weight)
  - 100–150 beats per minute
  - uninterrupted compressions when airway secured
  - avoid fatigue and do not miss compressions.
- Airway ventilation
  - ventilation rate should be 30 compressions to 2 breaths
  - tidal volume considered – normal
  - too much can lead to:
    - hyperventilating the patient ↓ in CO_2 and so will not breathe when consciousness returns

- ↑ in interthoracic pressure and a ↓ in cardiac output.
- ventilate between 10 and 22 breaths per minute or 1 every 6 seconds.

Automated electronic device (AED)

An AED will give a controlled electric shock to convert abnormal cardiac rhythm back into SR:

- switch the machine on
- attach leads
  - colour coded
  - remove chest hairs (older boys only, if applicable)
  - configure to Lead II
  - analyse rhythm (AR)
- shockable rhythms:
  - Ventricular tachycardia (VT) – is a shockable rhythm
    - Broad complex rhythm
    - Rapid rate
    - Constant QRS morphology
  - Ventricular fibrillation (VF) – is a shockable rhythm
    - Bizarre irregular waveform
    - No recognizable QRS complexes
    - Uncoordinated electrical activity
    - Two types: coarse or fine
    - Exclude any artefact
    - Movement
    - Electrical interference.
- Non-shockable rhythms
  - Asystole
    - Absent ventricular (QRS) activity
    - Atrial activity (P waves) may persist
    - Rarely a straight line trace.

Pulseless electric activity

- Clinical features of cardiac arrest
- ECG normally associated with an output.

There are a variety of makes of crash trolleys. The trolley is checked every day or each shift. Learn how the trolley works in your area.

- Ambu bag and mask, oxygen – know how they work/fit together
- IV access – needles, lines, fluids, ampoules
- Airways, intubation (ETT) – variety of sizes, tapes
- Laryngoscope – check light works
- Suctioning, catheters variety of sizes
- Drugs.

Post-resuscitation care

- During CPR:
  - Check electrode position, airway/ oxygen, IV access (variable rates of absorption from sites, e.g. radial CVP)
  - Give uninterrupted compressions
  - Give epinephrine (adrenaline)
  - Consider amiodarone, atropine, magnesium
- Consider potential reversible causes (4 Hs and 4 Ts)
  - 4 Hs
    - Hypoxia
    - Hypothermia
    - Hypo/hyperkalaemia
    - Hypovolaemia.
  - 4 Ts
    - Tamponade
    - Tension pneumothorax
    - Toxins
    - Thrombosis.

Know your own skills:

- How to:
  - open and maintain an airway
  - insert an oropharyngeal airway
  - assist in passing endotracheal tube / laryngeal mask

  - fit together, use Ambu-bag, mask and attach to oxygen (move clear away from the bed during the administration of shock)
  - connect and work the monitor (leads on chest), defibrillator (where to put the pads)
  - perform compressions: location, depth, rate and ratio of breathing
  - prepare the drugs
  - assist in gaining IV access and preparing the line.
- Know when to stand clear.
- When to stop CPR.

Remember: Do not resuscitate orders (DNR) are generally clearly documented in the child's notes. Nurses must know if DNR orders apply.

Shock (hypovolaemia, anaphylaxis, septic, cardiogenic, neurogenic)

Shock is a condition whereby the cardiovascular system fails to perfuse body tissues adequately with oxygen and nutrients which results in functional disturbances to vital organs and tissues (Edwards 2005a). The causes of shock are generally any factor, which affects blood volume, blood pressure or cardiac function. There are five forms of shock: hypovolaemic, anaphylaxis, septic, neurogenic and cardiogenic.

Hypovolaemic shock

This is the most common type of shock (Fig. 1.2). It is the state that results from a decrease in blood volume

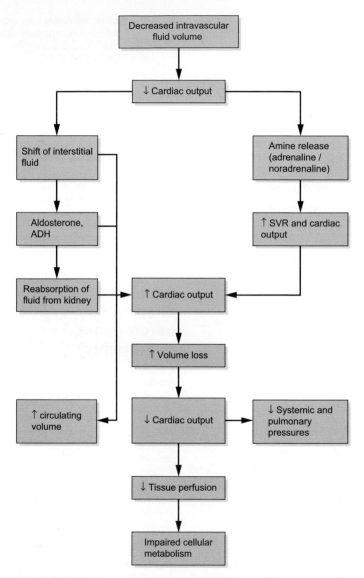

Fig. 1.2 Hypovolaemic shock

produced by continued bleeding, plasma loss, or water or so large that the body's metabolic needs cannot be met (Edwards 1998). The degree of hypovolaemic shock depends on the amount of blood lost, the rate at which it was lost, the age and general physical condition of the child, and the child's ability to activate compensatory mechanisms.

Anaphylactic shock

Anaphylaxis occurs when a sensitized child is exposed to an antigen, to which s/he is allergic. An antigen–antibody reaction occurs, which induces the release of histamine and prostaglandins into the blood (Fig. 1.3).

This can result in:

- Bronchospasm
- Oedema formation in the glottis and pharynx
- Oedema in the lungs and in subcutaneous tissue
- Changes in cardiac function.

Septic shock

Septic shock (Fig. 1.4) is caused by an overwhelming infection and may be the result of a suppressed immune system, a massive burn injury, or anything else that can introduce an infecting organism into a compromised victim. The result of septic shock is tachycardia and a high cardiac output. In this state the child may feel warm, have a high temperature. If this persists, cardiac output will decrease and the skin will become cool.

Neurogenic shock

Neurogenic shock may be the result of a severe brain stem injury at the level of the medulla, an injury to the spinal cord, or spinal anaesthesia (Fig. 1.5). Indications include severe hypotension, inadequate cardiac output and reduced tissue perfusion.

> **!** Neurogenic shock may mask signs and symptoms of other types of shock. If neurogenic shock is present, there should be a heightened suspicion for an undetected source of haemorrhage.

Cardiogenic shock

Cardiogenic shock (Fig. 1.6) occurs when the heart, due to impaired myocardial performance, cannot produce an adequate cardiac output to sustain the metabolic requirements of body tissues. Myocardial infarction (MI) is the most common cause of cardiogenic shock. Indications include a decrease in blood pressure and an increase in heart rate.

It is important to note that children may have components of more than one forms of shock. To identify the different types of shock in a child see Fig. 1.7.

Stages of shock

Shock is a very complex syndrome as the problem not only concerns the amount of blood volume, but also delivery in terms of blood flow to organs and cells of the body. The cellular changes in all forms of shock are shown in Fig. 1.8. The end result is always the same, whatever the cause of shock: the tissues fail to receive

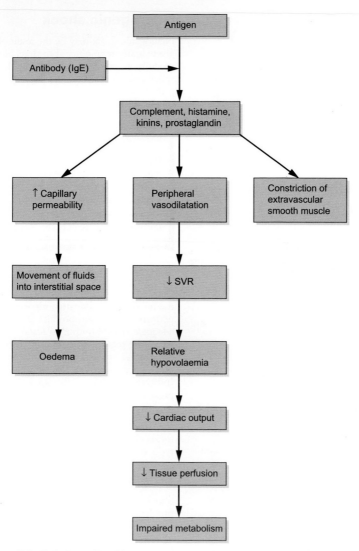

SVR = Systemic vascular resistance

Fig. 1.3 Anaphylactic shock

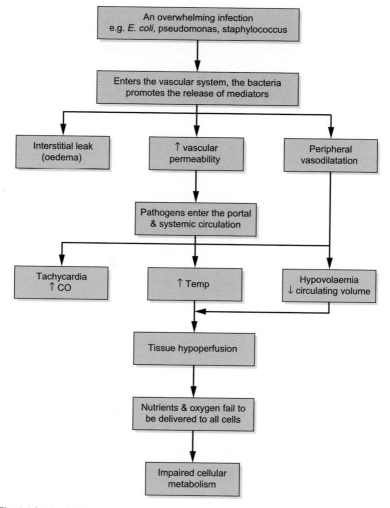

Fig. 1.4 Septic shock

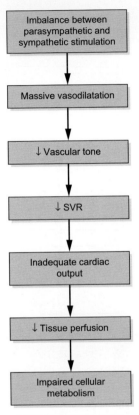

SVR = Systemic vascular resistance

Fig. 1.5 Neurogenic shock

oxygen and nutrients and to rid themselves of waste products. It is the responsibility of the children's nurse that the development of shock must be prevented. This includes early interpretation of observational and measurable data to recognize its early development.

The easy understanding and recognition of shock can be divided into three stages: compensated, progressive, or uncompensated and irreversible. These stages are not distinct and should be regarded as a continuum.

Compensated shock

The body's compensatory mechanisms are able to maintain circulation and blood pressure in the face of whatever defect is causing the shock. These mechanisms in very young children will cease to function quickly whilst in older children you have longer time, but if no intervention is given circulatory failure will ensue.

Generally, the clinical picture of a child in the compensatory stage of shock is:

- Tachycardia, narrowing pulse pressure
- Increases in temperature and blood glucose level
- An increase in blood pressure and rate and depth of respiration
- Pale skin colour and cool to cold skin
- Decrease in urine output
- Absent bowel sounds
- Mental state alterations ranging from restlessness to coma
- Complaining of thirst.

Progressive or uncompensated shock

Once shock has developed, the course it takes is complex. Once shock has progressed into the second stage the outcome is no longer as predictable. Why some children take a progressively downward course despite best efforts at treatment is not fully understood.

As shock progresses, there are deleterious changes that occur:

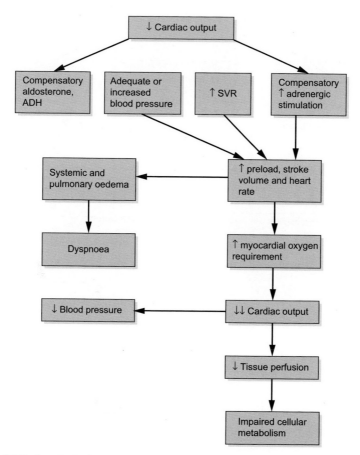

Fig. 1.6 Cardiogenic shock

An inadequate flow of nutrients and oxygen to the cell will occur. Eventually, cells become damaged as they cannot produce sufficient amounts of energy to survive.

An inflammatory response as the body will send nutrients, fluids, white blood cells, and clotting factors to repair the damaged site to repair tissue, prevent infection and if necessary stem blood loss. This leads to localized swelling and lymphatic blockage.

Hypercoagulability occurs as a result of the stimulation of the inflammatory immune response, which can produce drastic problems for the child.

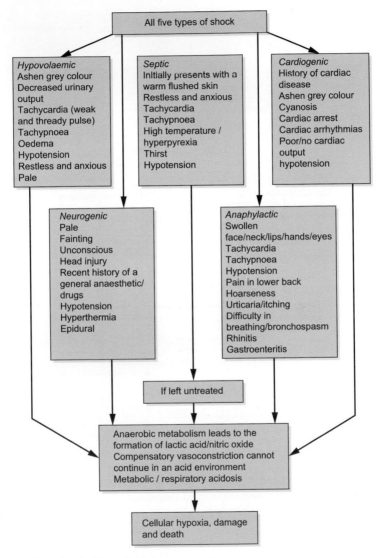

Fig. 1.7 Overview of all types of shock

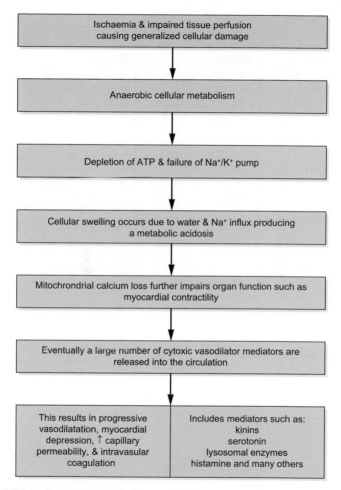

Ischaemia & impaired tissue perfusion causing generalized cellular damage

↓

Anaerobic cellular metabolism

↓

Depletion of ATP & failure of Na⁺/K⁺ pump

↓

Cellular swelling occurs due to water & Na⁺ influx producing a metabolic acidosis

↓

Mitochrondrial calcium loss further impairs organ function such as myocardial contractility

↓

Eventually a large number of cytoxic vasodilator mediators are released into the circulation

↓

| This results in progressive vasodilatation, myocardial depression, ↑ capillary permeability, & intravasular coagulation | Includes mediators such as:
kinins
serotonin
lysosomal enzymes
histamine and many others |

Fig. 1.8 Cellular changes common to all forms of shock

Refractory (irreversible) shock

- This is the final stage of shock, and is where severe cellular and organ dysfunction leads to general decline and death. The major organs affected are the kidneys, liver, GIT, heart, lungs and brain (Table 1.7).

- In this stage it may be possible to return arterial pressure to normal for a

Table 1.7 Effects of shock on specific organs

Organ	Effect	Result
Kidneys – the most important and apparent organ affected early in shock.	Renal blood flow is reduced early, as the total renal blood flow falls, the GFR is reduced and the kidney will release renin. The GFR is preserved for a time, but oliguria nevertheless occurs, due to ADH and aldosterone secretion.	When there is a reduction in oxygen and energy the re-absorptive functions for sodium and water are lost and the renal tubules undergo necrosis. ATN of the kidney commonly occurs in shock, and if severe may lead to acute renal failure, contributing to late deaths following resuscitation.
Liver – a highly complex organ having multiple functions.	Is sensitive to ischaemia, both hepatic arterial and portal venous blood flow are reduced in shock. Early in shock, the liver releases large amounts of glucose as the result of adrenaline-induced glycogenolysis and gluconeogenesis.	In uncompensated shock, all liver functions, including bile and cholesterol formation, protein synthesis, gluconeogenesis, lactate metabolism, detoxification, glycogen stores are depleted, and the phagocytic activity of the Kupffer cells are depressed.
The GIT – suffers an early reduction of oxygen in shock states due to ADH, angiotensin II and catecholamines.	There is, however, a threshold whereby the reduction in blood flow effects food/gut motility, absorption and produces lactate in large amounts. The gut is the major source of lactic acidosis in haemorrhagic shock.	In shock the gut mucosa barrier loses its integrity and is permeable to bacterial and endotoxins from the intestinal lumen, resulting in damage/necrosis of the intestinal wall by digestive enzymes. This may then allow pathogens to enter the portal and systemic circulation, causing infection and multiple organ failure.
Lungs – necessary for ventilation and perfusion for	In shock the reduced pulmonary blood flow results in an imbalance between oxygen supply	Ventilation and/or perfusion and gas exchange is poor or does not take place, resulting in progressive atelectasis, ARDS,

Table 1.7 Effects of shock on specific organs—cont'd

Organ	Effect	Result
oxygenation and removing waste gases.	and tissue demands. These are compensated for by hyperventilation due to chemoreceptor stimulation and thus arterial partial pressure of oxygen is well maintained.	respiratory muscle fatigue from respiratory muscle hypoperfusion, and respiratory failure may result.
Heart – early deaths are associated with unsupportable reductions in cardiac function.	The heart muscle relies on the delivery of oxygen and nutrients to its cells via the coronary arteries, and has a very high oxygen requirement. Thus, a major reduction in cardiac blood flow quickly renders the heart muscle ischaemic.	Blood flow during shock is relatively preserved due to homeostatic compensation. Myocardial dysfunction occurs if there is a reduction in coronary blood flow exceeding the limits of compensatory mechanisms. Eventually the heart ceases to function adequately as a pump, causing a decrease in cardiac output. Failure of the circulatory pump intensifies the deficient oxygen delivery throughout the remainder of the body, as well as to the heart itself.
Brain – most susceptible to hypoxic injury because it depends on glucose and oxygen to function.	Although protected by the homeostatic vasoconstriction and by its own autoregulation, if the systolic blood pressure falls below 60 mmHg, the capacity for autoregulation is exceeded.	Mental state abnormalities are associated with poor outcome, as respiratory alkalosis, hypoxaemia, electrolyte disturbances start to appear. If blood flow continues to deteriorate autoregulation can no longer maintain normal cerebral metabolism. Unconsciousness and irreversible brain damage rapidly occurs.

short while, but tissue and organ deterioration continue, and no amount of therapy will reverse the process.

Other considerations

There are a number of variables that affect the course of shock, such as the child's age; the general state of health of the child before the shock insult; pain and hypothermia.

Status asthmaticus

Asthma is the most common chronic childhood disease, affecting 5–10% of children and resulting in approximately 400 000 hospitalizations annually. Episodes are associated with obstruction that occurs in predominantly small-to-medium airways.

Status asthmaticus is an acute exacerbation of asthma that may be unresponsive to initial treatment with bronchodilators. The condition becomes progressively worse. In addition, the asthma may have been left untreated or with delay in medical treatment. Treatment with systemic steroids leads to a greater chance of dying. Status asthmaticus is an emergency and if left untreated can be life threatening.

Typically, patients present with the condition a few days:

- after onset of a viral respiratory illness
- following exposure to a potent allergen or irritant
- after exercise in a cold environment.

Mucous plugging and mucosal oedema or inflammation is the major cause for the delayed recovery in status asthmaticus.

Child assessment

- Evaluation should centre on the 'ABCs'.
  - Airway: Can the patient maintain their own airway?
  - Breathing: What is the degree of air exchange? Is the patient hypoxic?
  - Circulation: How is their perfusion?
- History taking and a more detailed examination
  - Is there any previous history of wheezing?
  - When did the exacerbation begin?
  - If they are a known asthmatic, what are their regular medications?
  - Is there any compliance?
  - When was the last bronchodilator used?
  - During previous hospitalizations, were they intubated?
  - When was their last course of steroids?
  - Are there any precipitating factors?
  - General medical history, including any medications.
- Use the clinical asthma score (Table 1.8) – the higher the score the more serious the asthma attack.
- Monitor vital signs
  - Temperature: fever may indicate upper respiratory tract infection
  - pneumonia, or other source of infection
  - Check pulse, respiratory rate and blood pressure.
- Respiratory examination
  - Check breath sounds and undertake chest examination
  - Is there symmetry of breath sounds?
  - Is there increased wheezing unilaterally?

Table 1.8 Clinical Asthma Score
The higher the score, the more severe the asthma

	0	**1**	**2**
Cyanosis	None	Room air (SpaO$_2$ <94%)	On 40% (SpaO$_2$ <94%)
Inspiratory breath sounds	None	Unequal	Decreased or absent
Accessory muscle use	None	Moderate	Maximal
Expiratory wheeze	None	Moderate	Marked
Cerebral function	Normal	Depressed or agitated	Coma

- Is there use of accessory respiratory muscles?
- Feel for the presence of crepitus in the neck or chest wall.
- Cardiac examination – heart rate and blood pressure, normal heart tones.
- Neurological examination – any confusion present?

Investigations

- Pulmonary function tests, chest X-ray, ECG, ABG.

Treatment

- Oxygen delivery
- Continuous monitoring
- Frequent assessment of work of breathing and breath sounds
- Physiotherapy – evaluate patient before and after
- An arterial line may be indicated if the attack is severe, this will allow for frequent ABGs and blood pressure monitoring
- Standard drug therapy includes steroids, beta-agonists, e.g. bronchodilators and possibly intravenous beta-antagonists. Additional therapy includes anticholinergic agents, e.g. Atrovent
- Additional therapies include magnesium, ketamine, antibiotics, and diuretics
- Intubation and ventilator assistance.

General management issues

- Fluids and electrolyte balance – maintain hydration with IV fluids. If patient is on steroids it may be appropriate to treat with H$_2$ blocker drugs to prevent ulcer formation.
- Antibiotics – used if a bacterial infection is the cause of the patient's asthma exacerbation.

- Chest physiotherapy – controversial, but if used evaluate patient before and after treatments.
- Hyperventilation should be avoided.
- Assessment of air trapping
  - Measure intrinsic PEEP.
  - Absence of pause between expiratory and inspiratory sounds.
  - Timing of audible expiratory wheeze following ventilator disconnection.
  - Increasing $PaCO_2$.

Convulsions

Convulsions are the most frequent neurologic disorders affecting children. A febrile convulsion is a brief generalized convulsion caused by a fever $> 37.8°C$. Febrile convulsions are not epileptic seizures because they are not caused by disrupted electrical activity in the brain. Febrile convulsions occur among children aged between 6 months and 5 years, with the peak age being 18 months. It usually occurs without warning.

Signs and symptoms

- Child becomes floppy or stiff
- Has jerky or twitching movements
- Difficulty breathing
- Unaware of surroundings
- Loss of consciousness.

Types of febrile convulsions

- Simple: isolated, generalized tonic seizure lasting less than 15 minutes.
- Complex: convulsion lasting 15–30 minutes, or are focal, and not followed by full consciousness with 1 hour.

Care and management

Most convulsions are brief and self-limiting, generally ceasing within 5–10 minutes. Most children who come to the hospital can be managed within the emergency department. However, there are criteria that indicate when a child needs to be admitted.

Criteria for admission

- Complex convulsion
- Aged under 18 months
- Signs and symptoms of meningitis
- Child was drowsy before seizure
- Cause of convulsion requires admission, e.g. poisoning, epilepsy
- Petechial rash (small red pinpricks on the skin)
- On antibiotics
- Child is irritable, unwell and cause of fever is unclear
- Parents not happy to take child home.

Immediate treatment:

- Remain calm and stay with the child.
- Maintain airway, breathing and circulation.
- Remove excess clothing and ensure neck is free from constraints.
- Remove any objects that could cause injury.
- Position on side with head supported.
- Check temperature.
- Check blood glucose.
- Observe type and duration of seizure.
- Observe level of consciousness.
- Administer rectal diazepam if seizure does not cease within 10 minutes.

Investigations

- Check for source of infection
- Obtain a sample of urine to check for UTI
- There is no need for an EEG after a first simple febrile convulsion
- Febrile convulsion is prolonged suspect a serious cause such as bacterial meningitis or epilepsy.

Advice for parents

It can be very frightening for parents to witness their little child having a febrile convulsion and they usually are very upset and anxious. It is essential to provide reassurance and support. Explain that convulsions:

- Are not harmful to the child
- Will not cause brain damage
- Will not cause the child to die
- Possibly will reoccur so parents need advice on how to prevent febrile convulsions
- Show parents how to take child's temperature and explain what medication can be given to reduce temperature, e.g. paracetamol or ibuprofen
- Explain that parents must only give recommended dose for child's age.
- Sometimes depending on child's condition, parents may be given a 6 week OPD appointment for review purposes.

Advice for parents on how to manage the child in the event of a reoccurrence:

- Stay calm as most stop within a couple of minutes

- Remove excessive clothing or bedding
- Time the length of the convulsion
- Stay with the child and lie them on their side
- Do not put anything in child's mouth or try to restrain the child
- Loosen tight clothing
- Remove any objects that could cause injury
- When convulsion has stopped call the doctor
- Advise parents to seek medical help immediately if child fits again
- If the convulsion does not cease or if child has difficulty breathing advise parents to call an ambulance immediately
- Advise parents to complete immunization schedules.

Status epilepticus

Seizures are caused by abnormal electrical discharges in the brain. A child is usually diagnosed as having epilepsy if they have had two or more seizures that started in the brain. When a seizure will not subside, this is called status epilepticus and is life threatening. Prolonged seizures require rapid and prompt treatment. Early treatment helps to reduce morbidity and mortality rates.

Early interventions mean the administration of antiepileptic therapy after the first 5–10 minutes of seizure activity. Rectal diazepam is quite effective in stopping acute seizures with minimal side effects. Buccal midazolam is the next drug of choice if rectal diazepam is not appropriate.

In some countries where intravenous access is unavailable, other routes of administration are used such as: intramuscular paraldehyde, buccal midazolam, rectal diazepam, intranasal lorazepam (The Status Epilepticus Working Party 2000).

Administration of therapy by families and carers

The administration of rectal diazepam by parents in the home has been shown to decrease the development of status epilepticus and admission to emergency departments. Rectal diazepam is safe for home use provided parents are shown how to administer the suppository.

Care and management in hospital

Stage 1: 0–10 minutes

■ Assess cardiorespiratory function
■ Secure the airway
■ Administer oxygen as hypoxia is usually severe
■ Start resuscitation if required.

Stage 2: 0–30 minutes

■ Perform neurological observations
■ Start emergency anticonvulsant therapy – usually a fast acting benzodiazepine
■ Establish intravenous access for drug administration and fluid replacement
■ IV lines should be sited in large veins as antiepileptic drugs cause phlebitis and thrombosis at the site of infusion
■ Monitor vital signs
■ Monitor oxygen saturation
■ Monitor heart rate through electrocardiogram
■ Blood tests for metabolic abnormalities
■ If hypoglycaemia is suspected, glucose solution should be administered intravenously.

Stage 3: 0–60 minutes

■ Establish the cause of the status epilepticus
■ Obtain medical history and duration of seizure
■ Obtain details of antiepileptic medication
■ Electroencephalogram (EEG) to record electrical activity
■ Blood tests to identify possible causes of seizures
■ CT scan which will show abnormalities in the brain
■ MRI scan which will show cerebral malformations.

Stage 4: 30–60 minutes

■ If seizures continue despite measures taken, the child needs to be transferred to intensive care unit
■ After 30 minutes compensatory mechanisms fail, resulting in cerebral oedema, cerebral damage and circulatory collapse
■ Continuous EEG monitoring may be required for comatose patients
■ Intracranial pressure monitoring may be required
■ Long-term anticonvulsant therapy must be given in tandem with emergency measures.

Airway obstruction

There are many potential causes of airway obstruction in children:

- Acute viral laryngotracheobronchitis, LTB (known as croup)
- Acute epiglottitis – inflammation of the structures above the glottis caused by bacterial infection commonly the Haemophilus influenza type b (HIB)
- Bacterial tracheitis – diffuse inflammation of the larynx, trachea and bronchi
- Retropharyngeal abscesses – serious infection of the retropharyngeal space
- Foreign body (FB) aspiration e.g. coins, toys, sharp objects, bones, and food
- Displaced tongue
- Trauma to head or neck area
- Chemical or thermal injuries
- Fluid e.g. vomit, blood
- Anaphylaxis due to contact with an allergen, e.g. peanuts, wasp sting, plant.

Prompt recognition and correct management of the condition are critical to achieving optimal clinical outcome.

Observation of the child

- Observe child for signs of respiratory distress, e.g. tachypitnoea, nasal flaring and use of accessory muscles
- Assessment of airway patency:
  - Use the look, listen and feel approach to assess airway patency
  - Look for movement of the chest, abdomen and use of accessory muscles
  - Listen for breath sounds or stridor (noise on inhalation)
  - Feel for expired breaths
- Ask child if able to speak to voice specific areas of discomfort
- Note child's level of alertness and response to surroundings
- Stridor is a key sign of narrowing of the airway and indicates the need for prompt attention
- Observe colour of lips and mouth – cyanosis (bluish tinge) indicates lack of oxygen
- The stable child with signs and symptoms of airway compromise needs a detailed history to establish the presence or absence of pre-existing conditions, ingestions, trauma, allergies, fever, and illnesses
- Check with the parent details on the onset and duration of signs and symptoms management

For foreign body aspiration

- Obtain history from parent or carer to determine type of foreign object
- If the foreign object is visible attempt to remove the object carefully
- Never use your fingers to explore child's mouth as you could cause further trauma
- Keep calm so you can help the child and parent to keep calm
- If child is able to breathe spontaneously maintain in upright position and administer 100% oxygen
- If the child is coughing, sneezing, wheezing, crying, bluish tinge to lips and mouth, the airway is partially obstructed

- Unconscious infants with witnessed foreign body obstruction should be straddled over the arm with the head lower than the trunk; five back blows should be delivered with the heel of the hand between the shoulder blades
- Older children can be given the abdominal thrust, which is a series of subdiaphragmatic thrusts with the purpose of forcing air out of the lungs
- Stay with child at all times as complete airway obstruction may occur
- Accompany child to radiology to check location of foreign body
- If the foreign object is unable to be removed, the child will need to be taken to theatre for removal under anaesthetic.

For children with anaphylaxis

- Obtain history from parent or carer to determine type of allergen
- Signs may include hives, pruritus or flushing, swollen lips/tongue and respiratory compromise
- Place in supine position
- Administer adrenaline usually via intramuscular dose
- Bronchodilator treatment may be required with continuous salbutamol and corticosteroids
- Administer IV fluids
- If the child is unresponsive resuscitation needs to be taken immediately.

Total airway obstruction

Total airway obstruction is a critical emergency and the aim is to restore airway function as soon as possible. Simple measures may be all that are required to open the airway.

Simple measures

- Suction the oropharynx if airway obstructed by fluid
- Insertion of a pharyngeal airway
- Head tilt and chin lift manoeuvre will work if the tongue is obstructing the airway
- Place your hand gently on child's forehead and slowly tilt the head backward
- Place the fingers of your other hand under the chin and gently tilt upwards
- If child has experienced a trauma to the neck or head this manoeuvre is not advised
- Administer high concentration of oxygen via bag-valve-mask technique
- A patent airway should be established
- Observe and record respirations as an open airway does not mean adequate ventilation
- Record oxygen saturations.
- Reassure the child and keep as calm as possible while delivering the treatment.

Advanced measures

- Direct laryngoscopy is most often used for insertion of the tube
- Straight blade used for infants and curved for children
- Tracheal tube size – 3–3.5 mm for infants, 4.0 mm for 1-year-olds, above 2 years use tracheal tube formula: $4 + $ age

- In children younger than 10 years the narrowest portion of the airway is below the vocal cords so endotracheal tube size should be based on the cricoid ring rather than glottic opening
- Post intubation X-ray is done to check tube is in correct position
- Child admitted to PICU until ventilator assistance is not required
- Intravenous line is inserted for fluid replacement and antibiotics
- Broad spectrum antibiotic is normally prescribed to control the inflammation
- Care and reassurance are vital as intubation is a frightening procedure
- Children are normally sedated whilst intubated.

> Children with airway obstruction due to suspected epiglottitis must never be placed in supine position as this may lead to complete airway obstruction. The child should be allowed to assume a position of comfort.

Diabetic emergencies

Hypoglycaemia

- Occurs when blood glucose falls below 3.5 mmol/l
- Does not occur in diabetics who are diet controlled, but may occur in type 2 diabetics on oral hypoglycaemics

such as tolbutamide or gliclazide; more common in patients receiving insulin
- Commonest cause of diabetic coma.

Causes

- Too much insulin (accidental or deliberate)
- Missing or delayed a meal or snack
- Excessive exercise with no reduction in insulin
- Alcohol binges may precipitate.

Clinical features:

- Pallor
- Trembling
- Sweating
- Feeling 'lightheaded'
- Blurred vision
- Tachycardia
- Increasing confusion – sometimes irritable or lethargic
- Incoherent speech.

Seek help immediately. Glucose or glycogen may be administered.

Diabetic ketoacidosis

- This occurs when there is insufficient insulin in the body, and the cells cannot utilize glucose and it accumulates in the blood
- Deterioration is generally slow and the patient may have been feeling unwell for months
- A hyperglycaemia is present; ketones are present in the urine in increased amounts and on the breath

- The condition is severe with acidosis due to production of ketones leading to a metabolic acidosis
- Nausea and vomiting may occur leading to electrolyte imbalance
- Dehydration will occur due to loss of excessive water, this lowers blood pressure and a rapid and thready pulse occurs
- Respiration becomes deep and rapid in an attempt to excrete excess metabolic acids
- Drowsiness and coma will occur if treatment is not instigated and indicates severe metabolic derangement.

Causes

- Untreated diabetes – undiagnosed condition
- Illness – as patient does not feel like eating so omits their insulin
- Vomiting and a total omission of insulin.

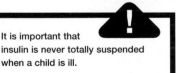

It is important that insulin is never totally suspended when a child is ill.

Treatment

- Assess consciousness level
- Have suction machine ready in case of vomiting
- Monitor vital signs
- Intravenous infusion of fluids to replace loss of water (normal saline); potassium may need to be added
- Check blood glucose level
- Monitor arterial blood gases
- Cardiac monitoring
- Insulin therapy (short acting such as Actrapid or Humulin S) may be titrated to the blood glucose measurement
- Once blood glucose has fallen to 11 mmol/l IV fluid will be replaced with a dextrose solution.

Pyrexia

A pyrexia is a body temperature between 37.6 and 40°C and hyperpyrexia is a temperature > 40°C. Infection and sepsis is the most common cause of pyrexia. Sepsis is the most common cause of hyperpyrexia. There are four stages associated with pyrexia:

1. The *chill stage* is the cold stage when the hypothalamic thermostat is reset to a higher level – the patient feels chilly, has goosebumps, is cool to touch and pale.
2. The *plateau* is the hot stage when the body temperature has been raised to a level equal to the hypothalamic set point – the patient feels hot, warm to touch, is flushed, and has raised heart and respiratory rates.
3. The *defervescence stage* is that stage when the temperature returns to normal, heat is dissipated through the heat loss mechanisms. The skin remains warm to touch and is flushed. Eventually there is a drop in body temperature to a normal level.
4. The *crisis stage* occurs if the temperature fails to respond to treatment and thermoregulatory mechanisms can no longer control heat loss; death may ensue.

Table 1.9 Patterns of pyrexia	
Pattern	**Description**
Intermediate	The elevated temperature returns to normal at least once in a 24 hour period. Temperature swings are usually rapid, multiple and accompanied by shaking chills, and leave the patient exhausted. An intermittent pattern is most often seen in intensive care units and is usually due to potent pyrogens, antigenic drugs and blood transfusions.
Remittent	The temperature patterns rise and fall throughout the day, but are less extreme than intermittent temperatures and do not return to normal. Often seen in endocarditis, and a variety of viral pulmonary infections, such as influenza and tuberculosis.
Recurrent	The temperature remains high for a few days then returns to normal, before the next episode of pyrexia (normal temperature can be observed for weeks or even months). This occurs in Hodgkin's disease, malaria, syphilis and parasitic infections.
Sustained	The temperature remains consistently high for more than 24 hours. Temperature readings do not vary by more than 1–2°C throughout the day. This pattern occurs in central nervous system disorders (hyperthermia) pneumococcal pneumonia and scarlet fever.

These stages account for the discomfort experienced by patients with high temperatures. They also explain why a patient with a high temperature may initially feel cold and want to wrap up rather than be uncovered. Different patterns of pyrexia, which exhibit recognizable changes in temperature over time, have been identified (Table 1.9).

Hyperthermia

Hyperthermia is defined as an increase in body temperature, with increased cellular metabolism, oxygen consumption and carbon dioxide production, but where the body fails to activate compensatory cooling mechanisms (Morgan 1990). This condition is caused by problems of the central nervous system and does not respond to antipyretic therapy. A temperature between 41 and 43°C produces nerve damage, coagulation, convulsions and death. Unless effective cooling measures are initiated, irreversible brain damage and death will occur (Holtzclaw 1993).

Hyperthermia also presents in five other conditions:

1. Heat cramps
2. Heat exhaustion
3. Heat stroke
4. Malignant hyperthermia
5. Neuroleptic malignant syndrome (NMS).

Heat cramps and exhaustion, even though they can be severe, do not generally warrant admission to hospital and those at risk can be taught ways to avoid it. However, heat stroke, malignant hyperthermia and NMS must be recognized quickly, as, untreated, they may be fatal.

> **!**
>
> Tepid sponging, baths and fans are not advised in lowering core temperature in a pyrexia as they result in:
>
> - A compensatory response by the hypothalamus, which will produce heat generating activities like chills and shivering.
> - Compromising an unstable patient by depleting their metabolic reserve and can create a new temperature spike.
> - The child may feel weak, especially during the early stages when the temperature is still rising.

Artificial cooling methods like tepid sponging and fanning are valuable in a hyperthermia (Thompson 1990), heat stroke and malignant hyperthermias, as they generally do not respond well to anti-pyretic therapy. Aggressive cooling should be commenced early, as temperatures of above 41°C causes coagulation, nerve damage, convulsions, cell, tissue, organ damage and eventually death.

The best way to treat a high temperature is by the use of antipyrexial drug therapy, in preference to cooling methods.

Common poisonings

There are a number of poisonings that may be encountered by the child: accidental, neonatal, deliberate. Usually, poisoned children are unable to say what they have taken, but the presence of signs and symptoms may help us to assess how severe the poisoning is.

Coma

This is one of the common signs of poisoning and is usually due to depression of the central nervous and respiratory centre system by:

- hypnotics
- antidepressants
- anticonvulsants
- tranquillizers
- opioid analgesics
- alcohol.

It is uncommon in acute salicylate poisoning (aspirin) and does not occur with paracetamol poisoning unless another drug has been taken as well, such as co-proxamol.

Convulsions

These are caused by CNS stimulation by anticholinergics, sympathomimetics, tricyclic antidepressants and monoamine oxidase inhibitors.

Respiratory features

- Cough, wheeze and breathlessness often occur after inhalation of irritant gases such as ammonia, chlorine and smoke from fires

- Cyanosis may be due to a combination of factors in the unconscious patient
- Hypoventilation is common with any CNS depressant. Usually respiration gets shallower rather than slower
- Marked reduction in rate is likely to be due to opioids
- Hyperventilation is most commonly due to salicylate poisoning and occasionally to CNS stimulant drugs and cyanide
- Pulmonary oedema may follow inhaled poisons and paraquat poisoning (contained in some weed-killers).

Cardiovascular features

- Tachycardia may be due to anticholinergics, sympathomimetics and salicylates
- Bradycardia may be caused by cardiac glycosides, e.g. digoxin and beta-blockers
- Dysrhythmias
- Hypotension may occur in any severe poisoning
- CNS depressants may lower the systolic blood pressure to 70–80 mmHg. The BP falls lower as the coma gets deeper
- Diuretics lower the blood pressure by depleting the blood volume
- Hypertension is uncommon in overdosage.

Pupil changes

- Very small and pinpoint pupils, especially if the respiratory rate is slowed, suggest opioid analgesics.

- Dilated pupils suggest tricyclic antidepressants or other anticholinergics or antihistamines
- Tinnitus is a very common feature of salicylate poisoning.

Antidotes

- Most important here is naloxone (Narcan), which is the antidote to all narcotic drugs. It may completely reverse a coma within 1–2 minutes and will increase the respiratory rate.
- Flumenazil is the antidote for severe benzodiazepine poisoning but is not always used in less severe cases.
- Acetylcysteine (Parvolex) is given in paracetamol poisoning and can prevent liver failure if given soon enough after the overdose.

Management

- About 90% of children have minimal symptoms and require little medical care. Half the remainder are seriously ill and recovery depends upon good care. Management of coma is a vital part of this care
- Ensure the airway, breathing and blood pressure are adequate (ABC)
- Assess the level of consciousness
- Screening for poisons identifies and quantifies poisons amenable to treatment. There is no point in doing an emergency screening if the result has no bearing on the treatment that will be given.
- Contact the poisons information services such as TOXBASE (www.spib.axl.co.uk) if there is any uncertainty about the toxicity of the substance or the management of the poison

- Consider whether an antidote is available or necessary
- Consider the need to prevent absorption of the poison
- Consider whether it is necessary to attempt to increase elimination of the poison.
- Minimize the absorption of ingested poisons:
  - Empty the stomach
  - Administer activated charcoal
  - Whole-bowel irrigation.

Emptying the stomach

There is an ongoing debate as to the usefulness of emptying the stomach.

There are always dangers involved and sometimes it may lead to more rapid absorption of the drug.

Gastric lavage is sometimes used, but be aware of the following points:

- Should never be attempted without intubation and an anaesthetist present if the patient is very drowsy or comatose.
- Should never be attempted when a corrosive material has been ingested.
- Gastric lavage is of doubtful value if it is conducted more than 1–2 hours after ingestion.
- Danger of inhalation of stomach contents.
- Petrol is more dangerous in the lungs than in the stomach and so gastric lavage should not be attempted.
- Syrup of ipecacuanha is the best agent for inducing emesis but is very rarely recommended as it can be dangerous and cannot be used alongside the administration of active charcoal.
- It causes excessive vomiting and if absorbed may have cardiac effects.

Activated charcoal

- There is a trend towards replacing the above methods with repeated doses of activated charcoal
- The charcoal is not absorbed and combines with some drugs in the stomach and intestine (adsorbs them) to prevent their absorption too
- Ten times as much charcoal is needed as the drug you wish it to combine with
- The sooner it is given, the more effective it will be
- It is best given within the first hour of ingestion but may be effective up to 2 hours after ingestion and longer if modified-release preparations are taken
- It is a tasteless, black, gritty slurry and patients do not like to take it
- It should not be given before ipecacuanha as it stops absorption of the latter
- It does not adsorb all toxins but is good for paracetamol, benzodiazepines, digoxin, paraquat, phenytoin, salicylates and quinine
- It is useful for poisons that are toxic in small amounts such as tricyclic antidepressants. It can enhance the elimination of some drugs when they have been absorbed
- Repeated doses are given for: aspirin, carbamazepine, phenobarbital theophylline, quinine.

Increasing the elimination of poisons

Methods include:

- forced diuresis (aspirin) – no longer recommended

- haemodialysis – salicylates, phenobarbital
- repeat-dose oral charcoal (gut dialysis).

> All children who have taken an intentional overdose should be admitted to hospital and given a child psychiatric referral as the overdose may be a 'cry for help'.

Chest drains

A chest tube (same as chest drain) is normally used to evacuate air or fluid that has accumulated in the pleural space. When fluid or air accumulates in the pleural space this reduces lung expansion and leads to respiratory compromise and hypoxia. The rapid diagnosis of lung collapse is essential.

Conditions requiring chest tube insertion

- Pneumothorax (collection of air in the pleural space)
- Haemothorax
- Pleural effusion (accumulation of fluid within the pleural cavity)
- Cardiac tamponade after open-heart surgery (accumulation of blood or fluid in or around the pericardial sac that causes compression of the heart muscle).

Signs and symptoms

- Decreased chest movement and breath sounds on the affected side of the chest on inspiration
- Difficulty in breathing (known as dyspnoea)
- Increased respiratory rate
- Increased heart rate
- Restlessness and agitation
- Cyanosis and chest pain.

A chest X-ray is normally done to confirm the diagnosis and then treatment begins with the insertion of a chest tube. The chest tube is a flexible plastic tube that is inserted through the side of the chest into the pleural space. Therefore it is a painful procedure for children. Additionally, the insertion of a chest drain can be a traumatic event for the child and family, therefore you need to ensure that the child and family are prepared.

Psychological care

- You provide adequate preparation and explanation prior to and during the procedure.
- It is essential to explain the procedure in simple, easily understandable terms to the child and parents before the procedure begins.
- Take time to answer any questions the child may have.
- Young children may take longer to agree to the procedure so please ensure that the doctor allows the child time to adjust to the need for the procedure.
- Ensure that the parent is allowed to stay with the child during the procedure.

■ The basic principle is to allow air and excess fluid to escape from the pleural cavity. The drainage tube is connected to a catheter, the end of which is submerged below a few centimetres of sterile water in a calibrated bottle.

Major principles of chest drain daily management

■ Position the drainage system in upright position, below the level of the chest. The drainage systems should be at all times at least 30 cm beneath the child's chest.

■ Drains should *not* be clamped during movement of the child.

■ The tubing should be securely attached to the child's skin with adhesive tape.

■ Check the chest tube for kinks as small soft drains are prone to kinking as the drain exits the skin, especially in young active children.

■ Record temperature, pulse, respirations and oxygen saturation levels regularly.

■ Nurse the child in a high visibility area and ensure suction and oxygen are available at the bedside.

■ Assess drainage collection system every 4 hours for fluctuations and air bubbles in the air leak indicator.

■ In a pleural drain observe the swings of fluid in the chest tube bottle. With inspiration water will rise up into the chest tube, with expiration, water will fall.

■ If the swing is less than 2 cm, the lung is not likely to be fully expanded and therefore suction may need to be increased.

■ Encourage the child to cough and deep breathe frequently to promote drainage.

■ Record volume of fluid drained regularly.

■ Ensure that extra drainage collection system is readily available in case of accidental damage.

It is important that children with chest drains are kept pain free.

■ The child's experience of pain should be assessed regularly using an appropriate pain score assessment tool.

■ Ensure that the child has regular oral analgesia prescribed to reduce the development of pain from the chest drain site.

■ If a child complains of continued pain with the chest drain (despite analgesia) this must be investigated to ensure it is not a symptom of an underlying condition or a complication.

Drains should never be milked or stripped. 'Milking' is where the chest tubing is either milked by hand or a specialized roller is used to compress the tube down its length of tubing. 'Stripping' is executed by running two pieces of alcohol gauze along the length of the tubing, each in their own turn, from top to bottom. In the past it was assumed that 'milking' or 'stripping' a chest tube would prevent the development of clots in the chest tubing. However, research has shown that milking will not prevent clot formation; instead it may cause lung damage since excessively high intrathoracic pressures may be created.

Compartment syndrome

Acute compartment syndrome is a common condition whereby there is a raised pressure within a closed fascial space (Edwards 2004). The increased pressure reduces capillary perfusion below a level necessary for tissue viability. This condition is serious. The ability for the patient not to identify pain may mask its progression.

The syndrome is fairly common following a soft tissue injury. Young men in particular are at risk of compartment syndrome.

The muscles of the legs are grouped into compartments that are formed by thick layers of fairly inelastic tissue called fascia. Within the compartments are the nerves and blood vessels that supply the limbs. The anterior compartment is the most frequent site If this condition goes unrecognized it can have devastating consequences for a critical care patient.

Causes of compartment syndrome

The compartment size may be decreased by crush injury, compression bandages or constrictive devices, such as a tight cast that has been improperly left in place for extended periods of time. Other causes include:

- fracture
- excessive exercise of a muscle group
- surgical procedures including closure of fascial defects
- major vascular surgery
- bleeding disorder
- snakebite
- burns
- IV drug abuse
- weight-lifting
- post-ischaemic swelling.

Pathophysiology of compartment syndrome

The initial injury, whether traumatic, haemorrhagic, surgical or vascular or a complication of another condition, leads to localized swelling in the muscle compartments. This is due to the stimulation of the inflammatory response (see Section 4). Further oedema forms when large amounts of fluid such as blood move into the compartments.

Compartment pressure measurement (Table 1.10) should be at the top of the list when compartment syndrome is considered. If the compartment pressure is greater than 40 mmHg, emergency treatment is needed. At this point blood flow through the capillaries stops. In the absence of flow, oxygen delivery stops. This may finally lead to irreversible cell damage, loss of limb and death. Necrotic muscle will never recover hence the seriousness of this condition and the importance of recognizing the warning signs. Another complication that can occur is myoglobinuria, which can lead to kidney failure due to excess of myoglobin causing dark pigmented urine.

Table 1.10 Measuring intracompartmental pressure

Type	Procedure	Advantages and disadvantages
Wick catheter	Uses polyglycolic acid suture wicks connected to a pressure transducer	It is an accurate method and allows continuous measurement; other methods require repeated insertion of needles. May lead to coagulation around insertion site, and wick left in the insertion wound.
Simple needle manometry	Uses an 18-G needle and a simple mercury manometer	The injection of saline is required into the tissues during the reading. Not as accurate as the wick method.
Infusion technique	Uses a syringe infusion pump to infuse 0.7 ml saline per day via a 19-G needle and allows continuous measurement	The insertion of saline can increase pressure 2–4 mmHg.
Slit catheter	Made from epidural catheter tubing, slits are used to reduce clotting problems	Continues to use an infusion system but easier than the wick method.
Central venous pressure manometer	An 18-G needle is attached to a simple CVP manometer	It is quick, no special equipment is needed. It suffers from some inaccuracies similar to the simple needle manometer technique.
Side-ported needle	Allows the measurement of several compartments using the same needle	This method cannot be used for continuous monitoring.
Fibreoptic transducer	This method is very expensive and only available in specialist units	It is easy to use, allows continuous monitoring.

Patient management

For early recognition more subtle skills and knowledge are required:

- Pain (out of proportion to the apparent injury) in conditions where the risk of compartment syndrome is high. High doses of morphine can mask the symptoms.
- Paraesthesiae.

- Sensory deficit – numbness occurs because the excess pressure within a compartment hampers the activity of sensory nerves carrying messages toward the brain.

However, all of these signs can only be identified in a fully conscious patient and are also present following vascular injury. A nurse has to be vigilant in clinical observation and examination.

Section 2

Assessment and investigations of a child

2.1 Identification of problems and scoring systems

Early warning scoring (EWS)

Children admitted to the ward often have abnormal physiological values present in the previous 24 hours. Most common observed is tachycardia, an altered level of consciousness, derangement in heart rate, blood pressure, arterial oxygen saturation and urinary output.

The EWS is used to aid early detection of a child's deteriorating condition and is a simple scoring system based on routine observations. This system to identify children at risk of worsening condition uses the child's physiological parameters:

- pulse
- blood pressure
- respiratory rate
- urine output
- temperature
- sedation level.

Combining these with observations of the airway, breathing and circulation (ABC), measures of fluid balance and neurological status forms the basis of this simple system of early detection. Deviations from the normal score points allows a total to be calculated (Table 2.1). A total score of 3 or more generally results in the patient's condition being reviewed by the nurse in charge or the ward medical staff and help sought from the outreach team or medical emergency team (MET) if appropriate.

Assessment of a deteriorating child

Assessment of a child is necessary when their condition is deteriorating for example, becomes breathless or level of consciousness decreases. In some instances assessment and treatment must be administered before a diagnosis has been made. A rapid systematic approach to the assessment process is essential so a child can receive simple life supportive treatments as soon as possible.

A standardized assessment for life support practice is now in place when dealing with multiple trauma or cardiopulmonary/respiratory arrest using the ABCDE style approach (see Section 1). This approach can also be used when assessing the deteriorating patient. The aim of this assessment is to halt the deterioration in the child's condition and prevent cardiac/respiratory arrest.

A = airway

Without a patent airway oxygen cannot reach the lungs, enter the bloodstream or be transported to the cells and tissues of the body:

- Determine if the airway is clear/ obstructed/either:
  - Partial obstruction – identify the cause of the obstruction:
    - Can you hear a wheeze during expiration or snoring sounds which may indicate a partial obstruction?
    - Gurgling may indicate secretions, vomit or blood in the mouth or upper airways.

Table 2.1 Paediatric early warning system criteria

	0	**1**	**2**	**3**
Behaviour	Playing appropriate	Sleeping	Irritable	Lethargic, Confused Reduced response to pain
Cardio-vascular	Pink or capillary refill 1–2 s	Pale or capillary refill 3 s	Grey or capillary refill 3 s Tachycardia 20 above normal rate	Grey and mottled or capillary refill 5 s or above Tachycardia of 30 above normal rate or bradycardia
Respiratory	Within normal parameters No recession No tracheal tug	10 above normal parameters Using accessory muscles 30 + % FiO$_2$ or 4 + litre/min	20 above normal parameters Recessing tracheal tug 40 + % FiO$_2$ or 6 + litre/min	5 below normal parameters with sternal recession, Tracheal tug or grunting 50% FiO$_2$ or 8 + litre/min

Scoring
Score 2 extra for quarter hourly nebulizers or persistent vomiting following surgery
Score 2: inform nurse in charge
Score 3: increase frequency of score and observations, inform outreach co-ordinator, inform nurse in charge
Score 4: or if score increases by 2 following intervention, call medical staff and inform outreach co-ordinator medical should respond within 15 minutes
Score more than 4 or red column: immediately call senior registrar, anaesthetist and outreach co-ordinator. Consider transfer.
Brighton PEWS 2005.

- Stridor may indicate an obstruction above the larynx – generally on inspiration.
- Complete obstruction may display:
  - Paradoxical chest and abdominal movements or seesaw respiratory pattern (the abdomen moves outwards during inspiration and the chest is drawn inwards, and vice versa during expiration).
  - Place the back of the hand in front of the child's mouth to detect any airflow; no airflow may indicate complete obstruction.
- Protected – normal breath sounds will be present.

- Check for the use of the accessory muscles, e.g. neck and shoulders or tracheal tug.
- Observe the pattern of the chest movement and are they expanding symmetrically.

Call the MET immediately, if prescribed, then administer oxygen and secure the airway, which may include head lift, chin lift or jaw thrust.

B = breathing

Assessment of breathing should be undertaken when the child's airway is secured, managed and before progressing to a full assessment of the child:

- Is there any distress observed in the child?
  - Are they using accessory muscles?
  - Is there any central or peripheral cyanosis?
  - Look for symmetry of the chest movement.
  - If of an age, are they talking in clear sentences?
- Check if the respiratory rate is normal for the child's age range; if this is very high the child will become exhausted very quickly.
  - Note the colour of the child, e.g. if cyanosed, check their oxygen saturation level.
  - A stethoscope may be used to determine:
    • any rattling noises, which may be a sign of secretions
    • bronchial breathing; are normal breath sounds present, absent or reduced – if no breath sounds or air entry are heard this may be a pneumothorax and is an emergency.

A pneumothorax is a medical emergency. Call for help immediately, as treatment with a large bore cannula through the second intercostals space in the midclavicular line on the same side as the pneumothorax needs to be instigated.

- Palpation of the chest may indicate surgical emphysema.
- Percussion may reveal differences in note:
  • hyper-resonance pneumothorax
  • dullness consolidation or pleural effusion.

If oxygen is prescribed then it should be administered immediately.

C = Circulation

Assessment of circulation should take place after the airway is secure and treatment has been instigated for breathing.

- Look at the child carefully – are they distressed, pale or cyanosed?
  - Peripheral veins may have collapsed making it difficult to cannulate.
  - Are there any obvious signs of haemorrhage.
  - Check abdominal or chest drains.
- What is the consciousness level?
- Check fluid balance for documentation of any urine output.
- In the initial stage of shock blood pressure is not a good indicator so use:

- pulse pressure (different between systolic and diastolic blood pressure (see haemodynamic monitoring)
- capillary refill > 2 seconds.
■ Is the pulse bounding (sepsis) or weak (reduced cardiac output)? ECG may be indicated if it is available.

Immediate management with an IV cannula, and if there is no evidence of cardiogenic shock, hypovolaemia should be suspected and fluid bolus administered according to age and weight of the child. If there are concerns about cardiac function the bolus should be reduced. Bloods should be taken for analysis.

D = Disability

The priority of ABC is paramount, but rapid assessment of disability now needs to be observed.

Check consciousness level using the AVPU method (alert, vocal stimuli, pain, unresponsive).

Check glucose level (BM).

Check pupil reactions to light:

- bilateral pinpoint may indicate drug overdose, e.g. opiates, brainstem stroke
- unilateral dilated unresponsive to light indicates brainstem death, cancer lesion or cerebral oedema.

Glasgow Coma Scale (GCS) if time (see section on assessment).

E = Examination

Assessment has taken place of the airway, breathing and circulation and any compromise in these areas has been corrected. Assessment of the child warrants further investigation:

■ Hypothermia – has the child recently been to theatre where loss of body heat may occur?
■ Electrolytes – urea, creatinine, potassium, sodium levels.
■ Fluids – check fluid balance chart over the past few days:
  - receiving IV fluids, what type, how much?
  - enteral feeding regimes – check absorption.
■ GIT – examine patient for any abnormalities:
  - check abdomen
  - recent surgery
  - drains excessive drainage or blood loss
  - wound infection
  - bowel sounds, bowel opened recently.
■ Haematology – clotting factors, haemoglobin, white blood cell count (WBC), full blood count (FBC).
■ Infection – do not forget to check for:
  - source of infection
  - temperature
  - recent microbiology reports, e.g. cultures from wounds, urine, sputum, drains, blood.
■ Lines – check if they are source of infection/sepsis:
  - drains, catheters
  - when inserted, how long have they been in place – remove or replace, send for culture where necessary.
■ Medication – check the drug chart:
  - prescribed drugs given
  - has usual medication been given
  - nephrotoxic drugs – have drug levels been monitored

- drug interactions – check with
  pharmacist if unsure
- allergies.

> **!**
>
> It is important to
> document your findings and the
> management of the child in the notes;
> it will assist with reviewing the child's
> condition later.

2.2 Assessment of a child – scoring systems

There are many scoring systems
available to assess different aspects of
care ranging from: developmental, pain,
nutritional status, neurological, wound
and pressure sores.

Developmental assessment

Children undergo biological and
psychological changes from birth to
eighteen years of age. Understanding
normal child development is essential to
assess a child and identify any deviations
from the normal.

Child development may be grouped
into five domains (areas):

1. Physical (physical growth and
   maturation)
2. Language (ability to speak and use
   words)
3. Cognitive (the ability to reason, think,
   perceptions, attention, memory)
4. Psychological/emotional (feelings and
   emotions)
5. Social (interactions with others).

Children's development occurs
simultaneously in all domains, so all are
closely linked and interdependent. It is
important to stress that children develop
in an integrated manner. If a child's
physical development is delayed, this may
hamper their psychological and social
development. If a child has a speech defect,
this may hamper their emotional and social
development. For example a 2-year-old
may show problems with speaking or
linking small words. When compared to
the age-specific ability, this may indicate
developmental delay and so should be
investigated. The speech delay may be
due to hearing problems or a physical
problem which once rectified may help the
child to develop normally. Alternatively,
the speech delay may be due to neglect and
lack of stimulation from the parents, which
would need to be assessed. The family
social circumstances may need to be
assessed and appropriate help and support
provided.

Early identification of developmental delay and disorders

Early identification of developmental
delays and disorders is crucial and many
can be identified before the child is
2 years old. Delays or disorders that are
not diagnosed and treated place children
as risk for later poor physical, academic,
and social progress. The importance of
assessing child development early allows
identification of developmental problems
and can result in better developmental
outcomes and better child health. Early
diagnosis leads to appropriate treatment
which facilitates the development of

skills that would otherwise lag behind or fail to develop. Although development is assessed using normative measures (how a child performs compared with the norm or average), you need to be aware that this method can be judgemental, resulting in children being labelled as 'backward' or 'deficient' in some way. Children develop at different rates and so it is essential to consider norms of development as linked broadly to the age of the child. For example some children walk at 12 months whilst other children prefer to crawl and do not walk till 15 months. So the key points are:

- Children grow and develop through various stages
- There are critical time periods when a child is ready to develop a particular skill
- Children develop at different rates, so assess development broadly
- Assess and document child's stage of development
- Deviations should be investigated and documented
- Provide support and stimulation for children's developmental needs.

Roles of professionals in developmental assessment

The promotion of normal development and the prevention of developmental delay are predominantly the role of the following professionals: public health nurse, health visitor, paediatrician, general practitioner, school nurse in the community. The health visitor or public health nurse usually performs the developmental checks in well child clinics, but this can vary between countries. When babies are born they are usually examined by a paediatrician and a midwife. Most babies and children are then assessed at specific time periods, which can vary between countries, but most checks are at:

- 1 week to 10 days after birth
- 6 to 8 weeks old
- 3 months
- 7–9 months
- 18–24 months
- 3–4 years
- 5 years
- 12 years.

Developmental assessments should focus on five key areas:

1. Gross motor development and locomotion
2. Fine motor development and manipulation skills
3. Hearing and speech
4. Vision
5. Social development.

Developmental tests and scales

Developmental screening tests have been used for nearly three decades to identify children in need of more assessment or interventions. The measuring of intellectual, social and motor abilities is called psychometrics. Sheridan's Developmental Progress Scale (1975) consists of an inventory of abilities and milestones. It can be regarded as a simple form of psychometric test whose method of administration is not rigorously standardized and whose normative data consist only of approximate mean ages at which the various milestones are reached. The Denver Developmental Screening Test (DDST) developed by Frankenburg and Dodds (1967) has been administered to millions of children and so is the most frequently used screening instrument. However, caution is advised in using screening instruments unless the scale has acceptable levels of sensitivity and specificity. Screening instruments should only be used by skilled and experienced clinicians who can link the findings from the test into a broad developmental context. A scale should be used primarily as a guide to normal development. Developmental screening should not occur in isolation because it is one component of a process. It should take account of the relationships between:

- Results of the screen/assessment
- The environment where test has taken place
- Area of function assessed
- Age of the child
- Child's medical history.

Developmental screening should consist of the following:

- Take a detailed history from the parents
- Use suitable age-appropriate materials for the assessment
- Create varied and near natural situations for eliciting behaviour
- Make close observations of the child's responses
- Combine personal observations with that from the parents

- Consider quality of performance across the domains
- Monitor child's progress over time as child may 'catch up' if there is a delay evident.

Developmental milestones

While the rate of development varies from one child to the next, the sequence is virtually the same for all children, even those with marked physical or intellectual disabilities. The development of a child from birth to 18 months can vary but there are approximate milestones that help distinguish the deviations from normal.

Developmental milestones for infants 0–6 months

Newborns have little day–night rhythms (circadian rhythms); they sleep about equal amounts at any given time of the day. By 6 weeks most have established a pattern, although they still spend about 15–16 hours sleeping each day. At 6 months babies are sleeping about 14 hours per day, but the regularity and predictability of the sleep increases over the months. These are average figures as babies vary a lot in their sleep patterns. Irregularity in sleep pattern may be a symptom of some disorder or problem. Often, babies born to drug-addicted mothers and brain-damaged infants are unable to establish a sleep pattern.

Crying is a crucial sign that babies use to tell the care-giver that they require care. Infants have a whole repertoire of cry sounds – different cries for pain, anger, hunger. Crying seems to increase over the first 6 weeks of life and then decreases. Initially the infant cries most in the evening, later shifting their crying before feeding times; 15–29% develop a pattern called colic. Many groups of babies with known medical abnormalities have different-sounding cries (e.g. Down's syndrome, encephalitis, meningitis).

- Babies are born with a large collection of reflexes which are physical responses triggered involuntarily by a specific stimulus.
- Newborns are light sensitive, can feel pain and seem to prefer the human face.
- At 1 month babies can recognize different speech sounds and can smile.
- At 4 months, babies can link familiar sounds with objects.
- At 5 months babies begin to respond to their name.
- At 6 months babies can:
  - pick up objects
  - pass objects from hand to hand
  - enjoy bright colours
  - can laugh and scream
  - can sit with support
  - bear weight on feet when held standing and bounce up and down
  - not follow an object with the eyes when it falls out of the visual field.
  - recognize and respond to mother's voice
  - have clear night-time sleeping patterns
  - begin to nap during the day at more predictable times.

Developmental milestones from 8–24 months

- At 8 months they can sit without support.
- At 8–9 months they begin to crawl on hands or knees or buttocks.
- At 12 months they can stand and some can walk. They develop a pincer grip. They can recognize familiar people and turn when their name is called. They can drink from a cup and can hold utensils for feeding.
- When toy falls out of visual field, they look for the toy in the correct place
- At 18 months they can walk safely, backwards and sideways. Can use delicate pincer grasp to pick up small objects.

Developmental milestones from 3–8 years

- At 3–4 years can walk and run easily, walk upstairs, and pedal a tricycle. Holds pencil between thumb and fingers. Can draw and name primary colours. Can cut paper with scissors. Can sing nursery rhymes and enjoys doing jigsaw puzzles.
- At 5–8 years can ride a bicycle easily, undress and dress self, balance, skip, climb, play ball games and dance.

Growth and development

Infants grow very quickly in the first year of life, adding 20–30 cm to their height and doubling their birth rate by the age of 5 months (Table 2.2A).

Table 2.2 Height and weight gain by age

A Height gain by age

Age	Height
Birth–6 months	2.5 cm per month
6–12 months	1–5 cm per month
12 months–4.5 years	7.5 cm per year

B Weight gain by age

Age	Weight
Birth–6 months	140–200 g per week (doubles by end of 5 months)
6–12 months	85–140 g per week (triples by end of 1 year)
12–4.5 years	2–3 kg per year (quadruples by end of 2.5 years)

There is a rapid increase in size by the age of 2 years. From 2 onwards the child usually gains about 5–7.5 cm in height each year and approximately 3 kg in weight per year. Weight has a similar growth curve to height (Table 2.2B). When the child reaches adolescence, usually from 10 years onwards, there is a rapid growth in height, called a 'growth spurt'. The hands and feet grow to full adult size earliest, followed by the arms and legs, and the trunk. Children will grow at different rates depending on genetics, nutrition, environment and illness conditions. So these are broad parameters which are a guide to assessment of growth and development.

Measuring growth

- To measure an infant's length, the infant is placed supine on a measuring board with the head firmly at the top of the board and heels at the foot of the board.

- To measure a child who can stand, use a wall-mounted stadiometer. Remove footwear and ask child to stand tall, with head in the mid-line and child looking straight ahead (parallel to the floor).

- To weigh an infant, undress the infant, ensure the room is warm, and the weighing machine is calibrated and then record the weight.

- To weigh a child, remove only shoes and stand child on weighing machine.

Language development (ability to speak and use words)

- Infant – cooing, babbling, laughing, gurgling
- 1 year – can say few words, imitates sounds, recognizes some words
- 2 years – can use 2–3 words in phrases and knows about 200–300 short words, e.g. 'want my teddy'
- 3 years – can use 4–5 words in sentences and has a vocabulary of 800–900 words

- 4–5 years – can use complete sentences clearly and has a vocabulary of 1500–2500 words
- 5–6 years – has a vocabulary of about 3000 plus words.

Deviations from normal

Pre-schoolers (< 5 years)

Communication delay or disorders may be present with preschoolers who:

- Have atypical comprehension of commands or requests
- May have few words or exhibit unintelligible speech
- May omit many speech sounds or produce unusual combinations of speech sounds
- Have limited vocabulary
- May grunt or point to items rather than attempt to produce words
- May show disinterest in toys or games suitable for their age group
- May be withdrawn or prefer to play alone if speech disordered
- May display aggression (e.g. tantrums, biting, kicking) because of frustration with communicating needs

Children who display these behaviours need appropriate referrals (e.g. speech and language therapist for necessary investigations, therapy, early intervention programme, early childhood education programme).

- Language delay may be due to undiagnosed hearing loss or an infection such as otitis media (infection of middle ear) with effusion.

- Language delay may be due to adverse social circumstances (e.g. neglect, parental depression or substance abuse) rather than a cognitive disorder.

Late talkers

Late talkers may display similar behaviour outlined above but the distinction is they generally:

- Have better comprehension of spoken language and tend to understand age-appropriate commands
- Develop normal language skills during early school years
- Have normal hearing
- Have age-appropriate non-verbal problem-solving skills e.g. can assemble age-appropriate puzzles and games.

Cognitive development (the ability to reason, think, perceptions, attention, memory)

Children who have cognitive delays or disorders usually display delays in problem-solving skills, memory skills, and general learning skills:

- Problem-solving may be seen in delayed development of basic concepts such as object permanence
- Memory can be demonstrated by inability to remember an event or words that were previously known
- General learning skills can be seen in reduced ability to acquire new skills, learn simple tasks or to apply skills to new events
- May play and interact with younger children

- May have poor social skills and poor ability to assess social situations (e.g. autism)
- May have age-appropriate language skills but display cognitive deficits (e.g. high functioning autism)
- May display impulsivity, hyperactivity, and inattention (e.g. attention deficit hyperactivity disorder, ADHD).

Nutritional assessment

Nutrition relates to the physical and mental development of a child, their health and individual well-being. The energy supply of the body is obtained from nutrients to carry out vital functions to sustain life, to form new body components for growth and repair and to assist in the functioning of various body process, such as breathing and physical activity. The energy supply must be constantly replenished.

It is important to ensure that children have food while in hospital, whether it be solid oral food, enteral or parental feeding. Food contains nutrients digested by enzymes, which are regulated and controlled by hormones. There are six principal classes of nutrients:

- minerals
- vitamins
- carbohydrates
- fats
- proteins
- water.

It is important to remember that nutrients are often separated for study purposes, but are always interacting as a dynamic whole to produce and maintain the human body, providing energy, building and rebuilding tissue, and regulating metabolic processes. The essential function of minerals and vitamins is their regulation of physiological processes. The energy-yielding nutrients are carbohydrates, fats and proteins, which provide primary and alternative sources of energy. Water is the overall vital nutrient sustaining all life processes.

Guidance on the adequacy of nutrition is required and standards have been devised against which measured intakes can be compared. These standards are known as Recommended Daily Amounts (RDA).

The assessment of a child's nutritional state is given high priority and most children's nurses will already be familiar with the use of assessment tools and protocols in their daily management of a child.

Nutritional assessment in a children's ward may vary from basic to complex nutritional requirements. Information collated to assist with the overall nutritional assessment should include:

- child's history
- psychological and social status
- physical examination
- diet history
- current dietary intake
- anthropometric measurements
- biochemical and laboratory data.

The above factors will all play an important role in assessing a child's level of nutrition and hydration.

History, psychological and social status

A concise history provides the first clues about existing or potential undernutrition. Ascertain if the child has:

- Been ill at home or on the ward for a long period of time prior to admission to hospital
- Has recently suffered a bad experience (death of close family member, friend)
- Is the family on income support, one parent family
- The type of accommodation the child lives in

Observe the child:

- Do they look thin or pale
- The appearance of their skin in terms of colour and condition
- Check nails: are they brittle
- Look in the mouth: are the gums swollen, teeth discoloured
- Are their clothes loose
- Are their eyes sunken
- Check their tongue for hydration, colour and condition.

These will all send warning signals to the trained eye that a problem with nutrition may exist, and may also give information about any recent loss of weight.

Physical examination

A physical examination involves observing the child's general appearance and should include the following assessment:

- Check the oral cavity – is there a sore mouth or lips?
- Check for the presence of difficulty in chewing and swallowing or any physical difficulties with feeding.
- Is there any nausea, vomiting, diarrhoea; this results in reduced absorption and appetite.

- Any constipation will affect nutritional intake and can lead to a feeling of fullness, discomfort, depression and confusion, thereby reducing food intake.
- Simple respiratory function tests can be recorded, such as vital capacity, maximum inspiration and maximum expiration, to determine respiratory muscle strength.

Diet history

A diet history should be obtained by asking the child and his/her parent or carer about their eating habits and consists of questions about:

- Likes and dislikes, e.g. fruit and vegetables, meat
- Religion – are there any long periods of fasting in the family – are they vegetarian?
- Changes in weight; loss of subcutaneous fat, apathy or lack of energy
- Type, quantity and texture of food eaten since the onset of illness, as disease often alters appetite
- Have there been any changes in taste and the ability to obtain food?
- Ask to recall food intake over the previous few days
- If an infant consider if:
  – they were breast or formula fed
  – they are being weaned, e.g. solids, types, variety, feeding him/herself
  – the milk the child is drinking now, e.g. semiskimmed (not recommended) or whole milk
  – they have any allergies
  – the infant's bowel patterns, frequency and consistency
  – are they in childcare during the day.

- If an older child consider:
  - if they eat breakfast, lunch and dinner
  - their favourite foods, drinks, snacks, school lunch
  - where they eat their meals, e.g. in front of the television
  - if they clean their teeth after meals
  - if they take any exercise.
- Consider issues related to the parents/ carers:
  - Does the family eat meals together at the table?
  - Preparation of food, eating in restaurants/takeaways.
  - Is the child a fussy eater – loss or gain of weight recently?

All these factors should be noted and recorded in the child's assessment and care plan. A food diary may be necessary to record total intake over a number of days / weeks.

Anthropometric measurements

One of the most important anthropometric measurements in determining nutritional status is weight, and changes in body weight do give an indication of the severity of malnutrition. All children that have been admitted to hospital or attended a healthcare clinic should have their weight measured and plotted on an appropriate centile chart. Accurate measurement of babies', infants', and children's weight is vital for calculations of medications and fluids. Different skills are required for weighing a baby and an older child:

- A baby or infant should be weighed naked (any additions e.g. splint/ medical equipment should be noted in the notes)

- Do not leave a baby/infant unattended in the scales
- Always record exact weight, do not round the figures up or down.
- Dress the baby/infant quickly

Height can also be used to determine if a child is growing at an optimal rate. Any reduction in growth rate may indicate a pathological disorder requiring possible diagnosis and intervention. The differences between measuring a baby's/ infant's length and a child height is detailed in Table 2.3.

Head circumference is used to monitor the growth of a child, especially those under 2 years, but continues to be useful after this age as it may detect abnormalities such as hydrocephalus, craniosynostosis or microcephaly. Any baby, infant or child with suspected neurological or craniofacial abnormality will need their head circumference measured more frequently, as this may indicate a raised intracranial pressure.

Biochemical measurements

Biochemical measurements can also be used, the most common in use are:

Serum albumin: with a level of less than 35 g/l being indicative of protein-energy malnutrition, it can be inaccurate as conditions such as stress, nephrosis and burns also exhibit hypoalbuminia. This makes the measurement often misleading and not altogether reflective of nutritional deficiency in the short term. In the chronic situation, serum albumin remains a simple and reliable indicator of malnutrition.

Serum transferrin: levels could be considered a better marker of acute

Table 2.3 Measuring a baby's/infant's length and a child's height

Baby's / infant's length	Child's height
The baby/infant should be lying down perfectly flat on a solid even surface	A child may require some input from a play specialist or nurse prior to the procedure
With assistance of another nurse/parent/carer position the baby on the measuring mat	Remove shoes and in some instances socks as well, hair clips
Baby/infant's head should be touching the top of the mat	Position the child with their feet together, flat on the floor, legs straight, back against the wall, arms by their side, their head should be facing forward
The body should be in alignment	Put pressure on the child's mastoids and take the reading of the height after full expiration
Record the baby/infant's length	Record the reading viewed at eye level

nutritional depletion. Interpretation of serum levels is complicated by factors such as iron deficiency, which directly affects transferrin production and so may not be wholly appropriate as a predictor of malnutrition.

Serum haemoglobin: measurements will highlight the presence of anaemia, which has been correlated with pressure sore development. Anaemia can occur for a variety of reasons, but may be directly related to dietary inadequacy and questioning of dietary intake should always follow this up.

Promising results have been demonstrated when nutritional assessment has resulted in initiation of pre-operative feeding regimes. This method of identifying the high-risk patients results in an optimization of their nutritional status and may help to ensure an uneventful recovery. The patient in critical care not only has an increased demand for energy, but also, due to periods of reduction or cessation of nutritional intake, has a reduced supply of energy-containing nutrients. As a result, under-nutrition, or in severe cases, malnutrition may occur.

Malnutrition

The maintenance of health depends upon the consumption and absorption of appropriate amounts of energy and all the necessary nutrients. A shortfall of one or other over a period of days or weeks may lead to malnutrition.

Malnutrition itself is defined as a state that occurs when there is an imbalance between nutritional intake and nutritional requirement. When nutrition ceases during periods of fasting, there is a resulting loss of energy stores and malnutrition occurs.

Physiological effects of malnutrition

Carbohydrates are the first source of energy utilized by the body and are needed to maintain a normal blood glucose level. During starvation, carbohydrates are not available directly from the gut but the body uses carbohydrates stored as glycogen in the liver and skeletal muscles as a source of energy.

■ During the first day of fasting, low glucose levels stimulate glucagon secretion by the pancreas. As a result, glycogen is converted to glucose and released from the liver. This restores blood glucose levels to normal. Glycogen can be lost without any physiological consequences.

■ These mechanisms supply blood glucose but cannot sustain blood glucose for a long period of time.

■ Fat stores may be used for energy. This method requires a major body adjustment, as all other body tissues must reduce their oxidation of glucose and switch over to fat as their energy source.

■ As the liver metabolizes fat, ketone bodies are produced in large quantities. These are oxidized by the body into carbon dioxide, water and adenosine triphosphate (ATP).

If fasting continues, the brain has to gradually adapt to the use of ketone bodies as its major source of energy.

When this occurs, depression of the central nervous system may ensue, leading to coma.

Since other body cells are also limited in the amount of ketone bodies they can metabolize, excess ketone bodies appear in the blood resulting in ketosis, which if not reversed by taking food can lead to a metabolic acidosis.

When fat reserves are completely depleted, the body will break down large quantities of muscle protein as a source of energy, to maintain cellular function. Large amounts of amino acids can be released and converted to glucose in the liver by gluconeogenesis or the amino acids may be oxidized directly. It is estimated that once protein stores are depleted to about one half of their normal level, death occurs. During fasting, amino acids contribute to blood glucose only after liver glycogen and fat stores are depleted.

Within the dietetic arena, promising results have been shown when a detailed nutritional assessment has taken place to ensure early feeding regimes. This method of early assessment results in an optimization of child's nutritional status and can be seen as promoting a speedy and uneventful recovery. It is important to note that malnutrition reduces the body's ability to:

■ Heal wounds, which increases risk of pressure sore development

■ Manufacture haemoglobin, which reduces the oxygen carrying capacity of the blood

■ Produce white blood cells, causing suppression of the immune response and reducing child's defence mechanisms

■ Maintain adequate respiratory drive due to the reduction in pulmonary diaphragmatic muscle mass and strength, predisposing patient to respiratory failure.

Consequences of malnutrition in children

■ Higher incidence of pneumonia due to impairment in respiratory function.

■ Catabolism and weight loss are accelerated

■ There is impaired gut integrity.

■ Delayed wound healing; this can lead to reduced healing of surgical sites.

■ Have an increased susceptibility to wound or systemic infections.

■ There are decreased visceral proteins.

■ May reduce the metabolism of drugs.

Information should be based on nurses' observations of the child

Pressure area risk assessment

Pressure ulcers are potentially an avoidable complication of bed rest and decreased mobility. Children who are at more risk of developing of pressure ulcers include:

■ those who are in a poor state of health and have numerous medical, surgical problems

■ the malnourished

■ babies, infants, children who have some degree of immobility, e.g. those nursed in intensive care, neonates, those undergoing prolonged surgery, spinal injury.

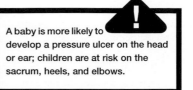

A baby is more likely to develop a pressure ulcer on the head or ear; children are at risk on the sacrum, heels, and elbows.

The pathogenesis of pressure ulcers is complex, since it is affected by so many predisposing factors. However, there are three major factors identified as significant:

1. Pressure greater than 25 mmHg will occlude capillaries. The tissues are thus deprived of blood, and if the pressure is maintained for a sufficient length of time, the tissues die.

2. Friction is a combination of pressure and friction caused by dragging children up the bed, which seriously damages the micro-circulation.

3. Pressure and strain to structures so great that they tear the muscle and skin fibres from their bony attachments cause shearing forces.

A child suffering from a combination of predisposing factors is more susceptible to developing pressure ulcers. Predisposing factors can be subdivided into two main groups:

1. Intrinsic factors – aspects of the patients' condition, mental, physical, and medical states, e.g. malnutrition, age, altered consciousness, immobility.

2. Extrinsic factors – external effects of drugs, treatment regimes, manual handling techniques, personal hygiene, and weight distribution.

Those children at greatest risk from developing pressure sores may be identified using a pressure risk assessment. There are two examples of paediatric tools:

1. The Braden Q tool – used for children between the ages of 21 days to 8 years, contains the same six criteria for use with adults, which have been modified to make them developmentally appropriate for children. There is the addition of tissue oxygenation and perfusion:
   - Intensity and duration of pressure
     - mobility
     - activity
     - sensory.
   - Tolerance of the skin and supporting structures
     - moisture
     - friction and shear
     - nutrition
     - tissue perfusion and oxygenation.
2. The Glamorgan Scale – developed especially for children and takes into consideration:
   - Mobility
     - cannot move without difficulty
     - unable to change position without assistance / cannot control body movement
     - some mobility, reduced for age
     - normal mobility.
   - Equipment/objects/head pressing or rubbing
   - Significant anaemia
   - Persistent pyrexia
   - Poor peripheral perfusion
   - Inadequate nutrition
   - Low serum albumin
   - Weight less than 10th centile
   - Incontinence
   - Risk score:
     - 10+ at risk
     - 15+ high risk
     - 20+ very high risk.

It is important to note that both scales are over-cautious and potentially over-predict pressure sore risk, a criticism made of many risk assessment scores. Yet, it is better to over-predict than under-predict risk, as the cost of treating pressure sores is high, while the cost of preventing them is considerably less.

> **!** It is important to realize that a risk assessment score is not a definitive answer to the question of whether an individual will develop a pressure sore. The calculator is an aid to professional and clinical judgement in determining what resources are needed.

If used effectively, these tools can be used to justify a request for resources, such as specialized beds and/or efficient moving and handling equipment. Specialized kinetic beds can be used to facilitate in the turning process, relieve pressure and prevent pressure sore formation. These beds are very expensive and are not used routinely or to replace quality nursing care.

Wound assessment

Wound assessment is a complex task that requires concise information before deciding on a strategy for treatment. Using a measurement tool to assess wounds encourages consistent intervention irrespective of who assesses the wound at any time.

A good wound assessment should include:

1. A body diagram to record the child's wound sites and in the case of multiple wounds these should be numbered individually.
2. A separate assessment sheet should determine the site of each wound and/or the number identified from the initial body diagram.
3. Consider the major areas in relation to the condition of any wound (Table 2.4).
4. The maximum dimensions should be traced and recorded, giving the length, width and depth of the wound in centimetres, in order to have a standard method of measurement.
5. Consider the child's age and weight and take into account current diagnosis and any medications.

Charting wound healing facilitates accurate recording of observations and wound treatment. Which wound assessment documentation tool used is

Table 2.4 Major areas that should be included in a wound assessment

Record of wound site	Body diagram from different angles: Back Front Legs Front Back Medial Lateral
Condition of wound	Wound dimensions Nature of wound bed Exudate Odour Pain (site, frequency, severity) Wound margin Erythema of surrounding skin Condition of surrounding skin infection
Dimensions/drawing	Length Width Depth Outside tracking Health granulating tissue Sloughy areas
Documentation	All these points need to be taken into consideration when documenting nursing observations and wound treatments in relation to wound care

largely a matter of personal preference, so long as the user is aware of the tool's limitations. It is of paramount importance that the child's wound(s) are assessed as soon as possible after admission, and that the risk is re-assessed whenever there is a significant change in his/her condition. Accurate and on-going wound assessment is a prerequisite to planning appropriate care and to evaluate its effectiveness.

The process of wound assessment identifies the expanding nature of nursing practice in nurse prescribing of wound-care dressings. The full implementation of the prescribing powers for nurses is to review nurse-prescribing practices to include all health professionals.

Neurological assessment

Neurological disease may produce systemic signs and systemic disease may affect the nervous system and there is a need for close neurological observations. For a quick neurological assessment the alert, vocal stimuli, painful stimuli, unresponsive (AVPU) can be used:

Alert responds to vocal stimuli, responds to painful stimuli or unresponsive to all stimuli. Alternatively, use the Glasgow Coma Scale.

The Glasgow Coma Scale (GCS)

The GCS assesses two aspects of consciousness, arousal and cognition:

1. Arousal: involves being aware of the environment:
2. Cognition: demonstrates an understanding of what the

observer has said through an ability to perform tasks.

The GCS was designed to:

- Record consciousness level and the activity of the ANS or mental state.
- assess consciousness with ease and standardize clinical observations of patients with impaired consciousness.
- Monitor the progress of head-injured patients, and children undergoing intracranial surgery.
- Monitor any other neurological disorder (cerebral vascular accident, encephalitis, meningitis).
- Minimize variation and subjectivity in the clinical assessment of children.
- Provide a neurological assessment that might indicate the level of patient dependency and subsequent need for nursing interventions.

The GCS has been modified for use in infants and children (Kirkham et al 2008), and accounts for different motor and verbal responses of children, particularly those under 5 years old. Only carry out neurological observations when injury or illness affecting the CNS is suspected and each assessment should be individual, according to the child's condition.

Assess the infant/toddler/child from afar; note their interaction with parents or carers, involve them, discuss your observations and ask them if they are happy with the way the child is behaving. You will need to use your knowledge of normal development landmarks (see Section one). The GCS is based on three aspects of brain function:

1. Eye opening – tests a primitive response managed by the reticular activating system, which extends from the brain stem through the thalamus

into the cerebral cortex.
Consciousness depends on the
interactions between them.

2. Verbal response – tests higher
   functions of the brain in the cerebral
   cortex; the most likely stimulus to
   initiate a response is the sound of the
   child's mother's voice or the sound
   of their name.

3. Motor response – tests higher
   functions of the brain in the cerebral
   cortex; this varies with age.

The rating for eye opening based on a four-point scale (1–4)

Assessing eye opening response in infants:

- If the child is not opening their eyes
  spontaneously, ask the parents to speak
  to the infant or child by calling his/her
  name, they may need painful stimuli
  to initiate a response (see later).

- If there is no response to speech,
  attempt to wake him or her up by
  touch by rubbing or stroking the
  infant's limbs.

- If there is no response to speech or
  touch use painful stimuli. This will
  depend on local hospital policy and
  the age of the infant; the principle is to
  do no harm. The ear lobe is often used
  in infants; it is not very painful but
  may provide enough stimulation to
  arouse an infant.

- For best results the stimulus should
  last between 20–30 seconds.

Assessing eye opening response in a child:

- As applied to an infant, involve the
  parents or carers and check with them
  if they are happy with the child's
  behaviour.

- If the child is not opening his/her eyes
  spontaneously, ask the parent to call
  the child's name, if there is no
  response then attempt to wake them
  up with touch e.g. rubbing or stroking
  limbs.

- If there is no response to speech or
  touch use a painful stimulus:
  - pressure point just behind the ear
  - trapezium squeeze
  - supraorbital pressure (not to be
    used in facial fractures)
  - sternal rub.

These can all lead to bruising so
alternate stimuli points to prevent
unnecessary bruising.

Best verbal response on a five-point scale (1–5)

Assessing the best verbal response in an
infant:

- This varies with age, and best
  elicited by the sound of their
  mother's voice.

- Are they babbling or cooing, if the
  child is crying is this appropriate.

Assessing the best verbal response in a
child:

- To get the best verbal response from
  an older child, ask them their name,
  where they think they are and what
  time of day it is.

Best motor response on a six-point scale (1–6)

Assessing the best motor response in an
infant:

- Encourage the parents to assist in the
  assessment.

- Observe while they play from a distance – are they handling toys in a normal way.
- If there is no response to verbal or touch use painful stimuli; this may involve pinching the ear lobe or applying fingernail pressure. If they are responding to pain they will purposefully move an arm in an attempt to remove the cause of the discomfort.

Assessing the best motor response in a child:

- You can give an older child simple commands to assess their motor responses e.g. ask them to stick out their tongue, touch their nose or move their legs.
- If there is no response to verbal commands you will need to use painful stimuli. In this instance for peripheral stimulation it is appropriate to use the fingernail pressure to determine localization to pain; this can be undertaken for the arms and legs to determine:
  - normal flexion to pain – arms bent upwards
  - abnormal flexion to pain – the arms flex, but are rotated
  - extension is an abnormal response to pain – the arms are extended and the shoulders and hands rotate internally.

A score for each parameter is recorded from a predetermined choice of options. The scores are then added together to give an overall assessment of the child's neurological status. A score of 15 represents the most responsive while a score of 3 is the least responsive.

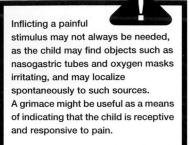

Inflicting a painful stimulus may not always be needed, as the child may find objects such as nasogastric tubes and oxygen masks irritating, and may localize spontaneously to such sources.
A grimace might be useful as a means of indicating that the child is receptive and responsive to pain.

Therefore, it is important to remember that the nurses' goal is to assess the brain's best response to stimulation in order to catch early deterioration, not to 'cause pain' for no reason.

Assessing arm responses:

- Lie the child in the semirecumbent position on the bed.
- Hold the child's hands and ask him/her to pull arms towards their shoulders against you pulling in the opposite direction.
- Ask the child to do the opposite and try to push you away while you provide the force in the opposite direction.
- Check both times for equal strength in both arms.
- Detect mild weakness:
  - if you ask the child to raise both arms about their head and shut their eyes
  - they should be able to hold their arms in the air if they have normal power
  - if there is a mild weakness the effected arm will drift slowly downwards.

Assessing leg responses:

- Lay the child in the semirecumbent position on the bed.

- Ask the child to raise his or her leg off the bed and hold it there.
- Then try and push the lower leg downwards with your hands.
- Perform this on both legs and assess whether the child has equal strength in both limbs.
- You can also ask the child to bend his or her leg by drawing the heel back towards the buttock, while you attempt to gently straighten the leg.

Pupil size and reaction to light

Pupil size and reaction to light is done by shining a torch onto the infant or child's eye. It is important to note whether the child has any pre-existing irregularities with their pupils, which are normal for them such as a previous eye injury or blindness in one eye. It is important to first reduce the environmental light by dimming and note:

- the pupil size – average pupil size is 2–5 mm (Fig. 2.1)
- the pupil reaction to light was brisk, sluggish or fixed
- the shape of the pupil - should be round
- if both pupils react equal to light and are equal in size.

Special care considerations when undertaking the pupillary response:

1. The light should not be shone directly into the child's eyes; a torch should be shone from the outer aspect of the eye towards the pupil, which will constrict quickly.
2. There should be a reaction in the other pupil, which should constrict simultaneously.
3. On removal of the light source, the pupil should dilate to its original size.
4. Repeat in the other eye.
5. It is best to carry this out in dim lighting or should be agreed among staff to eliminate any inconsistencies in the patient's score', (discrepancies of not dimming the light could occur during the night).
6. Progressive dilatation and loss of pupil reaction on one side occurs as a result of pressure on the third cranial nerve, on that side, indicating an enlarged intracranial mass (haematoma).
7. Progressive cerebral oedema eventually leads to compression of the third cranial nerve on the other side, so neither pupil then reacts to light (severe brain injury).
8. Some drugs e.g. atropine dilate the pupil, opiates e.g. morphine, constrict the pupil.

Observation of vital signs

The last section of the GCS is the observation of vital signs. Alterations in neurological function can result in changes to vital signs. Measurement is important and can provide essential additional information:

1. A high temperature can be due to damage to the hypothalamus, which

Pupil sizes in mm

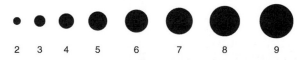

Fig. 2.1 Pupil size observed during the Glasgow Coma Scale (GCS) assessment.

increases cerebral metabolic oxygen requirement, an unwanted complication when oxygenation of the brain may already be depleted.

2. Control centres for blood pressure, heart rate and respiration are all located in the brain stem. Damage to this area of the brain can affect their control, and can lead to changes in:
   - rate, depth and pattern of breathing, due to increases in carbon dioxide
   - other changes occur in breathing, hypoxia, deterioration of brain stem function (Cheyne–Stokes respirations and/or central neurogenic hyperventilation)
   - decreases in heart rate due to hypoxia, deterioration of the brain stem (bradycardia)
   - increases in blood pressure when there is an increase in intracranial pressure; cerebral resistance occurs and to maintain cerebral perfusion, blood pressure is raised
   - a widening pulse pressure.

3. Neurological observations should be recorded at frequent intervals, 1 hour being the maximum time allowed in between measures. Following a head injury carry out observations (NICE 2007):
   - half-hourly for 2 hours
   - hourly for 4 hours
   - then 2 hourly
   - if GCS score drops at any point, revert to half hourly observations.

4. Always carry out a full assessment with the HCP you hand over to.

The GCS provides a quick guide for evaluation of the acutely ill child. The primary purpose of the GCS is to alert medical and nursing staff to deterioration in a patient's neurological status.

Signs of deterioration in a neurological patient are:

- increased drowsiness, restlessness, confusion
- fits
- changes in speech ability
- fixation and dilatation of one or both pupils
- increase in pupil size
- deterioration in motor power
- change in respiratory rate, pattern and depth
- increase in blood pressure, decrease in heart rate
- cardiac dysrhythmias
- increase in ICP
- nausea and vomiting
- changes in body temperature.

A complete general examination should accompany the GCS (Table 2.5).

Table 2.5 A complete general examination must accompany the central nervous system

Temperature
Blood pressure
Neck stiffness
Pulse irregularity
Cardiac murmurs
Cyanosis/respiratory insufficiency
Evidence of weight loss
Breast lumps
Lymphadenopathy
Hepatic and splenic enlargement
Prostatic irregularity
Skin marks, e.g. rashes, spots, purpura
Septic source, e.g. teeth, ears

The central nervous system is described systematically from the head downwards and includes:

- Consciousness level and higher centre functions:
  - cognitive skills
  - memory
  - reasoning
  - emotional status.
- Level of coma (Table 2.6).
- Cranial nerves 1–12.
- Upper limbs:
  - motor system – wasting, tone, power
  - sensory system – pain, touch, temperature, proprioception, stereognosis
  - reflexes
  - co-ordination.
- Trunk – sensation, reflexes.
- Lower limbs:
  - motor system – wasting, tone, power
  - sensory system – pain, touch, temperature, proprioception
  - reflexes
  - co-ordination
  - gait, stance.
- Sphincters – bowel and bladder.

Other signs and symptoms should be taken into consideration (Table 2.7).

Table 2.6 Levels of coma

Level	Presentation
Confusion	Inability to think rapidly and clearly Impaired judgement and decision-making
Disorientation	Beginning of loss of consciousness Disorientation to place Impaired memory Lost last is recognition of self
Lethargy	Limited spontaneous movement or speech Easy arousal with normal speech or touch May or may not be orientated to time, place or person
Obtundation	Mild to moderate reduction in arousal Limited response to the environment Falls asleep unless stimulated verbally or tactilely Questions answered with minimal response
Stupor	Condition of deep sleep or unresponsiveness May be aroused or caused to make a motor or verbal response only by vigorous and repeated stimulation Response is often withdrawal or grabbing at stimulus
Coma	No motor or verbal response to the external environment or to any stimuli, even deep pain or suction No arousal to any stimulus.

Table 2.7 Other considerations related to signs and symptoms of neurological conditions

Sign or symptom	Considerations
Headache	Onset (gradual, sudden), frequency, duration, severity Character (aching, throbbing) Associated features (vomiting, visual disturbances) Site (area affected right/left Relieving factors (analgesia) Precipitating factors (stooping, coughing) Timing (when it occurs, night/day, any time)
Visual disorder	Onset, frequency, duration Impairment (one/both eyes, total/partial, whole/partial) Diplopia (gaze direction where maximal) Hallucinations (formed images, unformed shapes) Precipitating factors
Loss of consciousness	Onset, frequency, duration Tongue biting, incontinence, limb twitching (epilepsy) Alcohol/drug abuse Head injury Cardiovascular or respiratory symptoms (chest pain, thumping in chest, breathlessness) Precipitating factors (stress, headache)
Speech disorder	Onset, frequency, duration Difficulty in forming words, expression or understanding
Motor disorder	Onset, frequency, duration Inco-ordination – balance (cerebellum, inner ear) Involuntary movement Weakness (progression, clumsiness, difficulty in walking and leg stiffness) Relieving factors (rest) Precipitating factors (walking)
Sensory disorder	Onset, frequency, duration Pain (lack of sensation, different types, severity) Numbness/tingling Site Relieving factors (rest) Precipitating factors (walking, neck movement)
Sphincter disorder	Onset, frequency, duration Difficulty in control (incontinence, retention) Anal Bladder

Table 2.7 Other considerations related to signs and symptoms of neurological conditions—cont'd

Sign or symptom	Considerations
Lower cranial nerve disorder	Onset, frequency, duration Deafness/tinnitus (uni/bilateral) Balance/staggering Swallowing difficulties Voice change Precipitating factors (neck movement, head positioning) Vertigo (rotation of surroundings)
Mental disorder	Onset, frequency, duration Memory intelligence deterioration Personality behaviour change

Anxiety

A person's response to anxiety is due to activation of the sympathetic nervous system, potentiated by epinephrine (adrenaline) and norepinephrine (noradrenaline) from the adrenal medulla. There are many factors in everyday life that provokes anxiety, and hospitalization can be counted as one of them. Anxiety is difficult to define, mainly because it is often explained as a vague, uneasy feeling, the source of which is often non-specific or unknown to the individual.

Anxiety may be both positive and negative:

1. Positive in relation to learning ability, as a high anxiety level may have a motivating function
2. Negative in relation to particular experiences, e.g. hospitalization.

Coping with the anxiety of hospitalization can sometimes lead to aggressive behaviour as a result of anger and frustration. Alternatively, the coping may take the form of escape from the anxiety-provoking situation, resulting in withdrawal due to the person's feelings of helplessness and the inability to gain control over events.

Anxiety is present in at least some hospitalized children. This means there is a need for nurses to be able to make an accurate assessment. The assessment of anxiety relies on listening and talking to children, questioning, and discussion through interview, observation or the use of tools such as the:

■ linear analogue scale (LAS)
■ visual analogue scale (VAS)
■ graphic anxiety scale
■ hospital anxiety and depression scale (HAD).

Nurses may already be familiar with their use. However, these may be relevant for older children, but are not specific for the use of infants. The Liverpool infant distress scale (Horgan et al 2002) is a behavioural assessment tool for infants following surgery and consists of eight categories:

- facial expression
- sleep pattern
- cry quantity
- cry quality
- spontaneous movement
- spontaneous excitability
- flexion of fingers and toes
- tone.

Each category includes a score from 0 to 5 and the higher the score the more pain or distress the baby is in. It is very detailed and takes time, but the cues given can help to identify anxiety and distress in infants.

Stress

Stress is seen in terms of an individual's interactions with events. The concept of 'stress' is seen as an interaction process, between the individual and his or her environment, rather than a single event or set of responses. Stressors, make physical and psychological demands, which require individuals to assess and understand the situation and then to respond to it.

In situations when a person can understand and react to the circumstances in a satisfactory manner (e.g. studying for exams) it is unlikely to be perceived as stressful by that individual. However, if the stressors demand new responses or ones which are undeveloped (e.g. illness), then it is likely that the experience will lead to stress.

Hence 'stress' is taken to be an absence of, or a deficiency in, the individual's ability to cope with current environmental demands. The resulting

illness caused by stress is linked to increased sympathetic nervous system arousal. The body's response to a stressor is reflected by a reaction, which involves the whole body and generally consists of three distinct response phases 1–3:

1. The alarm reaction – widespread physiological response, which includes a large outflow into the bloodstream of adrenal hormones in an attempt to defend the body from the stressor.
2. The stage of resistance or adaptation – where an attempt is made by the body to re-establish equilibrium and to regain control to maintain homeostasis. If the body is unable to re-establish homeostasis because of persistent exposure to the stressor then the third phase will result.
3. Exhaustion – ending in death.

The older acutely ill child in hospital is exposed to many stressors simultaneously. These act synergistically rather than cumulatively.

There are a number of events that make significant emotional demands upon the child while in hospital, for example:

1. For an older child hearing the initial diagnosis may be a difficult and stressful process; the fear and anxiety generated by the news may be disruptive and debilitating to its recipient, making it more difficult to absorb further information or to make informed choices.
2. Children also worry about their parents and family and how they may react to diagnosis or bad news.
3. Perception of the situation itself is an intricate concept, which may in turn be affected by past experiences, genetic predisposition, values and beliefs, self-concept and the level of anxiety at the time the stressor is perceived.

4. Some treatments use powerful drugs, accompanied by side-effects that may include nausea and vomiting.

5. Continued exposure to stressors can result in the development of stress ulcers, reduced wound healing, cardiac function, and a reduced immune response to infection, amongst other physiological and psychological sequelae.

6. Coping with specific life-events in the family – changes that occur through choice (marriage or divorce) or be totally unforeseen (bereavement, redundancy, accidental injury or long-term illness).

Therefore, the implications of stress for the nurse in caring for children in hospital is that they understand the relationship between the individual and his or her environment, life-events and acute illness, and as such take the following into consideration:

- Assessment of recent and current major life-events and/or crisis, as these may have accumulated to predispose to the acute illness.

- Assessment of the child's normal coping mechanisms and support networks, so that these can be enhanced, reinforced and/or improved.

- Recognition that the present acute illness may cause stress in itself, particularly with regard to:
  – potential impact on schooling
  – other family members.

- Stress can make a child more vulnerable to infection, depression and slower recovery.

- The need to assist the child's family members with positive coping mechanisms in a situation that may be perceived as stressful for them.

The ANS controls many other body functions and the physiological responses to stress can influence the measurements frequently undertaken by the nurse during his or her daily work. The physiological responses to stress involve neuroendocrine activation and increased sympathetic activity, which stimulates:

1. The cardiovascular system
2. A highly complex series of events that leads to stimulation of the peripheral sympathetic system;
3. The adrenal medulla resulting in the release of numerous substances into the circulation (Table 2.8):
   – catecholamines
   – noradrenaline
   – glucocorticoids
   – mineralocorticoids
   – anti-diuretic hormone (ADH).

The secretion of these stress hormones prepares the body for fight or flight from the insult, and can influence measurements such as: temperature; pulses; ECG; blood pressure; central venous pressure; respiration; urine output; blood analysis; oxygen saturation; pain. The nurse needs to be aware that ultimate control lies with the brain, and as such a reduced level of consciousness, anxiety and/or stress, can lead to inaccurate measurements, which can affect their assessment of the child's true condition.

Pain assessment

Pain is one of the main symptoms that cause parents of children to seek medical advice. The presence of pain can interfere with obtaining accurate and reliable measurements, which can often lead to

Table 2.8 Substances released during stress

Substance	Action
Catecholamines	Epinephrine (adrenaline) – increases heart rate, cardiac output, metabolic rate and blood glucose levels, causes dilatation of bronchioles Norepinephrine (noradrenaline) – peripheral vasoconstriction, increases blood pressure
Glucocorticoids	Cortisol, from the adrenal cortex of the adrenal gland, leads to gluconeogenesis, glycogenolysis, proteolysis and lipolysis, enhances adrenaline's vasoconstrictive effects
Mineralocorticoids	Aldosterone, which increases sodium reabsorption in the renal tubules, resulting in the reduction in urine output and increase in intravascular volume, providing compensation for stress and fluid/ blood loss
Antidiuretic hormone (ADH)	Targets kidney tubules and inhibits or prevents urine formation, results in less urine being produced, blood volume increases, the thirst response will be aroused

the acquisition of false and inaccurate readings; therefore, pain should be treated at an early stage for all ages of children. However, pain is one of the most common symptoms that is not assessed or treated adequately in paediatrics. Pain presents itself and follows a number of pathways, and includes characteristics that are essential to understanding pain in children.

Pain pathways

- Pain is a sensation that is difficult to measure objectively.
- Pain is a sensation that is evoked by the excitation of nerve cells in the brain.
- Pain alerts us to damaging forces in and around the body.

- Pain is associated with emotion more than many other sensations, e.g. anxiety, fear, alarm.
- The character of pain differs – it may be sharp, burning, crushing,
- The location of pain stimulates the reticular activating system, which is the area of arousal, and pain will prevent sleep.
- Character and location depends on:
  - the type and situation of the receptors stimulated
  - the pathways through which they are transmitted
  - their ultimate destination within the brain.

Internal causes of pain

- Pain is innervated by autonomic and somatic nerve fibres.

- Pain arises if there is:
  - local ischaemia, e.g. angina
  - chemical damage, e.g. leakage of enzymes in the pancreas
  - spasm of smooth muscle, e.g. colic
  - overdistension of a hollow organ, e.g. the bladder
  - irritation of the peritoneum, pleura or pericardium
  - stimulation of the inflammatory immune response and release of mediators.
- Some tissues, e.g. the alveoli and the liver parenchyma, are insensitive to pain.
- Others such as the bronchi and liver capsule are also sensitive.
- Brain tissue itself is largely insensitive to injury but the meninges are innervated.

Pain receptors – nociceptors

- Several million bare sensory nerve endings weave through all tissues and organs of the body, except the brain.
- They respond to noxious stimuli (those that are damaging to normal tissue – nociceptors):
  - injured tissue releases chemicals such as bradykinins, histamine and prostaglandins
  - ATP released by damaged cells also stimulates pain receptors.
- Nociceptors are located on A delta and C nerve fibres (Table 2.9); examples include:
  - back and neck pain
  - musculoskeletal pain
  - headache
  - osteoarthritic pain
  - rheumatoid arthritic pain
  - post surgical and trauma pain.

Pain receptors – neuropathic

- Neuropathic pain is caused by a functional or anatomical abnormality of the peripheral or central nervous system.
- Damaged nerves lead to pathophysiological changes resulting in a distortion or amplification of naturally generated signals.
- Usually described as burning, or shooting pain.
- Examples include:
  - phantom limb pain
  - neuralgia
  - fibromyalgia
  - peripheral neuropathy
  - complex regional pain syndrome (previously known as reflex sympathetic dystrophy).

Classification of pain

- Deep somatic pain:
  - arises from the skin, muscles or joints
  - can be superficial or deep
  - differs from superficial pain, which is sharp, pricking, usually brief and localized
  - is transmitted along finely myelinated A delta (δ) fibres at a rate of 12–80 m/s
  - is usually burning, itching or aching
  - stimulates nociceptors in deep skin layers, muscles or joints
  - is more diffuse and long-lasting than superficial somatic pain
  - always indicates tissue destruction
  - impulses are transmitted slowly along small, unmyelinated C fibres (0.4–1 m/s).

Table 2.9 Pain receptors – nociceptors

A delta fibres	Fast pain (A fibres)	C fibres	Slow pain (C fibres)
These are small myelinated axons 1–4 μm in diameter They conduct at a speed of 6–30 metres per second This is **fast pain** and can be localized much more exactly but still probably within 10 cm of the spot.	Sharp Piercing Acute Electric Needle to skin Cut to skin Electric shock Not felt in most deep fibres Duration predictable and limited Tends to get better Has meaning and purpose Can localize exactly	These are un-myelinated They are 0.1–1 μm in diameter They conduct at a speed of 0.5–2.0 m/s This is **slow pain** – localization poor and may only be to one limb and not any part of that limb They travel up to the brain via the reticular system With a low concentration of local anaesthetic, the C fibres can be blocked. This can relieve the slow, chronic type of pain	Burning Aching Chronic Throbbing Nauseous Usually associated with tissue destruction Skin and deep tissues Duration unpredictable Tends to get worse No meaning/ obscure Cannot localize

- Visceral pain:
  - results from noxious stimulation of receptors in organs of the thorax or abdomen
  - is usually a dull ache, burning sensation or a gnawing pain.
  - results from stimuli including stretching of tissue, ischaemia, irritant chemicals and muscle spasm
  - follows the same pathways as somatic pain and leads to referred pain.

A regular assessment of pain contributes to the quality provided by children's nurses and is beneficial in the treatment and monitoring of pain levels.

Effective treatment of pain is essential in the children's ward but is undoubtedly compounded by the fact that often a child may be unconscious or too young to understand. Therefore, it is often difficult to adopt an applicable and working pain assessment tool in a sick child, because often child participation is absent.

Many conditions can cause considerable pain for children, for example: otitis media, tonsillitis, lacerations, headache, abdominal pain, head injury, fractures, and burns. Children and infants in particular have been identified to have inappropriate treatment of painful conditions and may needlessly experience pain with minor illnesses and injury. Pain is a subjective experience so children's reports of pain are a reliable indicator of pain and should be treated appropriately. Young children may have difficulty verbalizing or communicating pain because of their level of development. Compared with older children, infants have less pain score assessment and treatment. This may occur because infants cannot verbally express their pain other than crying and so may have untreated pain symptoms.

It is nevertheless important that the same tool is used throughout and that the tool used is the most appropriate for the patient's needs at that particular time. Also, when assessing a child's pain, it is vital to listen to what the child and parent(s) are saying about their pain. Interestingly, nurses generally rate patient's pain lower than it actually is.

Recognition of pain and assessment of its severity is essential to improve the management of pain. Communication of pain may be altered in critically ill children if they are intubated, receiving paralytics and sedatives, or have an altered level of consciousness. These children almost always experience pain and should be assessed and managed appropriately. For critically ill children, vital signs are often misleading because of associated physiological events, so observation of non-verbal behaviour is essential.

It is important that children's pain is assessed and documented as lack of pain scores is linked to underestimation of pain and under treatment with inadequate analgesic prescription. Sometimes nurses do not use tools to assess and score pain, preferring to assess pain visually. Sometimes nurses assess pain scores but do not document the

scores and this is equally problematic as it contributes to communication breakdown. Children's pain can be difficult to measure but there are many tools available to help assess and measure pain. What is important is that the pain scales and assessment tools are valid and reliable, able to accommodate the needs of the child and easy to use. The decision about which tool to use can be determined broadly by the child's age and condition.

In children younger than 3 years of age

This includes behavioural assessment scales are the primary tools used by health professionals for assessing pain. These scales frequently use facial expression, motor responses and physiological indicators to assess pain.

- The Faces, Legs, Activity, Cry, and Consolability scale (FLACC) is suitable for use with infants from 2 months to 7 years of age.

- The Neonatal Infant Pain Scale (NIPS) includes observations of neonates' facial expressions, crying, breathing patterns, tone, movement of arms and legs, and state of arousal.

- For premature infants the Premature Infant Pain Profile (PRIPP) includes 7 pain measures, each evaluated on a 4-point scale.

- For assessment of neonatal postoperative pain, there is the CRIES scale (crying, requires oxygen to maintain saturation more than 95%, increased vital signs, expression and sleepless).

- There are other behavioural assessment tools such as the

Toddler-Preschooler Pain Scale (TIPPS) and the Preverbal, Early Verbal Pediatric Pain Scale (PEPPS), which can be used for toddlers.

In children between 3 and 8 years of age

Self-rating scales are commonly used. Examples of these are:

- Face interval scales – set of faces with varying expressions. The Wong–Baker Faces Pain Rating Scale (FACES) consists of six faces with word descriptors and numbers from 0–5. It is easy to use for children aged 4 upwards.
- Oucher scale – 6 colour photos from no hurt to biggest hurt.
- Hester's Poker chip tool – 4 chips with one chip a little hurt and 4 most hurt. Children 4 years and older can usually use this tool.
- Pain colour matching – pick colour that represents the pain – most picked red for intense pain, orange for milder pain and yellows for little or no pain.
- Eland colour tool – colour in part of body where the pain hurts.

For children aged 8 years and above

They can usually use unidimensional tools such as:

- Numerical rating scale (NMS) uses numbers 0–10 to reflect increasing degrees of pain. To use this scale the child must know number concepts.
- Graphic rating scale (GRS) – a series of words along a continuum of

increasing value (e.g. no pain, moderate pain, severe pain).
- Visual analogue scale (VAS) – a scale modified with five word anchors. Usually children 6 years of age and older can indicate the intensity of pain by using this tool.
- Pain thermometer – thermometer graded on a numerical scale (0–10 or 0–100) with zero indicating no hurt and the highest number the most possible hurt.

Assessment process for children younger than 3 years

- Ask parents to help with the assessment as parents know their child very well and will be attuned to non-verbal signs of pain and discomfort.
- Observe behaviour for indicators of pain, e.g. irritable/fussy, grimacing, whimpering, crying, and wrinkling of forehead, tenseness/rigidity, squirming, drawing up legs and mobility.
- Observe for physiological changes, e.g. increased heart, respiratory rate and blood pressure; palms are sweating, decreases in oxygen saturation and raised intracranial pressure.
- Use the pain scoring tool most appropriate for age group to assess and document the severity of pain, e.g. NIPS, PRIPP, CRIES scale, TIPPS and PEPPS.

Assessment process for children aged 3 upwards

Pain is a subjective experience and self-report of pain should be obtained whenever possible. Children are usually able to use an assessment tool to convey pain but it does depend on the cognitive maturity of each child as abilities can vary. Children who are very ill may not be able to respond to a pain assessment tool and may need help from parents and professionals to adequately assess their level of pain.

- Ask parents to help with the assessment as parents know their child very well and will be attuned to non-verbal signs of pain and discomfort.

- Consult with parents as to the best method for assessing their child's pain as parents usually know their child's behavioural response to pain and can identify behaviours unique to the child that can help in the accurate assessment of pain.

- Explain behavioural scales to parents and encourage them to actively participate in identifying pain and in evaluating their child's response to analgesics.

- Observe behaviour for indicators of pain, e.g. irritable/fussy, grimacing, whimpering/moaning, tenseness/rigidity, squirming, drawing up legs, touching painful area and mobility.

- Other signs of pain may include sleeping, withdrawal, lack of expression and lack of interest in surroundings.

- Observe for physiological changes, e.g. increased heart, respiratory rate and blood pressure; palms are sweating, decreases in oxygen saturation and raised intracranial pressure.

- For children who can verbalize pain, you can use pain scoring tool to assess and document the severity of pain such as: FLACC, Hester's Poker Chip Tool, FACES, VAS.

Key points about pain assessment

- All children are capable of experiencing pain and should be assessed and given adequate pain relief.

- Encourage parents to contribute to pain assessment.

- Parents' knowledge of child's typical behavioural response to pain can help identify behaviours unique to their child and so is essential in the accurate assessment of child's pain.

- Assessment of behavioural indicators is essential for children with limited verbal and cognitive skills.

- Children who are in obvious pain and who are unable to focus on the pain scale should receive immediate treatment.

- Assessing pain with a reliable tool provides specific evidence on severity of pain and ensures pain will be treated.

- Use a pain assessment scale that is appropriate for the child's verbal and cognitive ability and circumstances (e.g. illness condition).

- Explain the tool simply and clearly to the child so the child understands how to score their pain.

- Use a pain scoring tool and document the severity of pain.

- Pain should be assessed at regular intervals and treated appropriately.

- Never disregard or disbelieve children's expressions of pain.

- Cultural beliefs can influence expressions of pain so be aware of this.

- Be aware that children may under report pain if they are afraid of injections so reassure children about different routes for receiving pain medication.

Steps to pain assessment

Obtaining the pain story

Assessment of the physical component of the pain, including:

- initial assessment – pain assessment tools
- ongoing assessment
- the severity of the pain
- response to treatment
- assessment of the non-physical aspects of pain:
  - anxiety about treatment and meaning of pain
  - helplessness and depression
  - social worries.

It is important that the practitioner assesses the location, type and intensity of a child's pain in order to select the appropriate treatment. Once assessed it is imperative that the pain is treated, a failure to relieve pain is morally and ethically unacceptable (see section 5 for pain relief). Pain can have a detrimental effect on patients' condition and can significantly slow recovery.

The undertreatment of pain can lead to:

- Decreased tidal volumes and alveolar ventilation, leading to decreased oxygen delivery to organs.
- Prevention of the patient from coughing, resulting in an increase in the collection of secretions contributing to atelectasis and chest infections.
- Avoidance of movement, leading to an increased risk of deep vein

thrombosis and pulmonary embolism.

- Increased stress response and sympathetic stimulation, resulting in vasoconstriction and tachycardia, raising blood pressure, increasing the workload of the heart.
- Interference with intestinal smooth muscle function and an increase in metabolic rate, leading to difficulties in meeting nutritional needs and may lead to loss of weight.

Good pain relief can reduce these responses to pain, and lead to a safer and improved recovery.

It is paramount that the children's ward nurse takes pain assessment to the child. In order to to do this the nurse must be adequately equipped to take into account and interpret the child's physiological parameters as an early indicator of pain such as elevated blood pressure, tachycardia and sweating.

There is no doubt that pain in children can be avoided, leading to better satisfaction and quality of care. Children's nurses must move towards effective care in this important area of clinical practice.

Respiratory assessment

Respiration is an essential body function necessary for the diffusion of gases between the alveoli and blood as well as the maintenance of blood pH. Ventilation is the mechanical movement of gas or air in and out of the lungs. The respiratory rate is the ventilatory rate and is recorded in breaths per minute. Effective respiration is dependent on many factors, both nervous and chemical in nature; including the chemoreceptors and lung receptors, which control depth, quality and pattern of breathing.

Rate

A child's respiratory rate is measured in breaths per minute and is the number of times the child's chest rises and falls (counted as one) in one minute. Respiratory rate varies with age:

- newborns: 30–50
- early infancy and childhood: 20–40
- late childhood: 15–25.

Changes in the rate of breathing are defined as tachypnoea, a decrease in respiratory rate or bradypnoea.

Depth

This is the volume of air moving in and out with each respiration, normally measured as the tidal volume, which is constant with each breath and varies with age. Normal relaxed breathing is effortless, automatic, regular and almost silent. Dyspnoea is breathlessness and an awareness of discomfort with breathing.

Pattern

The pattern of breathing should be easy without any distress or struggle; it is normally regular and consists of inspiration, pause, longer expiration and another pause. It usually makes little noise, so listening and looking for changes may indicate deterioration in condition. In disorders of the respiratory control centre and in certain diseases, the pattern changes:

- *Hyperventilation* – an increase in both the rate and depth of respirations.
- *Apneustic* – a pattern of prolonged, gasping inspiration, followed by extremely short, inefficient expiration.
- *Cheyne–Stokes* – periodic breathing characterized by a gradual increase in depth of respiration followed by a decrease in respiration, resulting in apnoea.

Undertaking a respiratory assessment

1. Sight, hearing and touch, all play an important part in undertaking a respiratory assessment: Read and familiarize yourself with the child's past medical history and critical care admission notes. This will give you useful information and underpin your respiratory assessment strategy.
2. Observe the child:
   - If they are breathing spontaneously, note their respiratory rate, rhythm, depth and equality of movement from both sides of the chest.
   - Note whether the child appears comfortable or not.
   - Are they able to speak coherently?
   - What is their central and peripheral colour?
   - If the child is mechanically ventilated, note whether the ventilator settings correspond to the recorded settings.
   - Check and record the length of the tracheal tube at the lip.
   - Check $SpaO_2$ recordings and interpret ABGs.

- Listen to (oscillate) the lung fields using a stethoscope.
- Check for equal air entry, sounds and note if they are absent.

The rate, rhythm and depth are informative indicators of how a patient is breathing. Irregular breathing or the appearance of excessive respiratory muscle effort can both be considered as indicators that the patient is not oxygenating effectively. Symmetry in the child's chest movement is paramount in the effectiveness of oxygenation as an asymmetrical movement may indicate an underlying problem with ventilation; for example, tension pneumothorax.

> It is important to note that these indicators alone are not conclusive and without the change in other vital signs, oxygen saturation or deterioration in ABGs they cannot alone be seen as guaranteed indicators of potential respiratory failure.

Interpreting auscultation of the chest

Auscultation is the skill of listening to a child's breathing and heart sounds through a stethoscope. You should ensure that you can hear air entry to both sides of the chest.

In a normal chest, you are likely to hear three types of air entry sounds as you move around the chest. These are:

- *Bronchial.* These sounds are loud and high pitched and sound like air being blown through a hollow pipe. The expiratory phase is longer and

louder than the inspiratory. Normally they are heard only over the upper part of the sternum. They are only heard elsewhere in the lungs when there are respiratory problems.
- *Bronchovesicular.* These sounds are a combination of vesicular and bronchial and are heard mainly in the first and second intercostal spaces near the sternum. The inspiratory and expiratory phases are about equal and like bronchial sounds they are not normally heard elsewhere when there are respiratory problems.
- *Vesicular.* These sounds are normally described as relatively soft and low pitched, with sighing or gentle rustling sounds heard over the peripheral parts of the lung. Another characteristic is that the inspiratory phase is longer than the expiratory phase and there is no pause between each of these phases.

Children often present with an abnormal chest X-ray and this will make auscultation of the chest important in aiding chest diagnosis. Chest sounds can be divided into two main groups and these are:

- Abnormally transmitted sounds – bronchial breathing is caused by the transmission of bronchial sounds through consolidated lung tissue to a part of the lung where they are not normally heard. It is commonly associated with atelectasis or acute respiratory distress syndrome (ARDS).
- Adventitious sounds
  - Crackles:
    - Are caused by sputum in the bronchi and trachea and can be either coarse or fine.

- They can vary in quantity from scanty to profuse and can occur during either inspiration or expiration and can be heard early or late in the respiratory cycle.
- Coarse crackles are often found with bronchiectasis.
- Fine crackles are often associated with pulmonary fibrosis.
- Early inspiratory crackles are often scanty and can be heard at the lung bases. They tend to be indicative of severe airway obstruction e.g. chronic bronchitis, asthma and emphysema, coughing and postural changes do not affect them.
- Late inspiratory crackles are usually present in restrictive diseases, e.g. pneumonia, right sided heart failure and are more numerous than early inspiratory crackles and do vary with patient position.

- Wheezes:
  - Are associated with musical noises; these can consist of monophonic (single), multiple short or long 'notes' (polyphonic) of a high or low pitch and can occur during inspiration or expiration.
  - Monophonic wheezes start and end at different times, and often present with asthma symptoms or pulmonary obstructions, e.g. bronchial tumours.
  - Polyphonic wheezes consist of different notes starting and finishing at the same time and often associated with acute and chronic obstructive airways disease.

- Stridor:
  - Is a particular type of wheeze, which originates from a laryngeal or tracheal obstruction.

- Is distinctive and can be heard without the aid of a stethoscope, from a distance.
- Is commonly heard post-extubation in children who have developed laryngeal oedema, but it can also be heard in patients with a partial upper respiratory obstruction.

- Pleural rubs:
  - Are present in patients whose normally smooth and well-lubricated pleural membranes have become inflamed or thickened and can no longer pass easily and silently over one another.
  - The sound is often longer and lower pitched, in comparison to a crackle.
  - Pleural rub sounds vary depending on whether a large section of the chest wall is involved and they have the ability to reverse their sounds between inspiration and expiration.

Assessment of the skin

Loss of homeostasis in body cells and organs reveals itself on the skin. The skin is an organ from which a great deal of information can be obtained:

- nutritional status
- fluid balance
- circulation
- emotional state and age.

The skin can provide clues leading to the diagnosis of a child's health problems and to an evaluation of the effectiveness of a child's care. Assessment of the skin involves consideration of:

- Age
- The general state of grooming, e.g. hair and nails
- The physical or mental state
- General areas of neglect
- Skin lesions, e.g. rashes, itching, abrasions, bruising.

Observation of the skin:

- Indicates the child's physical condition
- It may indicate signs of shock, anaemia, high temperatures, reduced oxygen or a particular disease or condition.

Skin colour is of great importance in assessment of the skin in a child:

- Pallor:
  - This will occur due to vasoconstriction because skin is dependent on blood flow through the surface vessels.
  - Pallor occurs in exposure to cold.
  - Pallor occurs because during stress epinephrine (adrenaline) causes selective vasoconstriction and norepinephrine (noradrenaline) causes the blood vessels of the systemic circulation to vasoconstrict.
  - Pallor may be the result of anxiety and pain.

- Anaemia:
  - Surface vessel blood flow is adequate, but the haemoglobin concentration of the blood is low.
  - Oxygen saturation monitor is not a good estimate – all haemoglobin present in the blood will be fully saturated, giving a normal reading.
  - Look at the mucous membranes, e.g. inside the lips or lower eyelid –

blood vessels lie nearer the surface so colour can be observed.

- Flushing:
  - An increased blood flow of normal haemoglobin content to the surface of the skin gives a red appearance to the skin.
  - In hot weather, cutaneous vessels will dilate to facilitate heat loss from the skin surface.
  - In inflammation vasodilatation occurs over the affected area, and redness is a characteristic feature.

- Cyanosis:
  - Is a blue coloration and occurs relatively frequently in children with polycythaemia but is rarely seen in those who are anaemic.
  - Is difficult to assess in black children whose skin pigments may obscure the condition. The inside of the lips, palms of the hands and soles of the feet may give some indication of the problem.
  - Occurs in individuals suffering from diseases which result in a reduced amount of oxygen being carried by the blood (hypoxaemia), which may be:
    - central and occur over the face or lips
    - peripheral, where the extremities are affected – usually indicates inadequate or sluggish blood flow in the peripheral tissues.

- Jaundice:
  - Is an abnormal yellow skin tone – a sign of a liver disorder caused by the accumulation of bilirubin in the blood.
  - Bilirubin is the waste product of red blood cell breakdown by the spleen – 99% is excreted as bilirubin in bile; the other 1% is excreted in the urine as urobilinogen.

- If bilirubin cannot be excreted in bile due to an obstruction any excess is excreted in the urine or deposited in body tissues.
- The earliest sign of jaundice can be detected in the urine.
- A yellow discoloration of the skin is most easily recognized in the conjunctiva, before changes in skin colour.
- A slightly yellow appearance may be apparent in the skin in the later stages of malignant disease when cachexia exists.

■ Scars:
- The presence of scars, striae and bruising on the skin can be significant.
- Injection marks may give a clue to drug abuse or to conditions requiring prophylactic medication by injection, such as diabetes or haemophilia.
- Small bruises like dark purple purpura, which are evident in septicaemia, should be considered in relation to the child's condition.

Palpation of the skin

■ The feel of the skin can give information about the child's fluid balance, state of nutrition and health.

■ Palpation can show up moderate and severe dehydration.

■ Hydration is assessed by gently but firmly pinching up a fold of skin on the back of the hand or on the inner forearm.

■ In a well-hydrated child, it will immediately return to its normal position.

■ In a child who is in an advanced state of dehydration, the fold of skin may stay pinched for up to 30 seconds.

■ Oedema:
- is an abnormal collection of fluid in the tissues – the causes are varied
- is a problem of fluid distribution and does not necessarily indicate fluid excess
- is usually associated with:
  • weight gain
  • swelling and puffiness
  • tight-fitting clothes and shoes
  • limited movement of an effected area
  • symptoms associated with an underlying pathological condition.
- is recognized by pressing firmly over a bony prominence such as the medial malleolus of the ankle for about 5 seconds – waterlogged tissue retains the imprint of the finger (pitting oedema).

■ Obesity:
- can be assessed using skinfold calipers to measure superfluous subcutaneous fat.
- obese skin feels flabby and may wobble when pushed
- an obese child who has experienced rapid weight loss may have folds of skin on the abdomen and buttocks.

■ Temperature:
- A relative temperature can be obtained by feeling the skin:
- The skin will feel warm over an inflamed area or over an area of increased blood flow.
- When circulation to a specific area of the skin is increased – e.g. swelling and pain in the calf of the leg, a DVT may be provisionally diagnosed.

- Skin will feel cool or cold over an area of skin that is shut down due to reduced blood flow.
- It is usual to employ the back of the hand for testing skin temperature – this area has a more constant blood flow.

The skin can be a powerful observation tool when assessing a child. It requires no invasive technology just the experience and knowledge of the nurse undertaking it.

Sedation assessment scoring

Children often receive sedative agents and analgesics to induce sedation in order to relieve pain, reduce anxiety, body's stress responses, and supportive measures. Sedation is used to facilitate both diagnostic and therapeutic procedures in children (e.g. electrocardiography, bone marrow aspiration or biopsy, chest tube placement, renal biopsy). Sedation may be light for children undergoing imaging procedures, moderate for invasive procedures and strong for children requiring prolonged procedures and ventilation.

The availability of non-invasive monitoring, short-acting opioids and sedatives has led to more diagnostic and therapeutic procedures being done outside of the operating room and intensive care unit. It is important that sedation is appropriate to ensure that procedures are done safely without over-sedation or under-sedation occurring. The ideal sedation would be one at which the procedure can be successfully achieved with as little distress to the child

as possible and with cardiopulmonary stability and retention of protective airway reflexes (Krauss and Green 2006). Assessing sedation is essential if the complications associated with excessive or inadequate sedation are to be prevented.

States of sedation

1. Minimal sedation (anxiolysis) – drug-induced state during which patients respond normally to verbal commands. Respiratory and cardiovascular functions are unaffected.
2. Moderate sedation – drug-induced depression of consciousness during which patients respond purposefully to verbal commands, either alone or accompanied by tactile stimulus. Respiratory and cardiovascular functions are usually unaffected.
3. Dissociative sedation – a trance-like cataleptic state induced by the dissociative agent ketamine and characterized by profound analgesia and amnesia. Respiratory and cardiovascular functions are usually unaffected.
4. Deep sedation – a drug-induced loss of consciousness during which patients cannot be easily roused but respond purposefully after repeated or painful stimulation. The ability to maintain respiratory function is compromised and patients usually require assistance with maintaining a patent airway. Cardiovascular function is usually unaffected.
5. General anaesthesia – drug-induced loss of consciousness during which patients are not arousable, even by painful stimulation. The ability to maintain ventilatory function is often impaired and usually require assistance with maintaining a patent

airway. Positive pressure ventilation may be required because of depressed spontaneous ventilation or drug-induced depression of neuromuscular function.

Risks associated with sedation

Excessive sedation during procedures can result in depressed respiratory mechanisms. Excessive sedation in PICU patients could result in excessive mechanical ventilation, ventilator associated pneumonia, ventilator associated lung injuries, and neuromuscular irregularities. Under-sedation in PICU patients can result in ventilatory asynchrony, increased oxygen needs, unwanted removal of devices, increased use of resources and post traumatic stress. Under-sedation during invasive procedures can result in pain, anxiety, and resultant stress responses that are detrimental both physically and psychologically.

- Monitoring the level of consciousness is essential to ensure optimal sedation and prevention of complications.
- In clinical practice, validated sedation scales should be frequently used in measuring (i.e. scoring) the level of sedation.
- The goal of sedation scoring is to avoid subjective impressions.
- The desired level of sedation should be identified for each child and frequently reassessed.
- Administered doses of sedative agents should be titrated according to fluctuating requirements to ensure optimal sedation.

- Sedation monitoring must be accompanied with specific protocols or clinical guidelines as to what action to take when sedation is not optimal.
- Nurses can play an essential role in monitoring sedation and in cooperation with medical staff ensuring the correct amount of sedation for each child in their care.

Assessment scoring scales

Several different sedation assessment scoring scales have been developed. Although there are many scales available no standardized scale has been accepted (Cho et al 2007). Many scales have been used to measure sedation effectiveness in adult or paediatric ICU patients but few of them exhibit satisfactory clinimetric properties (De Jonghe et al 2000). None of these instruments have been evaluated with respect to their ability to detect changes in sedation status over time. Of the 25 plus sedation instruments around, only one, the COMFORT scale, was developed for paediatric patients.

COMFORT scale

The COMFORT scale was developed to assess the psychological distress of critically ill children under the age of 18 years. Additional research demonstrated that the scale is clinically useful when determining if a child is optimally sedated. The COMFORT scale is a subjective physiological and behavioural scoring system. It relies on the measurement of eight items: alertness, calmness/agitation, respiratory response, physical movement, blood pressure, heart rate, muscle tone and facial tension (Ambuel et al 1992).

The eight items have response options ranging from 1 to 5. This scale was developed to measure not only the level of consciousness but also parameters such as face grimacing, muscle tone, physiological values and the level of agitation. The tool requires observation of the patient for a 2-minute period of time, and during that time the child is scored on all items.

The advantage of the scale is that the scoring can be done without disturbing the child. Routine assessment using the COMFORT scale can be time-consuming and the scale is not appropriate when neuromuscular blocking agents are used. The COMFORT scoring system is the most widely used instrument in PICU in USA and is considered appropriate for assessing sedation in mechanically ventilated paediatric patients (Bear and Ward-Smith 2006).

COMFORT-B scale

Carnevale and Razack (2002) performed an item analysis on the COMFORT scale I in PICU and recommended omitting the heart rate and blood pressure parameters because although these were the most objective criteria, they had the lowest inter-rater reliability. Hence an adapted version, the COMFORT behaviour (COMFORT-B) scale was validated to assess distress and postoperative pain in young children under the age of three years (Carnevale and Razack 2002). The items to be assessed are: alertness, calmness, respiratory response (in ventilated patients) or crying (in non-ventilated patients), muscle tone, physical movement and facial tension. The response categories range from 1 'no distress' and 5 'severe distress', total scores

range from 6–30 (Ista et al 2009). It is a reliable alternative to the original tool, requiring less clinical time to complete.

Sedation assessment for light or moderate procedural sedation

Non-pharmacological interventions should be used in addition to sedative agents as careful attention to factors that promote comfort can reduce the amount of sedative required. Consider using interventions such as communication, continual reorientation, and reassurance to help reduce anxieties and attend to simple environmental factors such as warmth of the room and comfort from parents/carers.

- Assess level of consciousness.
- Assess airway compromise (young children desaturate more rapidly than adults because of their proportionally smaller functional residual capacity and greater relative oxygen consumption).
- Continuously monitor oxygen levels (pulse oximetry with audible signal).
- Assess and record vital signs, blood pressure and pulse rate every 10–15 minutes.
- Sedation area should include all necessary age appropriate equipment for airway management and resuscitation.

Sedation assessment in PICU

Sedation for the critically ill child can help minimize agitation, promote synchrony with the ventilator, and help prevent distress associated with the high technology environment of the ICU. Children may suffer pain and discomfort from procedures such as intubation, chest drain insertion, or from severe trauma and disease. The presence of an endotracheal tube and mechanical ventilation usually necessitates the use of sedation in many PICUs.

Physiological signs such as raised heart rate and blood pressure can indicate problems with sedation. But physiological parameters may be unreliable in critically ill children with poor cardiovascular function or on pharmacologic medication which affects heart rate and blood pressure. In PICU the pharmacologic agents may alter traditionally monitored physiological endpoints, and the use of neuromuscular blockade may preclude the use of clinical assessment (Grindstaff and Tobias 2004). Hence maintaining adequate sedation in the PICU can be a challenging and difficult task.

Key points for sedation in PICU

- Analgesia should be provided to all critically ill children irrespective of the need for sedation.

- Clinical protocols should be used to guide professionals in the use of sedation.

- Medical staff should document the desired level of sedation whilst ensuring sedative agents are prescribed at the lowest therapeutic rate.

- Nurses should assess each child's level of sedation using a validated scoring tool and take appropriate action.

- Behaviours indicating distress to pain may not be evident if the child is receiving neuromuscular blocking

agent. If it is feasible the neuromuscular agent could be ceased each morning until the child begins to move so that his/her level of sedation can be accurately measured. Once this is done the neuromuscular agent can be recommenced.

- Physiological indicators such as blood pressure and heart rate may be affected by factors other than the child's level of distress.

Sedation drugs

- Midazolam and fentanyl infusions are commonly used for prolonged sedation and analgesia in PICU.

- Midazolam through continuous infusion is the recommended agent for critically ill children requiring intravenous sedation (Playfor et al 2006). It is a short-acting benzodiazepine. The side effects include: respiratory depression and severe hypotension.

- Fentanyl is a relatively short-acting synthetic opioid with full agonist efficacy and minimal haemodynamic effects. Side effects include: nausea, vomiting and constipation.

- Oral chloral hydrate is one of the preferred drugs for non-invasive diagnostic imaging studies in children under the age of 3 years. It is quite unpalatable and should be given via nasogastric tube or rectally. It cannot be titrated so over sedation may occur and should be anticipated and the child carefully monitored.

Withdrawal of sedation

Tolerance and withdrawal are major concerns when opioid infusions (fentanyl and midazolam) are used for a prolonged period, for example over 7 days of continuous therapy. The abrupt cessation of medication can result in withdrawal phenomena:

- from opioids: pupil dilation, lacrimation, rhinorrhea, tachycardia, tacypnoea, hypertension, vomiting, diarrhoea, yawning, restlessness, fever, cramps, irritability, and anxiety.

- from benzodiazepines: agitation, restlessness, tachycardia, tachypnoea, diaphoresis, high temperature, vomiting, and convulsions.

- from combination of fentanyl and midazolam: tremor, clonus, ataxia, and choreoathetosis (abnormal movements of their extremities).

Managing sedation withdrawal

- Weaning from sedation should help prevent the distressing side effects of withdrawal.

- Doses of opioids should be routinely tapered to avoid withdrawal complications.

- Scoring of the child's physiological and behavioural signs and symptoms is a vital part of the weaning process.

- Scoring needs to be done consistently by all involved in the care of the child.

- Weaning regimens should be individualized to each child.

- Consider 'drug cycling' where each patient sedation regimen is reviewed regularly and sedation regimens changed are new initiatives being implemented to decrease the incidence of tolerance.

2.3 Haemodynamic monitoring of a child

Non-invasive cardiovascular haemodynamic monitoring

Temperature

A sound understanding of temperature measurement and influencing factors is essential for nurses who care for children. When taking the temperature, it is the temperature set by the hypothalamus, which is being determined.

Temperature sites

The sites that are in close proximity to the brain (axilla, sublingual, rectal and tympanic):

- The axilla temperature is accurate in neonates for detecting pyrexia, but less accurate in older children, as it is considered a skin temperature and not adequate as an indicator of core temperature. However, peripheral skin temperatures are used for determining vasoconstriction or vasodilatation to help assess a child's circulation status.

- The sublingual route (e.g. taking the temperature under the tongue).

- The tympanic membrane also reflects the brain's thermal environment.

- The rectal temperature is no longer routinely used.

Equipment

- The electronic thermometer is becoming increasingly popular to replace the traditional mercury-filled device, and uses the sublingual site for measurement of temperature.

- The single-use chemical thermometer is also available, which works by using a chemical that changes colour with increasing temperature.
- A tympanic membrane closer to the brain is the ear, a temperature site that is becoming increasingly popular in children:
  - uses tympanic membrane thermometry and is known as the infrared light reflectance thermometer
  - detects the temperature within the eardrum and has clear advantages:
    • the close proximity of the measurement site to the hypothalamus, convenience, comfort, rapidity and acceptance by the patient
    • registers in a matter of seconds with little inconvenience and no discomfort to the child.
  - inaccurate readings usually occur due to inconsistent measurement techniques by clinicians.

Temperature readings

It should be noted that there is a difference between sites in the body and often axilla temperature can be as much as 1°C less than actual core temperature:

- oral: 36.5–37.5°C
- tympanic: 36.9–37.5°C
- axillary: 35.8–36.6°C
- rectal: 37.0–37.8°C

Skin/toe temperature

When a patient's circulation is impaired there are changes to the peripheral circulation to the body's extremities (Edwards 2003). This will be reflected in the peripheral skin temperature, as it provides good indications of the presence and severity of a circulatory defect. The toe temperature gradient provides a valuable, inexpensive and non-invasive monitor of tissue perfusion.

Skin temperature can be used to determine the severity of shock:

- during hypovolaemic circulation to the major organs as central temperature needs to be maintained.
- under ANS control improves the circulation through:
  - baroreceptor activity – vasoconstriction
  - norepinephrine (noradrenaline) – receptors causes further vasoconstriction.

The end result is:

- heat conservation
- cool extremities that feel cool to touch
- an increase in BP
- improved circulation to the body's major organs.

Pulse

The rhythmic contraction of the left ventricle of the heart results in a transmission of a pressure impulse through the arteries. This pulse is customarily palpated at the radial artery in the wrist. The important factors to consider in relation to the radial pulse are:

- rate
- rhythm (regularity and character)
- pressure (volume or strength)
- deficits between pulse and apex rate.

Pulse rate is an important component of cardiac output and fluctuations of pulse rate in the well individual normally occur together with fluctuations in stroke volume to maintain optimum cardiac output for the activity being performed, for example, rest or exercise. Infants initially have a fast heart rate, which is necessary to produce adequate cardiac output. Cardiac metabolic needs in the infant whose small ventricular size cannot be compensated for by increasing stroke volume. The rate gradually declines with age, as the heart size grows; stroke volume increases so a higher rate is no longer necessary to produce an adequate cardiac output. Pulse rate varies with a child's age (Table 2.10) and between individuals of the same age.

A pulse rate can be felt:

- radial pulse – palpating the radial artery in the wrist

- apical pulse – listening directly to the heart, also heart sounds can be heard

- carotid pulse – last pulse to disappear in the event of a cardiac arrest

- brachial pulse – used when assessing manual measurement of blood pressure

- femoral pulse – used to assess cardiac output during cardiac arrest or to assess lower limb perfusion

- temporal pulse – easy to assess even when the infant is asleep.

In small children and neonates the pulse may be difficult to palpate at the radial artery, so the heart rate is counted by listening over the heart (apex area) using a stethoscope. In older children the pulse is taken using the radial. The first and second finger tips should be pressed firmly but gently on the pulse site until a pulse is felt and counted for 60 seconds.

An altered pulse does not produce signs of haemodynamic changes, but if the patient does show such signs (e.g. volume depletion), immediate treatment is indicated. This may include drug or intravenous infusion therapy or non-pharmacological measures can be used, such as the Valsalva manoeuvre, or the physician may perform carotid sinus massage.

The importance of using the pulse as an early reliable indicator of physiological change is often overlooked and a greater significance put on the blood pressure (BP). Yet, the pulse rate is less invasive and less time-consuming and the pulse is measured more accurately.

The pulse deficit

This is the difference between the heart rate counted at the apex of the heart using a stethoscope and the pulse rate counted simultaneously at the wrist. For the majority of patients the heart rate and pulse rate will be the same, but a deficit will occur in:

- atrial fibrillation,

- multiple ectopic beats.

This is sometimes observed in children with cardiomyopathy.

Table 2.10 Range of beats over 60 seconds

Age range	Beats per minute
Infants (resting) < 1	110–160
Child 1–2 years	100–150
Child 2–5 years	95–140
Child 5–12	80–120
Adolescent to adult > 12	60–100

Pulse pressure

This is a wave of pressure caused by a sequence of distension and elastic recoil in the wall of the aorta, which force blood rapidly down the systemic arterial system. It determines the strength of force of the pulse and it can be defined as the difference between the systolic and diastolic blood pressures.

When the pulse pressure is low (e.g. below 35 mmHg) the strength of the pulse may be feeble and thready suggestive of arterial vasoconstriction (e.g. in reduced cardiac output states in hypovolaemia and cardiogenic shock). When the pulse pressure is high (e.g. above 45 mmHg) the pulse strength may be bounding and the person experiencing this may feel palpitations or a pounding heart suggestive of vasodilatation, such as in sepsis. Taking into consideration the strength of a pulse can be difficult, but a grading chart such as seen in Table 2.11 may

Table 2.11 Determining pulse strength or amplitude

Grading	Description
0	Pulse absent
1+	Pulse difficult to palpate, weak or thready, easily obliterated
2+	Normal pulse, easily palpated, not easily obliterated.
3+	Strong, bounding, easily palpated pulse, cannot be obliterated

help to clarify what can be felt on palpation.

By feeling the pulse and taking notice of either a deficit or pulse pressure a nurse can determine if a pulse is present, absent, strong and equal, faint and equal. Any weakness or a bounding feeling as if there is a great pressure within the artery, whether it is fast or slow or irregular can be felt. These will all give the nurse indications as to whether perfusion is inadequate or over-supplied, each giving clues to the overall circulation of each individual area of the body.

Peripheral pulses

These include the pulses of the lower limbs, the popliteal pulse located behind the knee and the dorsalis pedis and posterior tibial pulses in the feet are important in determining adequacy of perfusion to the lower limbs. Sometimes they are difficult to locate and palpate and a Doppler may be used to hear the blood flow. They are invaluable when assessing the circulation to the lower limbs and because of this it should be undertaken in good light as any mottled or bluish discoloration to the feet may indicate a poor blood supply and ischaemia in the lower limbs.

Blood pressure

Blood pressure (BP) is the force exerted on the blood vessel wall by the blood as it is pumped around the body by the force of ventricular contraction. BP varies throughout the vascular system and is highest and most variable in the aorta and other elastic arteries, decreases through arterioles and capillaries. A number of factors, most significantly cardiac output, peripheral resistance, elasticity of vessels and hormonal and chemical control mechanisms determine it.

The arterial systolic blood pressure in children varies with age and on average the readings rise as the child gets older:

- < 1 year: 70–90 mmHg
- 1–2 years: 80–95 mmHg
- 2–5 years: 80–100 mmHg
- 5–12 years: 90–110 mmHg
- > 12 years: 100–120 mmHg

Another way to calculate a child's blood pressure is:

- In children aged between 1 and 10 years, you can calculate the systolic blood pressure using the formula age $\times 2 + 80$ (ALSG 2005)
- In adolescents, the formula is age $+ 100$; this will give an approximate expected systolic blood pressure.

For accurate blood pressure recording, a cuff of the appropriate size needs to be selected (Table 2.12). The width of the cuff needs to cover two-thirds of the limb. The length of the bladder within the cuff should encircle the limb without overlap (Hockenberry and Barrera 2003). It may be difficult to obtain an accurate manual blood pressure reading in infants and young children as they are often not willing to co-operate with the procedure or remain still for a sufficient period of time for a measurement to take place.

There are two types of blood pressure monitoring:

- Direct measurement is an invasive procedure involving cannulation into an artery and connection of a pressure transducer, which gives an arterial pressure waveform and a continuous read out of BP (see later).
- Indirect measurement is usually performed manually using sphygmomanometry, either electronically with a digital device or via auscultation with a stethoscope.

The accuracy and efficiency of the BP measurement is influenced by many factors:

- The equipment – the last time it was serviced, where it is positioned in relation to the patient's heart, e.g. too high will give an inaccurately higher reading, too low will give an inaccurately low reading.
- The patient – temperature, full stomach, and crossed legs will all affect the BP reading.

Table 2.12 Guide to cuff size, neonates to adolescents

Indication	Limb circumference (cm)	Cuff size (cm)
Neonates	3	6
	4	8
	6	11
	7	13
	8	15
Child	12	19
Adolescent	17	25

■ The nurse – favourite digits, e.g. systolic or diastolic, the positioning of the nurse in relation to looking at the reading, incorrect technique.

BP: Maintenance of an adequate blood pressure is essential to permit perfusion of the brain, and the coronary arteries, and the production of urine by the kidneys. A child's homeostatic mechanisms responsible for maintaining optimum blood pressure (Table 2.13) may be immature, stretched to their limit, fail to function, or be interfered with by drugs. The consequences of not being able to maintain an adequate blood pressure may lead ultimately to:

■ cerebral hypoxia
■ cardiac failure
■ acute renal failure
■ multisystem failure.

These states occur as a result of prolonged hypotension (a low BP) or hypertension (a high BP):

■ Hypotension will only occur when all of the homeostatic mechanisms are exhausted, which can be very quick in children. It may occur in hypovolaemia where there is a diminished circulatory fluid volume.

■ Hypertension is consistent elevation of systemic arterial BP, which can be equally harmful to a child, as it can affect the circulation by damaging the wall of the systemic blood vessels. Hypertension can also be indicative of raised intracranial pressure (when combined with a simultaneous decrease in pulse rate), and is a protective measure to maintain cerebral perfusion if the

Table 2.13 Summary of homeostatic mechanisms that govern BP

Control	Action
Control of resistance via the sympathetic nervous system, maintains vasomotor tone in all vessels	Directly via baroreceptors Indirectly via chemoreceptors
Chemical control	Epinephrine (adrenaline) and norepinephrine (noradrenaline) ADH Angiotensin II Atrial nutrietric peptide (ANP) Alcohol Inflammatory mediators
Renal autoregulation	Renin Aldosterone
Capillary dynamics	Pressures exerted within the capillaries: filtration absorption

intracranial pressure increases following head injury, anoxia or space occupying lesions.

Monitoring BP is an important facet of the nurse's role as systolic pressure reflects the adequacy of cardiac output, and diastolic pressure reflects the peripheral resistance exerted by the arterioles, measured in millimetres of mercury. Measuring the BP remains one of the most important and widely used assessment tools in hospital, as from this one test much information can be gleaned about the patient's state of health.

Respiration

Respiration is an essential body function necessary for the diffusion of gases between the alveoli and blood, as well as the maintenance of blood pH. Ventilation is the mechanical movement of gas or air in and out of the lungs. The respiratory rate is the ventilatory rate, or the number of times gas is inspired and expired per minute.

Effective respiration is dependent on many factors, both nervous and chemical in nature, but which generally include the chemoreceptors and lung receptors. When assessing respiration there are other important observations to make (in addition to rate) which will help identify the effectiveness of breathing. Observation of respiration itself can be considered in terms of quality, rate, pattern and depth.

The respiratory rate in infants is best observed using the abdominal movement as this is where the effort of breathing is observed. In older children the chest wall movements can be observed. Respiratory rate varies with age

and is measured in breaths per minute (bpm):

- < 1 years: 30–40 bpm
- 1–2 years: 25–35 bpm
- 2–5 years: 25–30 bpm
- 5–12 years: 20–25 bpm
- > 12 years: 15–20 bpm

The number of times the infant's abdomen or a child's chest rises and falls is observed and counted for the duration of 60 seconds. Counting should take place when the child is resting and unaware of the observation, since conscious awareness of breathing can lead to alteration in rate and pattern. This is because breathing is under the control of both the involuntary and voluntary nervous system.

Dyspnoea is an awareness of discomfort with breathing. The depth of respiration can be specifically measured using a spirometer, or observed by inspecting chest expansion for depth or shallowness at the same time as observing for equality and uniformity of movement. Noisy, gurgling and wheezing respirations are abnormal and imply an obstruction in the upper respiratory tract. The louder the noise heard at the mouth during inspiration, the greater the degree of airway obstruction present. Noisy breathing must be separated from other sounds superimposed on a normal breathing pattern, which are usually heard through a stethoscope. The noises are termed crackles (or rales) and wheezes.

In addition, observations should include:

- Cyanosis of lips, toes, fingers indicates lack of oxygen, or due to peripheral shut down (↓ tissue perfusion)

- Ability to talk is due to shortness of breath
- Use of accessory muscles (pectoral or sternomastoids); these are used to increase thoracic size in an attempt to improve ventilation
- Cough: effectiveness, sputum production, colour, consistency
- Chest movement:
  - is it bilateral?
  - can sputum rattle be felt?
  - is the patient confused?
  - signs of wheezing (expiration).

Urine output

The process of passing urine or emptying the bladder is called micturition (also known as voiding or urination). This should be regularly monitored by urine output, either from collecting the child's urine in a bedpan or urinal or by a catheter inserted into the bladder and collected in a bag, and charting it on a fluid chart. Fluid balance charts measure:

- Fluid intake (IV, oral, EF)
- Fluid output (urine, wound/chest drains, vomiting, diarrhoea, insensible loss)
- Urine output reduces during:
  - stress, to increase BP
  - loss of circulating volume
  - renal failure, hypoxic injury to the kidney (ATN), retention
  - heart failure (LVF, CHD, CHF, MI)
- Urine output increases:
  - in diabetes insipidus
  - in the diuretic phase of renal failure
  - following the administration of diuretics

  - in hypothermia (massive diuresis, due to extreme cold).

If there are concerns about kidney function, overall fluid and electrolyte balance, quality of urine and circulatory status, then urinary output should be measured at regular intervals, and accurately recorded. If urine output falls (in ml/kg/hr) for more than 2 hours, the medical team should be informed as fluid administration may need to be increased or diuretics prescribed. The measurement of urine output is measured at hourly intervals and accurately recorded. Interpretation of urine output is always considered as an overall fluid balance over a 24-hour period.

Oxygen saturation

Adequate tissue oxygenation depends on a balance between oxygen supply and delivery, and the tissue demand for oxygen. When oxygen demands exceed oxygen supply, hypoxia occurs. Most cells require oxygen to survive, function correctly and maintain tissues.

Hypoxia can occur from:

- a blockage whereby the tissues become hypoxic due to a reduced blood flow, as in arteriosclerosis
- from the loss of red blood cells which carries oxygen to the cells, often observed in haemorrhage
- the inability to get oxygen into the circulation, seen in patients with impaired respiratory function.

The nurse is frequently the first to observe the presence of hypoxia and the one who can intervene to correct the problem with oxygenation. Hypoxia may be observed in a number of ways.

There may be changes in behaviour and level of consciousness:

- the inability to think abstractly or perform complex mental tasks
- restlessness
- apprehension
- uncooperativeness
- irritability
- short-term memory may also be impaired.

Hypoxia can cause vasoconstriction of blood vessels and thus redistribute the circulating volume.

Oxygen saturation monitoring

Oxygen saturation is the monitoring of haemoglobin oxygen saturation, and is widely used in many patient care settings. The normal percentage of oxygen saturated with haemoglobin is 98%. Pulse oximetry is used:

- to estimate arterial oxygen saturation (SpO_2)
- to monitor changes in arterial oxygen saturation.

O_2 saturation monitoring uses pulse oximetry and reductions in this measure from normal may lead the nurse to extend his/her assessment of hypoxia, for example arterial blood gases. The oxygen saturation measurement is valuable as it allows nurses to evaluate the relative state of oxygenation, and can help to improve the care the patient receives. However, when using pulse oximetry in practice other observations should be undertaken in conjunction with it, if hypoxia is suspected, such as colour, pulse rate, breathing pattern and rate and arterial blood gases (will give partial pressure of oxygen).

Oxygen saturation monitoring can be measured on the:

- finger
- toe
- ear lobe.

There must be:

- a good flow of blood to the area (not effective if severe vasoconstriction is present)
- no mechanical movement of the probe – will cause interference
- no nail varnish – this will affect the normal haemoglobin saturation measured.

Limitations of O_2 monitoring

- It is important for practitioners to note that the oxygen saturation monitor can give misleading information regarding the true nature of the patient's oxygen status.
  - The oxygen disassociation curve plots the relationship between the amount of oxygen bound to haemoglobin (oxygen saturation) and the partial pressure of oxygen (PaO_2) in the blood.
  - The steep S shaped curve highlights that at a normal PaO_2 of 13.3 kPa, oxygen saturation is 100%.
  - If the PaO_2 drops 5.3 kPa to 8 kPa the oxygen saturation will remain within acceptable limits – 90%. At a further drop of just 1.7 kPa, the oxygen saturation will drop from 90% to 70%. At this level breathing is difficult and respiratory arrest may occur, requiring emergency intubation.

– An oxygen saturation of 90% may not indicate to the nurse that there is a low oxygen supply in the blood (determined by partial pressure of oxygen).

■ If the oxygen saturation falls below 85% the pulse oximeter may become progressively less accurate.

■ Pulse oximetry cannot be used in any form of carbon monoxide inhalation because the carboxyhaemoglobin will result in the oximeter over-reading the saturation level.

■ In anaemia there is a reduction in haemoglobin, those red blood cells available will be fully saturated.

An awareness of these principles will ensure that oxygen saturation monitoring is safe, and minimize the potential for unrecognized hypoxaemic episodes.

End tidal carbon dioxide ($P_{ET}CO_2$) monitoring

The $P_{ET}CO_2$ monitors exhaled carbon dioxide on both intubated and non-intubated patients. The normal range for expired $P_{ET}CO_2$ is generally between 4.5 and 5.7 kPa. This method of expiratory gas analysis can be undertaken through a nasal cannula and simultaneously deliver supplemental oxygen. In lungs where ventilation is uniformly distributed and evenly matched to perfusion end-tidal CO_2 ($P_{ET}CO_2$) reasonably reflects partial pressure of arterial CO_2:

■ Pulmonary embolism or decreased cardiac output is associated with a decrease in $P_{ET}CO_2$, because of decreased alveolar blood flow.

■ An increase in $P_{ET}CO_2$ reflects the presence of airway narrowing or other lung disease associated with respiratory changes in the mechanical properties of the lungs.

This method of expiratory gas analysis is not commonly used in all clinical practice areas, but studies are showing its benefits and value in respiratory management of patients.

Connected clinical observations

The vital signs detailed above should be accurately and clearly recorded at the time they were taken on the appropriate chart. These measures may over time begin to show patterns and identify any deterioration in an infant or child's condition. All of the observations detailed above are not viewed as isolated recordings, there is a relationship between them all and when one observation changes there will be a relational change in another. Therefore, a holistic assessment includes all the clinical observation before making a judgement about a child's condition.

Invasive cardiovascular haemodynamic monitoring

Invasive cardiac monitoring gives a much clearer picture of a patient's haemodynamic state; however, they are invasive and therefore have numerous complications attached.

Arterial blood pressure monitoring

This involves a needle being put into an artery, generally the radial or brachial artery. A cannula is inserted, attached to a pressure bag to prevent backflow and attached to a transducer, from this a continuous readout of systolic and diastolic BP is given on the monitor screen. In addition, the monitor calculates the mean arterial pressure (MAP) which is the:

- average pressure in main arteries
- heart spends more time in diastole.

MAP = diastolic pressure (P_D) + (pulse pressure [P_P] divided by 3)

This measure determines BP in a different way (BP is measured by the pressure exerted on the sides of the blood vessels) to manual BP. and therefore the two measures cannot be compared. Depends on:

- compliance (distensibility) of elastic arteries
- stroke volume
- rises during ventricular systole, decreases during diastole
- systolic pressure (P_s) – pressure in arteries during ventricular systole (cardiac contraction)
- diastolic pressure (P_D) – pressure in arteries during ventricular diastole (resting period).

The body maintains BP in many ways as summarized in Table 2.13. The mechanisms include neural and chemical controls alter distribution to meet

demands of various organs/tissues to maintain overall MAP through vasomotor tone (see Section 1).

Therefore due to the many mechanisms that control BP, it is a poor indicator of shock. For early detection of changes assess the following:

- Tachycardia, ↑ in temp. and blood glucose level due to stress and the release of catecholamines
- Pale skin colour, cool to cold skin due to redistribution of blood
- ↓ in urine output, due to selective vasoconstriction of the renal bed, actions of ADH and aldosterone
- Absent bowel sounds
- An ↑ or → in BP and rate and depth of breathing
- Mental state alterations ranging from restlessness to coma
- Complaining of thirst.

These are much more reliable, as the body will attempt to maintain BP at all costs.

Central venous pressure (CVP) monitoring

The CVP normally reflects the volume of blood returning to the heart, which exerts a pressure on the walls of the right atrium and measuring it can provide information about:

- the adequacy of the body's bloods volume in relation to circulatory capacity
- the effectiveness of the right side of the heart as a pump
- vascular tone
- pulmonary vascular resistance.

The measurement of the central venous pressure (CVP) provides haemodynamic information to guide the therapy of patients. Central venous pressure (CVP) is indicated:

- to obtain blood for laboratory estimation
- to administer parenteral nutrition
- administration of hypertonic or irritating solutions
- administration of vasoactive or inotropic agents and monitor effect
- as a venous access when all other routes exhausted
- where massive fluid replacement is required and monitor effect.
- in acute circulatory failure.

Measurements are usually made using a CVP placed within the subclavian vein or internal jugular vein attached to a transducer and then plugged into a monitor. However, a CVP line can also be placed in the external jugular or femoral vein. The insertion of a CVP is a strict aseptic procedure. For the measurement the patient should be in the supine position. If breathlessness occurs when lying flat, the CVP readings may need to be taken with the patient lying at a greater angle no more than 30 degrees, in which case the angle used should always be indicated alongside the recorded CVP measurement. The monitor has to be zeroed at regular intervals. The CVP is a dynamic measure and as such differs between individuals the average is between 4–12 cmH$_2$O for water manometers and 2–8 mmHg for mercury transducers.

It is not the single CVP reading that is important but the trend demonstrated by a series of readings over time.

Therefore, each time a CVP measurement is made, it is essential that it is made under identical conditions so that all possible variables (such as patient position) remain constant. Patient management should not result from the information received from CVP measurements alone. The wider clinical picture needs to be considered, for example blood pressure, cardiac output, heart rate, respiratory characteristics, urine output.

Complications of CVP monitoring

- Air embolism – the lines used to measure CVP are central venous lines and thus present the inherent danger of air embolism. All intravenous administration equipment should, therefore, possess Luer lock connections to minimize accidental disconnection.
- Pneumothorax – damage to the apices of the lungs, leading to pneumothorax.
- Damage to the ventricular muscles of the heart causing ventricular arrhythmias.
- Risk of infection and subsequent septicaemia, maintenance of asepsis is therefore essential.

Changes in the CVP reading

Generally, there is an overestimation as to the value of the CVP reading. If a fall in CVP occurs this is proposed to indicate a moderate fluid loss. For example, in patients who are bleeding following surgery, or because of extreme vasodilatation, whereby the capacity of the circulation is increased but the circulating volume remains constant, as in patients with pyrexia or from the excessive use of vasodilator drugs (Edwards & Manley 1998).

A consequent rise in CVP is thought to give rise to concerns about fluid overload. This can lead to circulatory collapse, whereby the left side of the heart becomes dysfunctional. The consequences being that the heart is unable to pump blood, leading to a low cardiac output and an increase in right and left ventricular filling pressures. It is presumed, therefore, that the CVP can be used as a guide to determine severity of both fluid loss and measure when too much fluid has been administered, and ascertain cardiac instability.

However, a reduction in CVP will occur in hypovolaemia due to fluid loss, and during fluid overload and left-sided cardiac failure due to the reduction in venous return. In the case of fluid overload it may take nearly 24 hours for events occurring in the left side of the heart to reflect through the lungs into the right ventricle, atria, and superior vena cava, and be mirrored as an increased CVP reading.

This implies that CVP levels are not completely reliable in estimating circulatory function. Therefore, a more accurate measure would be that which could determine the pressure in the left side of the heart.

Pulmonary artery pressure (PAP)

In the late 1960s the first flow-directed catheter measuring pulmonary right, and left heart pressures was developed.

■ When the balloon is deflated the pressure reflected is the pulmonary artery pressure (PAP), which is elevated in pulmonary hypertension caused by tension pneumothorax, haemothorax, COPD, fluid overload and tamponade, and is decreased in hypovolaemic shock.

■ Pulmonary artery wedge pressure (PAWP) is measured when the balloon is inflated and the pulmonary artery is blocked. The tip on the other side of the balloon reflects left-sided heart pressure. This pressure is elevated in pulmonary embolism, hypoxia, ARDS; and decreased in hypovolaemia.

■ Cardiac output (CO) is the amount of blood pumped by the heart per minute (L/min) and determines the function of the heart and cardiovascular system.

■ Systemic vascular resistance (SVR) is the average or total resistance to blood flow in the entire systemic circulation and lower values indicate vasodilatation (sepsis) while higher values indicate vasoconstriction (stress, hypothermia).

■ Mixed venous oxygen monitoring (SVO_2) is the percentage of saturation of venous haemoglobin, reflects the overall balance between oxygen delivery and oxygen consumption of perfused tissues. Normal is 75%.

– A decrease in SvO_2 is an early indication that oxygen transport and uptake may be inadequate and interventions may be necessary and result from increased oxygen demand or decreased oxygen delivery; usually an indication that oxygen delivery falls or tissue oxygen demand increases.

– Increased readings reflect a failure of cells to take up and utilize oxygen SvO$_2$ (> 80%); levels can be caused by high FIO$_2$ rates or decreases in oxygen demand, such as with hypothermic patients or those who are anaesthetized.

A special catheter tip (Swan Ganz or thermodilution pulmonary artery catheter) that sits at the distal port of the pulmonary artery and includes a balloon obtains these measurements.

The PAWP is a much more reliable measurement than the CVP in determining cardiac function:

■ If the PAWP is high and CO low, this may indicate fluid overload, giving rise to left ventricular insufficiency, and cardiac dysfunction.

■ If hypovolaemia is present both PAWP and CO would be reduced.

Fluid overload and hypovolaemia require different therapies to maintain adequate cardiac function. However, this method involves the threading of a catheter from a central vein, through the right atrium, right ventricle and into the pulmonary artery. It is indicated for:

■ acute cardiac failure

■ shock

■ diagnosis of tamponade

■ mitral regurgitation

■ ruptured ventricular septum

■ intra-operative and postoperative management of high-risk patient

■ when the CVP fails to give accurate or sufficient detail regarding cardiac function.

It is a highly invasive technique with a recognized risk of morbidity and mortality. Therefore its use in clinical practice is deteriorating. When in use the PAP monitor can measure CVP, SVR, CO and cardiac input.

There is an increase in the use of other techniques that adequately measure PAP, PAWP, CO, and SVR.

Intracranial pressure monitoring (ICP)

The skull and meninges contain three major components:

■ brain tissue (80%)

■ cerebral spinal fluid (CSF) (10%);

■ cerebral blood flow (CBF) (10%).

The pressure of these three components in the rigid skull is termed the intracranial pressure (ICP). The normal range of ICP is between 0–15 mmHg, above 15 mmHg is determined a raised ICP. The brain maintains this normal pressure by compensation mechanisms known as autoregulation, which occurs following an insult or injury leading to increased brain, blood or CSF volume. To compensate the following occurs:

■ Displacement of CSF from the cranial subarachnoid space, spinal and lumbar space.

■ CSF production decreases and CSF absorption increases.

■ Reduction in CBF, venous blood is shunted away from the affected areas. A widespread reduction in CBF to compensate can lead to further brain insult or ischaemia due to the reduced cerebral perfusion.

These compensatory mechanisms may become exhausted and an increase in ICP above 15 mmHg may occur. This may occur due to:

- trauma
- hydrocephalus
- infection
- tumours
- metabolic disorders
- cerebrovascular accident
- encephalopathies.

In certain injuries monitoring techniques can be employed to measure the ICP. There are three types of ICP monitoring devices, but only one can drain; these include:

- Fluid coupled systems with external transducers:
  - Ventriculostomy (intraventricular catheter, IVC), able to drain excess CSF
- Fluid-coupled surface devices:
  - subarachnoid (SA) bolts devised because of the concern for infection with IVCs – unable to drain CSF
  - are only monitoring instruments
  - can be inaccurate and tend to underestimate the ICP.
- Solid state systems include the fibreoptic system and cable:
  - can be combined with IVC to form simultaneous ICP monitoring and CSF drainage
  - solid state systems are not always directly compatible with common critical care bedside monitoring a separate system for recording and trending is necessary. Can be placed in the:
    • lateral ventricle
    • the brain parenchyma
    • epidural space.

Complications of IVC ICP monitors are the risk of infection such as meningitis or ventriculitis, which is related to the duration of catheter insertion.

Close records of observations need to be kept especially of mean arterial pressure (MAP). This is necessary to determine adequate CBF. Calculate and record ICP and cerebral perfusion pressure (CPP). CPP is the pressure needed to perfuse the brain, and the normal range is 80–90 mmHg. It is calculated by subtracting the ICP from the MAP.

$$CPP = MAP - ICP$$

CBF is compromised if the CPP is below 60 mmHg. Reduced CPP may result in irreversible brain damage or death. It is thought that the threshold for mechanical brain injury is an ICP between 20 and 30 mmHg.

Factors that reduce the ICP:

- Position – head elevated by 30°,
- Fluid restriction – slightly dehydrated state.
- Temperature control – hypothermia.
- Drugs:
  - diuretics
  - corticosteriods
  - anticonvulsants
- Hyperventilation – reduced partial pressure of carbon dioxide will cause cerebral vasoconstriction and a reduction in ICP – hypercarbia is important to avoid in patients with increased ICP.
- A reduced level of oxygen will increase ICP and hypoxia or cerebral ischaemia should be avoided.
- Removal of the cause, e.g. surgery.

2.4 Diagnostic procedures

Collecting specimens

Sputum specimen

This is often collected if a child has a respiratory problem to identify the presence of an infection. Involve the parents or carers or play specialist to ensure the child understands what needs to be done. There are different methods of obtaining a specimen:

Coughing up a specimen:

- If it is difficult for the child to do this practise coughing, particularly in the morning.
- Use a physiotherapist to assist.
- Ask child to cough into a sputum container, label and send to the laboratory.

Other methods of obtaining a specimen:

- Suctioning
  - Use the lowest suction pressure 60–120 mmHg.
  - In infants the pressure should be no higher than 100 mmHg
  - Do not insert the catheter too far and a premeasure should be taken from the child's nose to the top of the rib cage – the suction catheter should not be passed any further than this measure.
  - When using the nose or mouth if any resistance is met withdraw the catheter, attempt this twice and if resistance is still felt, use a smaller catheter.

- Nasopharyngeal aspirate (NPA)
  - Used in young babies under 6 months old and for the diagnosis of severe bronchiolitis (viral infection), chronic lung disease, immunodeficiency, neuromuscular disease.
  - Not commonly used as generally diagnosed by clinical symptoms.
  - A fine suction catheter is used with a sputum trap and sent promptly.
  - Infection control practices need to be enforced, e.g. goggles, gloves and aprons.
  - Normal saline is required to aid with the collection.
  - Oxygen and suctioning need to be available by the bedside in case of an emergency.
  - Result can be obtained within an hour.

The investigations that take place on the specimen:

- Bacterial – the culture will take around 24–48 hours, and then an antibiotic sensitivity test is undertaken. This is often referred to as MC&S (microscopy, culture and sensitivity test).

- Viral – these organisms do not survive for very long outside of the body and so it is important they are sent to the laboratory quickly; specimens should be kept in the fridge (not the freezer) to maintain; their survival.

- *Mycosis fungoides* and *Mycobacterium tuberculosis* – special medium is needed to grow these organisms.

- Protozoa – used if malaria is suspected, they are mobile so need to get to the laboratory quickly.

Other tests that accompany a sputum specimen:

- chest X-ray
- blood tests.

Stool specimen

The most common reason is for gastrointestinal tract (GIT) infections (Jasper 2008):

- Rotavirus
- *Giardia*
- *Escherichia coli*
- *Salmonella*
- *Shigella*

Another reason may be to test for occult blood, which indicates bleeding in the GIT and can be carried out on the ward. Infection control practices must be adhered to when handling faeces. Involve the parent or guardian and ensure the child understands what they need to do:

- The specimen sent needs to be fresh.
- Collected first thing in the morning if it is for threadworm or pin worm.
- Decide if the specimen is to be collected from:
  - nappy
  - clean potty
  - bedpan
    bedpan on the toilet.

Swabs

When observing a child's condition it is important to note any signs of weeping of fluid (exudates) or pus, redness, swelling, odour, or rise in temperature as this may denote an infection. This may be from the ear, eyes, insertion site of lines (feeding or intravenous), catheters (boy or girl) or wound sites. If any of these signs are present a sample of the exudates should be retrieved and sent to the laboratory to detect the infecting organism. Use the special implement available for this task – generally a cotton tipped swab contained within a sheath or capsule. Take the swab before cleansing of the area or changing of the line. Once removed or changed the tip of the catheter or IV line may also need to be sent to the laboratory, by cutting if off with a sterile pair of scissors and placing it in a clean specimen pot.

Urine sample

A urine sample will determine if there is an infection in the urine. Methods used to collect a sample:

- Toilet trained children can be requested to pass urine into a container.
- Non-toilet trained children may involve the use of urine collection bags or pads, but these are prone to contamination as they come into contact with the skin.
- Catheter insertion – a specimen can be obtained on insertion 10 ml in a specimen container.

A urine sample may also be used to detect any signs of blood, glucose, ketones or protein present in the urine (can be achieved by undertaking a simple urine test – see later). Other tests are used to determine the levels of other chemicals or proteins.

A 24 hour urine collection is used to determine if certain chemicals and what levels of proteins over a period of time are excreted. This may indicate a particular disease. The most common use is for creatinine (creatinine clearance in comparison to blood creatinine), estimation of glomerular filtration rate and the functioning of the kidneys.

Urine testing

The kidney has a prime role in maintaining normal healthy life and many early changes that occur in the body may be reflected in the urine well before they become clinically obvious. A nurse is usually the first person to deal with a patient admitted to the unit, and has the most opportunity of contact with, and a chance to observe, the patient. Thus, nurses are well placed to aid in the detection and diagnosis of disease, as they may be the first to be aware of the patient's clinical condition. Often there are some clues (Table 2.14), which can suggest a few simple preliminary tests that may easily show whether to pursue a particular line of investigation and these tests can be performed by the nurse on a urine sample.

Urine examination can yield important information about the early signs of disease, as many life-threatening conditions of insidious onset such as diabetes, cancer of the bladder or renal disease may be revealed by the analysis of the constituents of the urine and their interpretation (Table 2.15):

- specific gravity 1005–1035 (state of hydration)
- pH 4.5–8 (acid–base balance)
- blood (cancer of the bladder, stones, infection, trauma)
- protein (renal disease, UTI, hypertension, CHF)
- bilirubin and urobilinogen (liver disease, haemolytic anaemia)
- nitrates (UTI)
- glucose (diabetes mellitus, stress, Cushing's syndrome, acute pancreatitis)
- ketones (fasting, uncontrolled diabetes mellitus).

The measurements of routine urine tests help to provide valuable clues to the child's condition or the effectiveness of treatment. It is unfortunate that urine

Table 2.14 Clues suggesting preliminary urine tests are required

Symptom or sign	Possible diagnosis	Tests to consider
Weight loss	? Malnutrition	Look for ketones
Weight loss, perhaps with an increase in thirst	? Diabetes	Look for glucose and ketones
Frequency of micturition	? Infection	Test for bacteria (i.e. nitrites) or protein and blood
	? Renal disease	Test for specific gravity, protein, blood
Yellow tinge to skin	? Jaundice	Test for increases in urobilinogen and urine bilirubin

Table 2.15 Urine testing: significance of results

Measure	Interpretation	Significance in disease
Specific gravity Determines hydration and the amount of waste products to be excreted in relation to water dependent on state of hydration and the amount of waste products to be excreted. One way to determine if hydration is adequate.	SG gives a good indication of the net fluid balance and is of particular value in patients where there is an un-quantifiable loss, such as in burns cases, breathing difficulties, diarrhoea or fever. In healthy adults, SG varies between 1.005 to 1.035 (pure water is the standard, with a SG of 1.000).	Urine with a persistently low SG is suggestive of diabetes insipidus or renal damage. An increase in specific gravity will indicate dehydration, perhaps due to bleeding, vomiting, diarrhoea, reduction in fluid intake or fever.
pH Should reflect the acid–base balance of the body, as excess hydrogen or bicarbonate ions are excreted by the tubules to maintain the normal status.	Under normal circumstances, the urine has a pH of around 6 but it can range from about 5–8.5.	Metabolic acidosis from starvation, high protein diets or diabetic ketoacidosis will lead to an acid urine but diets including a lot of vegetables, mild or even bicarbonate-based antacids can cause an alkaline urine, when the pH will rise.
Blood A potentially serious sign and needs thorough and rapid investigation.	Positive results must be followed up to determine where the blood is coming from. False positive results may occur, from containers contaminated with bleach, skin preparation with povidine iodine, or from the use of stale urine.	Asymptomatic haematuria is usually the earliest sign of cancer of the bladder. It can also be due to trauma, infection or stones. The blood will disappear with resolution of the infection, or stone.

Protein

In early renal disease, the glomerulus and tubules may leak small amounts of protein into the urine.

As renal disease progresses, detectable levels of protein will be found in the urine.

A number of diseases associated with proteinuria including renal disease, urinary tract infection, hypertension, pre-eclampsia or congestive heart failure.
When testing for urinary protein, a morning specimen of urine is recommended to ensure sufficient concentration.

Bilirubin and urobilinogen

In normal health, bilirubin is not found in the urine as it is excreted via the bile duct into the gut.

When the liver is diseased or there is obstruction to the flow of bile into the gut, bilirubin or its metabolites are likely to be found in significant quantities in the urine.

Urobilinogen is normally present in urine, but elevated levels may indicate liver abnormalities or excessive destruction of red blood cells, such as in haemolytic anaemia.

Nitrates

Urine normally contains nitrates from dietary metabolites, and some of the common bacteria responsible for urinary infections will convert these nitrates to nitrites.

Nitrites are not normally present in urine, but are produced in increasing numbers when gram negative bacteria such as E. coli convert dietary nitrates (found in the preservatives in meat products and cheese and smoked food) to nitrites.
It would be appropriate to send the specimen to the laboratory for culture and sensitivity and refer the patient to the doctor for treatment.

As E. coli is responsible for 80% of urine infection the presence of nitrites is strongly suggestive of urinary tract infection.
Visible signs may also be present, for example is the specimen clear or cloudy? Cloudiness should be noted If the specimen is turbid and one or more of the four tests are positive, there is a 50% chance that the urine is infected.

(Continued)

Table 2.15 Urine testing: significance of results—cont'd

Measure	Interpretation	Significance in disease
Glucose Not normally found in urine.	There are two categories of urine tests for glucose, the Clinitest, and the impregnated test strips.	The presence of glucose may be due to raised blood glucose levels (hyperglycaemia). It can be associated with many medical conditions such as diabetes mellitus, stress, Cushing's syndrome, and acute pancreatitis.
Ketones When the body metabolizes fat waste, the breakdown products are the ketone - excreted in the urine. In good health they are not detectable in urine	There are two tests available for ketones: acetest which is a tablet test, and a strip test.	Usually ketones may be found in people who are fasting, but can also be present in excessive amounts in people with uncontrolled diabetes. Ketones are acidic substances and when present in excess can lead to metabolic acidosis, which, if untreated, can cause death.
Odour A urine specimen should be noted before further testing.	Normal, freshly voided urine has very little smell, but develops an ammoniacal smell on standing. Infected urine smells foul and may have a characteristic fishy smell on voiding and the smell worsens on standing.	Ketoacidosis of patients who have been starving or suffering from anorexia or diabetes, gives urine a characteristic smell. Eating fish, curry or other strongly flavoured foodstuffs can also make the urine smell.

testing is described as 'routine' and generally undervalued. Urine testing is a simple and cost-effective procedure. It is fast, easy to interpret and non-intrusive to children.

Appearance of urine and cause

- Colour
  - yellow–orange to brownish green – bilirubin from obstructive jaundice
  - red to red–brown – haemoglobinuria
  - smoky red – unhaemolysed red blood cells (RBC)
  - dark wine colour – haemolytic jaundice
  - brown–black – melanoma
  - dark-brown – liver infection
  - green – bacterial infection
- Odour – infection, diabetes, anorexia.

By taking note of some of the areas measured in routine urine test:

- fluid balance may be evaluated
- diagnosis may be aided
- circulatory status monitored
- valuable clues to the effectiveness of treatment are provided.

The results of a urine test should be recorded accurately in the child's records, as soon as possible after testing. A negative test result may not only point to an alternative diagnosis, but it is also a valuable baseline indicator to be referred to later in evaluating the progress of a child during the course of his or her illness. A negative result should always be recorded even if at the time it appears unimportant, or irrelevant.

Pleural effusion

This is an excessive collection of fluid in the pleural space. The fluid may be serous fluid, pus or lymph (for the removal of air and blood see emergency care and chest drain insertion in section one). A pleural effusion on a chest X-ray is best seen with the child in the erect position. A CT scan may help to identify underlying lung pathology and possible sites for diagnostic aspiration.

- Causes:
  - heart failure
  - infection following thoracic surgery
  - hypoproteinaemia
  - abscess secondary to pneumonia
  - pulmonary tuberculosis.
- Clinical features:
  - pallor
  - tachycardia
  - cyanosis
  - reduced breath sounds and air entry on the affected side
  - may be a drop in blood pressure
  - dyspnoea, which is variable dependent upon the size of the effusion.
  - dull chest pain
  - symptoms due to the underlying cause, e.g. abscess, tuberculosis.

The effusion will be seen on a chest X-ray as a water-dense shadow with a concave-upwards upper border. If the effusion is causing dyspnoea it should be drained. The drain is inserted into the pleural cavity through the fifth intercostal space in the mid-auxiliary line, on the side of the effusion. It is performed by an experienced doctor or health care practitioner using sedation or a general anaesthetic. If an emergency then a local anaesthetic may be used. The fluid is best removed slowly to allow the lung to re-expand. An indwelling chest drain may be inserted.

Lumbar puncture

In this procedure cerebrospinal fluid (CSF) is withdrawn following the insertion of a hollow needle into the lumbar subarachnoid space. It will give information on the presence of:

- meningeal inflammation
- meningoencephalitis
- cerebrospinal fluid cytology
- subarachnoid haemorrhage
- administration of intrathecal chemotherapy.

A lumbar puncture should not be undertaken if the child is too acutely ill or has an increased intracranial pressure. In these instances the child's condition needs to be stabilized as there is a risk of cerebral herniation. In addition:

- Children with papilloedema or deteriorating neurological symptoms, where raised intracranial pressure is suspected.
- In the presence of infection, as this may lead to meningitis or abscess formation, e.g. localized skin infection around the insertion site.
- The presence of frontal sinusitis.
- Middle ear discharge.
- Congenital heart disease or prosthetic heart valves.
- In children who are unable to co-operate or who are too drowsy to give a history.
- In children who have severe degenerative spinal joint disease.
- In those children undergoing anticoagulant therapy or who have coagulopathies or thrombocytopenia.

The child needs to be given a topical anaesthetic at least an hour before the procedure. A doctor carries out the procedure using an aseptic technique. The position of the child is vitally important and the nurse may be responsible for helping to maintain this position during the procedure:

- The child should be in the left lateral position, with maximum flexion of the spine and as near the edge of the bed as possible.
- There should be one pillow under the head.
- To gain maximum stretching of the lumbar vertebrae the client should flex the head to the chest and draw up the knees to the abdomen, holding them with their hands.
- The nurse may help by supporting the child behind the knees and neck, thus ensuring the widening of the intervertebral space.

Careful positioning is necessary so that the doctor can feel the lumbar spine more easily and so insert the needle accurately. It is imperative that the lumbar puncture is performed below the first lumbar vertebra where the cord terminates. The needle is usually inserted between the second and third or third and fourth lumbar vertebrae (L2 and L3 or L3 and L4). This is below the level of the spinal cord, which extends to L1 or L2, and is in the region of the cauda equina. The fluid obtained is examined for diagnostic purposes and may be required:

- To record the pressure of the CSF using a manometer.
- In suspected meningitis or encephalitis to look for bacteria in the CSF.

- In suspected malignant tumours to look for cancer cells (cytology).
- To aid diagnosis in subarachnoid haemorrhage when there would be blood in the CSF.
- To introduce intrathecal medication such as antibiotics or cytotoxic drugs.
- To introduce contrast media for radiological examination.

When the needle is in position the stylette is removed and a manometer attached to record the pressure of the CSF. The normal pressure of the CSF is 60–180 mmH$_2$O. For laboratory analysis approximately 5–10 ml of CSF is withdrawn. The nurse should note:

- the colour of the CSF – it should be colourless
- the presence of blood in the CSF – the first few millilitres may be bloodstained due to trauma following insertion of the needle but after this the fluid should run clear
- the consistency of the CSF – it should be like water
- the opacity of the CSF – it should be clear; cloudy CSF is typical in bacterial meningitis.

The Queckenstedt's test is done when an obstruction to the flow of CSF in the spinal pathway is suspected. Pressure is recorded using the manometer whilst jugular compression is applied. Normally the pressure of the CSF would rapidly rise when jugular compression is applied and just as rapidly released. If an obstruction such as a spinal tumour or dislocated vertebra is present the rise and fall of pressure will occur much more slowly. Pressure is applied for a maximum of 10 seconds and recordings taken via the manometer. Further

recordings are then taken for 10 seconds when the pressure is released. When pressure recordings are complete, the specimens of CSF will be collected in culture bottles.

> It is the professional responsibility of the nurse assisting with the procedure, to ensure that if the lumbar puncture has been undertaken unsuccessfully three times the performing doctor ceases and seeks assistance from another doctor before making another attempt.

Following the completion of the procedure:

- The needle is withdrawn and the wound sealed with a plastic sealant dressing.
- Neurological observations are carried out as the child's condition indicates.
- The child is asked to lie down flat in bed for 6–12 hours. This should prevent the development of a headache.
- Observation for leakage from the puncture site together with neurological observations should be continued for up to 24 hours.

Radiography (X-rays)

An X-ray can give a variety of information about the lungs, heart, pleura, bones and mediastinal structures. X-rays are electromagnetic vibrations of short wavelength produced by passing a high voltage through a cathode ray tube. The remnant radiation that leaves the child produces the photographic image on the radiographic film.

- *Radiolucent* materials allow X-rays to pass through them easily, air is radiolucent.
- *Radiopaque* materials do not easily allow light to pass, bone is a relatively radiopaque material.
- On a plain radiograph, gas and fat absorb few X-rays and appear dark.
- Bone and other calcified regions absorb most of the X-rays and appear white.
- Some foreign bodies such as metal and some glass are radiopaque but wood and plastic cannot be seen.

Chest X-rays

This is by far the commonest type of X-ray to be taken. The different types of chest X-rays are:

- Posteroanterior (PA) – standard department film, the plate is in front of the child's chest, with the X-ray tube 2 m (6 feet) behind the patient.
- Anteroposterior (AP) – usually a portable film, the plate is behind the child's chest, and the X-ray tube is closer to the child. The positioning of the child is often inconsistent and often the film will not show full inspiration.
- Lateral – departmental film, difficult to take as a portable film, due to the added difficulties in positioning the child. Helpful to show specific areas of consolidation.

Examination of a chest X-ray

The examination must be carried out in an orderly sequence, identifying normal anatomical structure and any abnormal shadows:

- Any abnormal shadow should be analysed for its anatomical site, size and shape of its margins.
- Consolidation – is the replacement of air in the lung by tissue or fluid of greater density? Chest infection may cause consolidation and/or collapse.
- Collapse – this is the absorption of air with loss of lung volume. The position of the tissues are often altered with possible displacement of the heart, trachea. The mediastinal outline may be obliterated.
- Pneumothorax – air in the pleural cavity seen as an area of no lung markings, which will result in reduction of lung size. Common features are a white, visible air lung interface, mediastinal shift to the opposite side.
- Pleural effusion – present as a uniform opacity, which extends up from the costophrenic angle. A large pleural effusion will cause mediastinal shift to the opposite side.
- Asthma – in asthma the X-ray is often normal except during severe attacks or long-term asthma, then the following will be seen:
  – over-inflation
  – low but curved diaphragms
  – vessels remain normal.
- Pulmonary oedema – may be cardiac or non-cardiac in origin, may see upper lobe venous

engorgement, fluffy shadows, pleural effusion may be present, cardiac enlargement may develop due to dilation of the left ventricle.

- Pulmonary embolism – generally to exclude other pathology, patchy areas of atelectasis are often seen in sub-massive PE, may be confused with consolidation or collapse. May see some vascular shadowing in the affected areas, other diagnostic procedures are more reliable e.g. nuclear imaging or pulmonary angiogram.

- Positioning of invasive devices to observe the tip and position during movement or following insertion:
  - endotracheal tubes (ETT)
  - naso-gastric tubes (NGT)
  - CVP and PAP
  - aortic balloon pumps.

Portable X-rays

Children in some instances cannot often go to the radiotherapy department to have their X-rays taken and require the radiographer to come to the ward critical care area. In this instance protection of the child and staff present on the unit at the time is imperative. Exposure to radiation always involves the risk of biological changes within the body. Therefore, the child should always be exposed to the lowest amount of radiation possible and all individuals coming into contact with radiation should be protected:

Protection occurs by:

- Minimizing the time the child is in the path of the X-ray beam.

- Maximizing the distance between the radiation source and the child.

- Shielding the reproductive organs of the child if they are within 4–5 cm of the beam. This is extremely important in children and young adults. The shields are made of lead, which absorbs X-ray.

- Improvement of X-ray machines so that there is less scatter of the radiation.

Time, distance and shielding are also used to protect staff:

- The time spent in the room where the radiation source is active should be as short as possible; the risk is only there when exposures are being made.

- Increasing the distance from the source of the beam greatly reduces the quantity of radiation that will reach the radiographer or nurse. This means that if the nurse has to hold the child while he is X-rayed there will be much greater exposure.

- If the nurse does have to support the child, a shield should be worn. Lead aprons or gloves are used where a fixed shield is not in place.

- Any worker regularly exposed to ionizing radiation must be monitored, usually by the use of a film bade. The film inside gets darker in response to the amount of radiation exposure and it is analysed, usually monthly.

- Contact with X-rays should be avoided in pregnancy as exposure can lead to malformations of the fetus. There is a safe limit of 5 mSv (0.5 rem) for a declared pregnant woman.

Computed tomography (CT) and magnetic resonance imaging (MRI)

These are generally used as a diagnostic test as an adjunct to the treatment regime in children with neurological conditions as they provide valuable information regarding their neurological state.

CT scan

This allows the visualization of the anatomy from various sectional planes by X-raying a series of thin transverse slices of the child's head or body that are then analysed by a computer. Very specialized equipment, which uses computerized digital imaging as does ultrasonography and MRI. A CT scan is very beneficial but children need to be carefully prepared and escorted by an experienced nurse.

A CT scan can:

- Determine pathological anatomy, which can reveal as much as an explorative operation, especially following injury to the brain – it enables appropriate surgical intervention only when necessary.

- Be very useful for areas where radiography is unsuitable:
  - the pancreas (deep inside the body)
  - the lungs and mediastinum
  - the brain and spinal cord.

- Be essential in the planning of radiotherapy or chemotherapy and staging tumours.

- Be essential in planning surgery, e.g. establishing the extent of invasion of oesophageal cancer.

- Assess damage in abdominal or thoracic trauma.

- Guide needles in biopsy, drainage of fluid or aspiration.

MRI

Strong magnetic fields and radio waves are used along with a computer in MRI to generate sectional images of the anatomy. It is a rapidly expanding diagnostic field and images are produced using sophisticated equipment that can be viewed in any plane:

- Lipids have a high hydrogen content and so are clearly seen on MRI.

- Very useful for examining the brain and spinal cord.

- Atheroma can also be demonstrated.

- Can be used to investigate blood flow and cardiac function without the use of contrast media.

Preparation for a CT or MRI scan involves:

- A simple explanation of the scan taking into consideration the child's level of understanding, previous experience and hospital procedures.

- Techniques such as guided imagery and therapeutic play can assist in preparing a child for diagnostic procedures.

- Information regarding pain during the procedure.

- This level of preparation will determine how well the child co-operates during the procedure and reduces their level of anxiety.

- Involve the family in the discussion as their anxiety can transmit to the child.

- Consent is needed from the parent/guardian.

- Sedation may be necessary but this depends on the age of the child and the type of imagery being performed.

CT and MRI both require the child to be still throughout and so chloral hydrate may be prescribed (not recommended for children who require CT or MRI scan due to decreased level of consciousness or increase in intracranial pressure).

- It is recommended the child should not eat if sedation is used.

- Observation of the child who has been administered sedation is commenced.

Echocardiography

In recent years a new technique has been developed where the cardiac output and cardiac function is estimated using an ultrasound probe. It is used to examine the heart and great vessels and is invaluable in cardiac diagnosis and treatment (Table 2.16). Its advantages include its portability, ease of performance and non-invasive nature.

Table 2.16 Echocardiography

Area of Importance	Role of echocardiography
Size of heart chambers	Assesses dimensions or volume of the cavity and the thickness of the walls.
	Helps identify certain types of heart disease that predominantly involve the heart muscle.
	Can determine left ventricular wall thickness and stiffness with long-standing hypertension.
	Serial studies can assist in gauging the response of medical treatment.
Pumping function	Can detect the pumping power of the heart and whether it is normal or reduced to a mild or severe degree. This measurement is known as an ejection fraction (EF).
	A normal EF is around 55 to 65%. Figures below 45% usually represent some decrease in the pumping strength of the heart, while figures below 30 to 35% are representative of an important decrease.
	Can identify if the heart is pumping poorly, e.g. due to cardiomyopathy.
	Can assess the pumping ability of each heart chamber, the movement of each visualized wall. The decreased movement can be graded from mild to severe. In extreme cases, an area affected by a heart attack may have no movement (akinesia), or may even bulge in the opposite direction (dyskinesia). The latter is seen with aneurysms of the left ventricle.

(Continued)

Table 2.16 Echocardiography—cont'd

Area of Importance	Role of echocardiography
Valve function	Echocardiography identifies the structure, thickness and movement of each heart valve.
	Can determine if the valve is normal, scarred from an infection or rheumatic fever, thickened, calcified and torn.
	Assesses the function of prosthetic or artificial heart valves. Can diagnose mitral valve prolapse.
Volume status	Low blood pressure, poor heart function, reduced volume of circulating blood, e.g. with diuretics.
	Confusion may be caused when patients have a combination of problems. Therefore, echocardiography may help clarify the confusion.
Other uses	Diagnosis of fluid in the pericardium.
	Can determine if problem is severe/potentially life-threatening.
	Other diagnoses made include congenital heart diseases, blood clots or tumours within the heart, active infection of the heart valves, abnormal pulmonary pressures.

Types of echocardiography

- M-mode records a one-dimensional view of the heart it can measure:
  - left ventricular wall thickness
  - cavity size
  - valve leaflet excursion
  - aortic root
  - left atrial dimension.
- Two-dimensional the ultrasound beam moves continually in an arc.

Other uses of ultrasound

Ultrasound examination is a non-invasive form of organ imaging, with considerable appeal. It uses high-frequency sound waves and used in diagnostic medical sonography to visualize structures in the body by recording the reflections of high-frequency pulses directed into the tissues. Ultrasound:

- Is painless and almost certainly safe.
- Uses a transducer, which both emits and receives the ultrasound.
- Is based on the emission of sound waves and the reflections of ultrasound echoes.
- The ultrasound probe containing a transducer is applied to the skin over the area of interest and the image is displayed on a screen.
- Jelly is used to exclude air and ensure a good connection to the skin.

- The probe is moved at different angles and in different directions to display any abnormalities.
- 'Spot' films are also taken to record any images.
- Minimal child preparation is needed.
- The bladder needs to be full of urine to examine the pelvis.
- The child should be fasted to minimize gas shadows in gall bladder studies.

Its advantages include minimal risk to children, no radiation exposure and good diagnostic specificity in selected types of pathology. Ultrasound is used to examine virtually all areas of the body. It:

- distinguishes solid from cystic lesions
- assesses abdominal masses (difficult to see on X-ray)
- detects abnormal material in an organ, such as metastases
- detects movement, as in the pulsation of an aneurysm
- can measure physical dimensions, such as the diameter of the aorta.
- detects stones in the urinary bladder or the gall bladder
- guides intervention procedures such as aspiration or biopsy.

Ultrasound may help identify pathology in the following organs with a high degree of accuracy:

- liver and biliary tree
- pancreas
- renal tract
- pelvic structures
- pleural, abdominal and pelvic fluid collections.

Now that portable ultrasound equipment is available means that these examinations may be carried out at the bedside, without the need to move the child out of the unit.

Limiting factors of ultrasound

- Bone completely reflects ultrasound and obscures any tissues beyond it. This means it cannot be used to examine the brain or the spinal cord.
- Bowel gas partly reflects the ultrasound and here starving the child or using laxatives may help.
- A thick layer of fat scatters ultrasound and so it may be better to investigate the gall bladder by other means in the very obese.

Doppler-shift ultrasound

This method is used to study blood flow. The beam is directed towards the artery and is reflected from the red cells. It can be used to generate an audible signal for detecting blood flow or may be processed to give information about the nature of the flow. Other uses include:

- Measuring systolic blood pressure when low. A portable Doppler is used to detect flow beyond a sphygmomanometer cuff placed around the arm or ankle.
- Detecting the fetal heart.
- Studying flow dynamics for example in carotid artery disease.

Duration of echocardiography

An examination in an uncomplicated case may be completed within 15 to 20 minutes. However, it may take up to an hour when there are multiple problems or when there are technical problems.

Transoesophageal echocardiography (TOE) versus standard echocardiography

A standard echocardiogram is obtained by applying a transducer to the front of the chest. The ultrasound beam travels through the chest wall and lungs to reach the heart. Because it travels through the front of the chest or thorax a standard echocardiogram is also known as a transthoracic echocardiography.

Often, closely positioned ribs, obesity and emphysema may create technical difficulties by limiting the transmission of the ultrasound beams to and from the heart. In such cases, a TOE may be used. In such cases, the echocardiography transducer is placed down the oesophagus. Since the oesophagus sits behind the heart, and runs parallel with the descending aorta at the level of the fifth and sixth thoracic vertebra.

TOE has the advantage of being continuous and relatively non-invasive; it involves no skin punctures and holds some advantages over pulmonary artery catheter insertion:

- a reduction in the risk of complications, which have been quoted up to 7.2% for the more invasive procedures

- ease and minimal expertise required for insertion of the probe and acquisition of signals

- negligible running costs after the initial capital expenditure with the transducer reusable after sterilization in a suitable detergent

- prolonged usage in the same patient

- continuous appreciation of circulatory changes, ventricular function, and the effects of therapies by both medical and nursing staff

- a pulmonary artery catheter may still be necessary in situations such as severe septacaemia.

How is a TOE performed

The child is made to lie on their left side. An intravenous sedative is given to help in relaxation and the throat is sprayed with a local anaesthetic to numb the area. The TOE transducer is much smaller than the standard echocardiography equipment and is positioned at the end of a flexible tube. The tube transfers the images from the transducer to the echocardiography monitor for ease of visualization.

On commencement of the procedure the child begins to swallow the tube if conscious. The tube goes down the oesophagus. Therefore, it is important that the child is cooperative and swallows the tube. If unconscious, the clinician advances the tube into the mouth and down the oesophagus and the procedure begins. The combined use of local anaesthesia and chosen sedative minimizes the child's discomfort and there is usually no pain experienced with this procedure.

The transducer at the end of the tube is positioned in the oesophagus, directly behind the heart. By rotating and moving the tip of the transducer, the clinician can examine the heart from several different angles. The child's physiological signs are continuously monitored during this procedure. Oxygen is given as a preventive measure and suction is used, as needed.

Risks associated with TOE

■ TOE is a relatively common procedure and considered to be fairly safe. However, it does require entrance into the oesophagus and stomach. On occasions, children may experience breathing problems; abnormal or slow heart rhythm, reaction to the sedative and minor bleeding. In extremely rare cases, TOE may cause perforation or an oesophageal tear.

Importance of TOE

A TOE is an extremely useful tool in detecting blood clots, masses and tumours that are located inside the heart. It can also gauge the severity of certain valve problems and help detect infection of heart valves, certain congenital heart diseases and an aortic tear. In addition, TOE is also very useful in evaluating children who have had mini or major strokes as a result of blood clots. In addition, TOE is used to determine:

■ cardiogenic shock –

■ severe fluid overload –

■ cardiac tamponade –

■ assessment of left ventricular function

■ myocardial ischaemia and infarction

■ complications of cardiac surgery

■ valvular heart disease

■ aortic dissection

■ suspected endocarditis

■ pulmonary embolism

■ thoracic trauma.

Doppler

Doppler helps to identify abnormal leakage across heart valves and determine their severity. Doppler is also very useful in diagnosing the presence and severity of valve stenosis or narrowing. Doppler follows the direction and velocity of blood flow rather than the movement of the valve leaflets or components. Thus, reversed blood direction is seen with leakages while increased forward velocity of flow with a characteristic pattern is noted with valve stenosis.

Electromyogram (EMG), nerve conduction velocity (NCV)

The EMG is used to measure electrical potentials of individual muscles, used to differentiate neuropathies and myopathies. A sterile needle electrode is inserted through the skin into the muscle tissue and the electrical activity is detected. The muscle activity is displayed visually and audibly and abnormal activity might indicate some nerve and/or muscle damage.

The NCV measures the speed and intensity of electrical signals travelling along a nerve and the time it takes to reach its destination. It is used to detect neuromuscular disorders.

Preparation for EMG or NCV is analgesia as they can be uncomfortable. Paracetamol or ibuprofen should be adequate in this situation.

Electroencephalogram (EEG)

EEG is used to aid the diagnosis of epilepsy and cerebrovascular diseases. Twenty-one electrodes are placed on the surface of the head and two electrocardiogram electrodes are placed to monitor the heart rate. The electrodes are connected to an EEG computer and the electrical activity of the brain is amplified and displayed. Deep breathing during the procedure may activate and show seizure patterns, which will record on the EEG trace.

The child and family require explanation of the procedure. No fasting is required for this procedure. After the procedure the child's hair will need to be washed thoroughly as the gel used is sticky and can leave residue on the scalp.

Endoscopy

An endoscopy is a minimally invasive diagnostic procedure, which is used to examine and evaluate internal surfaces and organs by inserting a small flexible or non-flexible tube. This not only provides an image for visual inspection and photography but also enables biopsies and retrieval of foreign objects. The endoscope has an internal camera and light, often, but not necessarily inserted through a natural body opening. Through the scope itself, lesions and other surface abnormalities or conditions can be identified.

The majority of endoscopic procedures are relatively painless and at worst associated with mild discomfort therefore the majority receive a sedative prior to commencement of the procedure. Any method of looking into the body uses an instrument. This can either be via an orifice, such as the nose or mouth, or via an artificial opening such as an arthroscopy. Endoscopies are now illuminated by the use of fibreoptics enabling accurate diagnosis to be made. There are a number of different areas that are investigated by the use of an endoscopy:

- Gastroscopy, oesophagogastroduodenoscopy (OGD) this enables the whole area to be viewed and abnormalities of the digestive system to be seen, e.g. pyloric stenosis.

- Duodenoscopy allows the injection of contrast into the common bile duct.

- Colonoscopy – large bowel endoscopy, can be used to diagnose Crohn's disease or ulcerative colitis or remove polyps and to biopsy suspicious lesions.

- Bronchoscopy enables inspection of the bronchi with a narrow fibreoptic endoscope.

- Cystoscopy, cystourethroscopy – inspection of the bladder and urethra is very important in both diagnosis and treatment of diseases of the urethra and bladder.

- Ureteroscopy can now be used to remove stones from the lower half of the ureter.

- Laparoscopy is used by gynaecologists to diagnose disorders of the reproductive system. The abdomen is inflated with carbon dioxide and a scope passed into the peritoneal cavity. Can also be used to obtain liver biopsies.

- Arthroscopy – looking at joints, range of movement
- Thoracoscopy is used to examine organs of the chest.

Risks associated with endoscopy

Complications associated with endoscopy are relatively rare but can include:

- infection
- punctured organs
- allergic reaction to dyes used in certain endoscopic procedures
- renal failure associated with dyes used in certain endoscopic procedures
- respiratory depression from over usage of sedative for endoscopic procedure
- nausea and vomiting.

Fibreoptic bronchoscopy

Indications

- Aid difficult intubations.
- Clearance of secretions and direct physiotherapy.
- Cleansing of bronchial areas.
- Collection of microbiological and/or cytological specimens.
- Identify cause of bronchial/lumen obstruction.
- Identify extent of inhalation injury.
- Diagnose concerns with trachea and or bronchus.
- Placement of catheters or balloon in pulmonary bleeding matters.

Complications

- Hypoxaemia
- Cardiovasular disturbances
- Bleeding
- Perforation.

Contraindications

- Severe hypoxaemia
- Coagulopathy.

Blood analysis

Taking a blood sample is often the role of the doctor or phlebotomist, but the results of blood tests have a prime place in assisting the nurse to gain a full detailed assessment of the child. Those a nurse may be interested in are: haemoglobin; plasma osmolarity; potassium; sodium; haematocrit levels; urea and creatinine; cardiac enzymes; arterial blood gases.

Sodium

- Major cation of extracellular fluid.
- Determines plasma osmolarity.
- Major role in the movement of water and electrolytes between body fluid compartments.
- Essential for:
  - nerve impulse transmission
  - muscle contraction
  - movement of glucose, insulin and amino acids.
- Normal range 50–125 mmol/l
- 2–4 g of sodium needed per day, usual intake is higher 6–10 g/day in the form of table salt.

Potassium

- A major intracellular cation.
- Essential for:
  - muscle contractions
  - transmission and conduction of nerve impulses
  - maintenance of normal cardiac rhythm – ECG changes if ↑ or ↓
  - skeletal and smooth muscle contraction resting membrane potential.
- Normal range 20–60 mmol/l
- ↑ Will stimulate an increase excretion in urine – renal failure K^+ ↑, if not treated death will ensue
- ↓ Will cause re-absorption in renal tubules to maintain homeostasis.

Chloride

- Is an extracellular fluid anion.
- Secreted by the stomach mucosa as hydrochloric acid assisting in digestion.
- Maintains acid–base balance and involved in the removal of oxygen and carbon dioxide from haemoglobin in red blood cells – the chloride shift.
- Normal levels 95–106 mmol/l
- Balance maintained by the kidney.

Calcium

- Calcium is a necessary ion for many fundamental metabolic processes (Edwards 2005b).
- The bones contain more than 99% of the body's calcium; the rest is in the serum and exists in two forms:
  - ionized or free calcium (found in foods, and only type that the body can use)
  - bound to albumin – which accounts for about half of the serum calcium.
- Serum levels of free calcium are 1–1.25 mmol/l, and total serum calcium including bound and free is 2.12–2.65 mmol/l.
- Regulated by two hormones:
  - parathyroid hormone (PTH)
  - calcitonin.

Phosphorus

- Primary anion or negative charged ion in intracellular fluid.
- If enough calcium is ingested then enough phosphorus is likely, as both electrolytes present in many of the same foods.
- Normal levels 0.8–1.45 mmol/l.
- Needed for:
  - Formation of stored energy in cells (ATP)
  - Assistance with the formation of bones and teeth
  - Interaction with haemoglobin to promote oxygen release to tissues
  - White blood cell activation
  - Metabolizes fats, carbohydrates and proteins.

Magnesium

- Most abundant intracellular positive ion.
- 53% in bones, 27% in muscles.
- Recommended daily amount is 280–350 mg/day.
- Normal level 0.75–1.05 mmol/l.
- Involved in:
  - enzyme reactions resulting in ATP production
  - right amount of excitability in nerves and muscle cells including the heart.

Non-electrolytes

Glucose

The final product of carbohydrate digestion and the chief source of energy in human metabolism.

The principal sugar of the blood, insulin is required for its use.

Lipids

Substance extracted from animal or vegetable cells, consisting of fatty acids, glycerides, glyceryl and phospholipids.

Creatinine

Waste product of metabolism, excreted in the urine, concentration increases in blood in renal impairment.

Urea

The chief end product of nitrogen metabolism. Excreted in urine, concentrations increase in blood in renal impairment.

Haemoglobin levels

The amount of red blood cells in the blood. It is contained in the erythrocyte's cytoplasm and is primarily responsible for carrying oxygen and carbon dioxide to the body's tissues. The normal range is 11–18 g/100 ml of blood. A low haemoglobin will indicate that red blood cells are being lost.

Plasma osmolality

A measure of the number of milliosmoles per litre of solution, or the concentration of molecules per volume of solution e.g.

the volume of water in relation to added solutes can be determined. The normal is 280–294 mOsm/l, an increased serum osmolality, greater than 295 mOsm/l, indicates a loss of fluid and dehydration or hypovolaemia is present.

Haematocrit

Haematocrit is a measure of the consistency of the blood, for example thick fluids move more slowly and cause a greater resistance to flow than thin fluids. This is expressed as the ratio of volume of red blood cells to the volume of whole blood. The haematocrit is elevated in dehydration, and haemorrhage. The haematocrit is a guide for determining if whole blood or some other intravenous fluid should be used for volume replacement in the haemorrhagic shocked child.

Arterial blood gas analysis

Blood can be taken from an artery and analysed to determine partial pressure of oxygen (pO_2) and carbon dioxide (pCO_2) to interpret a child's acid base balance (Fletcher and Dhrampal 2003). Arterial blood gas analysis is part of the medical and nursing care of a child who may have a related physiological disorder. Blood gas machines measure pH, pCO_2, pO_2, base excess (BE) and HCO_3^- (Table 2.17). For list of chemical abbreviations related to ABG analysis see Table 2.18. A BE is the change from normal of the concentration of bicarbonate (Woodrow 2004). With excess alkali in the blood there is a positive BE (excess bicarbonate), whereas with excess non-respiratory acid

Table 2.17 The measures obtained from arterial blood gas analysis and normal values

Measure	Normal range
pH	7.35–7.45
pCO_2	4.6–5.6 kPa (35–42 mmHg)
pO_2	12–14.6 kPa (90–110 mmHg)
HCO_3^-	22–26 mmol/l
BE (base excess)	0
O_2 saturation	94–98%

To convert from mmHg to kPa divide by 7.5.

Table 2.18 Chemical abbreviations

Abbreviation	Interpretation
O_2	Oxygen
CO_2	Carbon dioxide
kPa	Kilopascals
pO_2	Partial pressure of oxygen
pCO_2	Partial pressure of carbon dioxide
H^+	Hydrogen ion
HCO_3^-	Bicarbonate ion
H_2CO_3	Carbonic acid
Na^+	Sodium ion
K^+	Potassium ion
Cl^-	Chloride ion
NH_4^+	Ammonium ion

there is a base deficit, or negative base excess (reduced bicarbonate). By measuring partial pressure and other values in arterial blood a respiratory or metabolic acid–base disorder can be determined and whether the respiratory system or kidneys are compensating.

When attempting to analyse a person's acid–base balance, scrutinize blood values in the order shown in Table 2.19. Notice that pCO_2 levels vary inversely with blood pH (pCO_2 rises as blood pH falls); HCO_3^- levels vary directly with blood pH (increased HCO_3^- results in increased pH). If any changes occur in the partial pressures of O_2 or CO_2, for example due to respiratory disease (asthma, COPD, ARDS), metabolic disease (diabetes, renal failure), or because of symptoms of disease (vomiting and diarrhoea) then the changes will be reflected in these measures.

Respiratory disorders

- Acid–base disorders resulting from primary alterations in the pCO_2 are termed respiratory disorders.

- Any increase in concentration or retention of CO_2 (considered a volatile source of acid which evaporates rapidly in body fluids), i.e. production > excretion will produce an increase in H^+ through the generation of carbonic acid (H_2CO_3) (Box 2.1) is termed a respiratory acidosis:
  - This lowers the pH and is observed in conditions where CO_2 excretion is impaired.

- The pH will rise and a respiratory alkalosis results from a decreased concentration of free H^+.

Table 2.19 Measure of arterial blood gases

Measure	Normal limits	Interpretation
pH	7.35–7.45	This indicates whether the person is in acidosis (pH < 7.35) or alkalosis (pH > 7.45), but it does not indicate the cause
pCO_2	4.6–5.6 kPa (35–42 mmHg)	Check the pCO_2 to see if this is the cause of the acid–base imbalance. The respiratory system acts fast, and an excessively high or low pCO_2 may indicate either the condition is respiratory or if the patient is compensating for a metabolic disturbance
		The pCO_2 is over 5.7 kPa (40 mmHg), the respiratory system is the cause of the problem and the condition is a respiratory acidosis. The pCO_2 is below normal limits 5.2 kPa (35 mmHg), the respiratory system is not the cause but is compensating
pO_2	12–14.6 kPa (90–110 mmHg)	This does not reveal how much oxygen is in the blood but only the partial pressure exerted by dissolved O_2 molecules against the measuring electrode
HCO_3^-	22–26 mmol/l	Abnormal values of the HCO_3^- are only due to the metabolic component of an acid base disturbance:
		A raised HCO_3^- concentration indicates a metabolic alkalosis (values over 26 mmol/l)
		A low value indicates a metabolic acidosis (values below 22 mmol/l)
BE	$-2-+2$ mmol/l	Is the amount of acid required to restore 1 litre of blood to its normal pH, at a pCO_2 of 5.3 kPa (40 mmHg). The BE reflects only the metabolic component of any disturbance of acid–base balance:
		If there was a metabolic acidosis then acid would have to be added to return the blood pH to normal, the BE will be positive
		If there is a metabolic acidosis, acid would need to be subtracted to return blood pH to normal, the BE is negative

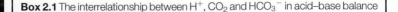

> **Box 2.1** The interrelationship between H^+, CO_2 and HCO_3^- in acid–base balance
>
> $$CO_2 + H_2O = H_2CO_3 = H^+ + HCO_3$$
>
> CO_2 = carbon dioxide, HCO_3^- = bicarbonate, H_2CO_3 = carbonic acid, H^+ = hydrogen ions, H_2O = water.
>
> The CO_2 /HCO_3^- buffer system is important in acid–base balance but the H^+ concentration of body fluids is influenced by both pCO_2 and HCO_3^- concentration. This demonstrates that the lungs and the kidneys largely determine acid–base balance. The lungs maintain acid base balance through control of pCO_2 and the kidneys through the excretion or re-absorption of HCO_3^-. It should also be noted that this equation is completely reversible. Therefore, increases in CO_2 can be converted into H^+, and H^+ can be converted to CO_2 for excretion – depending upon the presence of the enzyme carbonic anhydrase.

Modified from Marieb 2006.

- This is seen in conditions such as hyperventilation where CO_2 excretion is excessive.
- The lungs therefore play a major role in ensuring maintenance of H^+ ion concentration.

Metabolic disorders

- Disorders of acid–base physiology of non-respiratory origin are metabolic disorders and result from abnormal metabolism.

- Metabolic disorders may be due to excessive intake of acid or alkali or due to failure of renal function or diabetes mellitus.

- If non-respiratory acid production exceeds the excretion of acid from the body HCO_3^- decreases, and H^+ concentration increases as in a metabolic acidosis. The CO_2 yielded in a metabolic acidosis is lost via the lungs.

- This is achieved, as an increase in H^+ will reduce pH, immediately stimulating central chemoreceptors increasing rate and depth of respiration.
- This can be observed in conditions such as diabetic ketoacidosis (due to elevated H^+ production) and renal failure (due to inadequate H^+ excretion), and is referred to as 'respiratory compensation'.

- If acid production is less than the excretion of acid from the body, then HCO_3^- concentration increases and H^+ concentration decreases and a metabolic alkalosis result.
  - A decrease in H^+ will increase pH depressing central chemoreceptor response, reducing rate and depth of breathing. CO_2 is retained which generates H^+ and so reduces blood pH close to normal limits.

– This response is observed with severe vomiting when gastric acid loss depletes body fluid of H^+. This is another example of respiratory compensation. The rapidity of respiratory compensation is evident in these conditions, but it is also limited.

Renal compensation

The ultimate acid–base regulatory organs are the kidneys, which act slowly to compensate for acid base balance situations (Yucha 2004). The most important renal mechanisms for regulating acid–base balance of the blood involve:

■ Excreting HCO_3^- and conserving (reabsorbing) H^+ in an alkalosis

■ Excreting H^+ and reclaiming HCO_3^-, conserving (reabsorbing) bicarbonate ions, as in an acidosis (the dominant process in the nephrons).

This response to acid–base disturbances requires several days to be marginally effective.

Liver function tests (LFTs)

Serum bilirubin normal 5–21 µl/ml.

■ *Unconjugated bilirubin* – breakdown of red blood cells in the spleen produces bilirubin, in this form it is potentially toxic – significant in haemolytic anaemia where more is being produced or when being poorly taken up by the liver or poorly conjugated.

■ *Conjugated bilirubin* – converted in the liver to a water soluble compound which is less toxic and excreted in bile, to the intestine. Ninety-nine per cent is excreted in faeces as stercobilinogen (1% reabsorbed and excreted in the kidneys as urobilinogen) – significant when biliary vessels are obstructed in the liver, bile ducts are blocked, e.g. gallstones or tumour.

A rise in both, known as mixed hyperbilirubinaemia, occurs in liver disease such as hepatitis and cirrhosis, as bilirubin metabolism is impaired in several ways.

Serum enzyme levels

During liver disease many enzymes in high concentrations within liver cells leak across damaged cell membranes and can be detected in blood. These levels are not measuring function, but indicate damage.

Transaminases:

■ Alanine aminotransferase (ALT) – is liver specific

■ Aspartate transaminase (AST) – found also in muscle and lungs, if excessively high hepatocellular damage e.g.
   – acute infective hepatitis
   – hepatitis due to drugs
   – chronic hepatitis.

ALT is generally greater than AST, except in alcoholic liver disease.

Alkaline phosphate (ALP) is elevated in tumours, cysts, abscesses, because the locally obstructed bile canal makes more enzymes, increased in cirrhosis (2–10 times). Can arise from bone and intestinal damage. High levels generally indicate obstructive jaundice or carcinoma or tumour of the liver.

Gamma glutamyl transferase (AGT) is a microsomal enzyme, increased in hepatitis and other diseases damaging liver cells. Especially useful when found together with a raised ALP suggesting liver origin.

Serum proteins

Clotting factors (factors II, V, VII and IX synthesized in the liver) are abnormal due to deficiency of vitamin K; liver cannot synthesize factors if purely vitamin K deficient and will return to normal within 48 hours. Prothrombin time is lengthened by more than 3 seconds longer than the control (usually < 15 seconds); it is lengthened in obstructive jaundice as fat-soluble vitamin K cannot be absorbed properly from the intestine in the absence of bile. A vitamin K injection can return prothrombin to normal within 24 hours.

Serum albumin is synthesized only by liver cells, and is increased in liver disease.

Increase in serum immunoglobulin is generally unknown, maybe due to the stimulation of the inflammatory response or due to damaged liver.

- increase in IgG – autoimmune chronic active hepatitis
- increase in IgM – primary biliary cirrhosis
- increase in IgA – alcoholic cirrhosis.

Transport proteins fall to low levels when liver function is impaired.

Anti-mitochrondrial antibody (AMA) is present in children with primary biliary cirrhosis; absence excludes diagnosis.

Cardiac monitoring

A continuous read out of the ECG in Lead II is a record of the changes in electrical activity occurring within cardiac muscle. The cardiac cells involved in the contraction are specialized and are unlike any other cells in the body, as each individual cell can initiate its own electrical impulse (Edwards & Sabato 2009). Although cardiac muscle has this special property, hormones and chemical transmitters are important in producing the finer control of the heart and maintenance of homeostasis.

Bipolar and unipolar electrodes provide an ECG rhythm known as the PQRST waves, which detect the electrical charges within the cardiac cell. The ECG can provide information about the heart rate and rhythm, the effects of electrolytes or drugs on the heart and the electrical orientation of the cardiac muscle. The normal ECG trace should record complexes (PQRST) per minute according to whether the child is an infant or child (Table 2.10).

What is an ECG?

The action potentials transmitted through the heart during the cardiac cycle can be recorded on the surface of the body. The recording can be obtained by electrodes on skin surface and then connected to an ECG machine. The voltage changes are fed to the machine, amplified and displayed visually on a screen, graphically on ECG paper, or both.

Terminology

- Isoelectric line – baseline
- Positive – upward deflection
- Negative – downward deflection
- Voltage – height and depth of a wave
- Time – measured along horizontal axis, one second = 5 large squares
- Cardiac cycle – represented on ECG by P wave, QRS complex, T wave
- Biphasic – deflection which is both positive and negative.

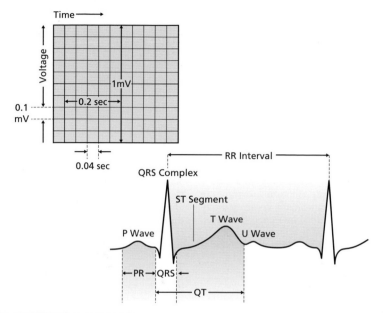

Fig. 2.2 ECG voltage and seconds.

ECG leads

The ECG leads provide a variety of views of the heart's electrical activity from different angles. An ECG lead consists of two surface electrodes of opposite polarity either one positive and one negative or one positive surface electrode and one reference point.

- Standard limb leads (I–III)
- Augmented limb leads (aVR, aVL, and aVF)
- Precordial leads (V1–V6).

These 10 leads produce different ECG tracings to make up the 12 lead ECG.

ECG paper moves at 25 mm/s and consists of small and large squares (5 small squares). ECG measures time and amplitude:

- time is measured on the horizontal plane
- small squares are 0.04 s in time, and 1 mm in voltage
- large squares are 0.2 s in time, and 5 mm in voltage.

Amplitude is measured on the vertical axis of the graph paper (Fig. 2.2):

- small squares equal 0.1 mV
- large squares equal 0.5 mV.

Methods of calculating heart rate

25 mm × 60
= 1500 divided by 5 small squares
= 300

Count the number of small squares between R waves, divide these into 1500, e.g. 18 small squares divided into 1500 = 83 bpm.

Count the number of large squares between the R wave and divide into 300, e.g. 4 large squares divided into 300 = 75 bpm.

During a period of acute illness the sequence of the ECG can be affected. The rate may increase due to: heart failure, hypertension, blood loss, pain, stress or anxiety or reduce its rate due to over-prescription of certain drugs or a lack of oxygen supply. Abnormal rhythms can occur from heart failure, coronary artery disease, myocardial infarction (Edwards 2002), and fluid overload (Edwards 2000) and fluid and electrolyte imbalance (Edwards 2001a).

ECG interpretation

Maturational changes occur over the early years of childhood, centred on heart rate and normal duration of intervals, as well as right ventricular dominance and increase in age (Table 2.20):

- gradual decrease in heart rate
- gradual lengthening of the PR interval
- gradual lengthening of the QRS interval
- shift from right to left ventricular dominance.

Because of the faster rate and shorter distances the electrical impulses have to travel through the smaller heart, the PR and QRS intervals are much shorter, but lengthen with age. This is key in identifying specific arrhythmias that use the interval as the criteria for abnormality (e.g. first degree heart block).

The P wave

- Refers to atrial depolarization and it is the first positive deflection seen.
- It should always be followed by a QRS complex, unless conduction disturbances are present.

Table 2.20 Rate and interval based on age

Age	Heart rate	PR Interval / sec	QRS Interval / sec
1–3 weeks	100–180	0.07–0.14	0.03–0.07
1–6 months	100–185	0.07–0.16	0.03–0.07
6–12 months	100–170	0.08–0.16	0.03–0.08
1–3 years	90–150	0.09–0.16	0.03–0.08
3–5 years	70–140	0.09–0.16	0.03–0.08
5–8 years	65–130	0.09–0.16	0.03–0.08
8–12 years	60–110	0.09–0.16	0.03–0.09
12–16 years	60–100	0.19–0.18	0.03–0.09

Modified from Allen et al (2008).

The PR interval

- Measured from the beginning of the P wave to the beginning of the QRS complex irrespective of whether the QRS complex begins with a Q or an R wave.
- It varies according to age (Table 2.10).
- Dependent on the heart rate and conduction of AV node
- Normal tracing indicates electrical impulses have been conducted through the correct conduction pathways.

The QRS complex

- Consists of three waves, Q, R and S.
- Should be narrow and sharply pointed.
- Represents ventricular contraction (depolarization), marking the beginning of ventricular systole, and can be:
  - Predominately positive (upright)
  - Predominately negative (inverted)
  - Biphasic (partly positive, partly negative).
- Varies according to age (Table 2.10).

The ST segment

- Is the resting period between ventricular contraction and the returning of the cardiac muscle to its resting stage.
- Early repolarization, should always return to the baseline, depressed or elevated in abnormalities.

The T wave

- Represents repolarization of the ventricular myocardial cells.
- Usually slightly rounded.
- Deep and symmetrical inverted T waves suggest cardiac ischaemia.

- T waves elevated more than half of the height of the QRS complex (peaked T waves) could indicate hyperkalaemia.

The QT interval

- Is the period from the beginning of ventricular depolarization (onset of the QRS complex) until the end of ventricular repolarization, or the end of T wave and highly influenced by heart rate and a faster heart rate will shorten the interval.
- During this period the heart is fully refractory (the absolute refractory period) whereby no other electrical impulse can be accepted by the cardiac cells.
- During the latter period of the interval (from the peak of the T wave onward), the conduction system is relatively refractory.
- Drugs may prolong the QT period:
  - digitalis
  - quinidine
  - procainamide
  - lithium
  - tricyclics
  - phenothiazides.
- The QT interval is also effected by an increase in blood electrolytes:
  - a high potassium (hyperkalaemia)
  - a low calcium (hypocalcaemia).

The diagnosis of arrthymias

Some of the important features which can be looked for in an ECG in its interpretation note the:

- Rate of discharge according to age of the child.

- Rhythm or regularity of the complexes.
- Duration of the PR interval.
- Whether each P wave is followed by the QRS complex.
- QRS complex – width, configuration, deep Q waves in leads.
- T wave – are they inverted throughout, only in certain leads, or more prominent in others?

Interpretation

Normal sinus rhythm (Fig. 2.3)

- Rate: varies with age (Table 2.10).
- Rhythm: regular.
- Pacemaker site: SA node.
- P waves: normal in shape, upright.
- PR interval: varies with age.
- QRS: normal: varies with age.
- Clinical significance: none, normal rhythm.

Sinus bradycardia (Fig. 2.4)

The normal rates of an infant and child are higher, thus definitions of a bradycardia are different for the paediatric population and this is defined as a heart rate lower than expected for age:

- aetiology: cardiomyopathy
- rate: varies according to age
- rhythm: regular
- pacemaker site: SA node
- P waves: upright, normal in shape
- PR interval: varies with age
- QRS interval: varies with age
- clinical significance: can result in reduced cardiac output, hypotension
- management: nothing if fit young person, atropine, internal pacing wires.

Sinus tachycardia (Fig. 2.5)

The normal rates of an infant and child are higher; therefore definitions of a tachycardia are different for the paediatric population and are defined as a heart rate higher than expected for age:

- aetiology: exercise, anxiety, homeostatic compensation, hypovolaemia, pain, fever, fear, cardiomyopathy
- rate: varies with age
- rhythm: regular
- pacemaker site: SA node

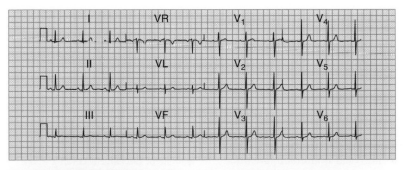

Fig. 2.3 Normal sinus rhythm.

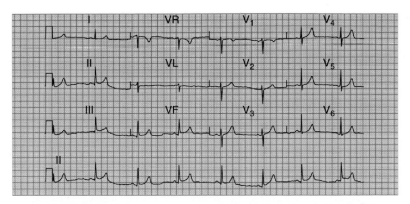

Fig. 2.4 Sinus bradycardia.

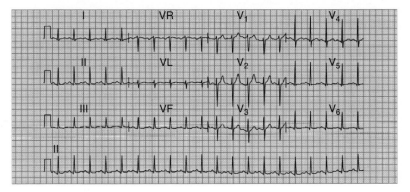

Fig. 2.5 Sinus tachycardia.

- P waves: upright, normal in shape
- PR interval: varies with age
- QRS interval: varies with age
- clinical significance: can result in decreased cardiac output, increases myocardial oxygen demand
- management: treat the cause, e.g. pain, hypovolaemia or fever, or normal compensatory mechanism to stress, anxiety and fear

The most common abnormal rhythm in children is bradycardia and sinus arrhythmia (see above) and supraventricular tachycardia (SVT).

Supraventricular tachycardia (Fig. 2.6)

This includes a variety of rhythms that emanate from the sinus, atrial or junctional areas of the heart.

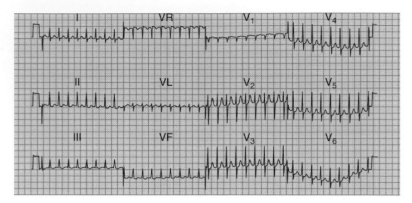

Fig. 2.6 Supraventricular tachycardia.

- Aetiology: it can occur in Wolfe–Parkinson–White syndrome (WPW) and re-entry tachycardia, circulate around AV node, occurs at any age, may have a history of being irritable, lethargic, and feeding poorly or signs of heart failure.
- Rate: very rapid > 220 in infants as high as 280–320.
- Rhythm: usually regular but can be too fast to count.
- Pacemaker site: may vary from SA node to AV node.
- P waves: may be upright, normal if pacemaker at SA, inverted if near AV junction.
- PR interval: usually shortened, possibly normal.
- QRS interval: varies with age (Table 2.20).
- Clinical significance: can occur in healthy hearts, can be well tolerated, and accompanied often by palpitations, dizziness, anxiety and nervousness. Cardiac output can be compromised, and may increase myocardial ischaemia.

- Management: vagal manoeuvres, Valsalva, adenosine, amiodarone, verapamil, cardioversion.

A very fast sinus tachycardia should be considered if the rate rises to 220 but falls to 170 with calming and rises again to 210 in a screaming child.

Atrial fibrillation, atrial flutter and heart block are rarely found in children; however ventricular tachycardia, fibrillation and asystole are classified as cardiac arrest and so will be mentioned.

Ventricular tachycardia
(Fig. 2.7)

Interpretation: three or more consecutive ventricular complexes occurring at rate over 100, which override primary pacemaker. The clinical significance:

- reduced cardiac output
- is life threatening

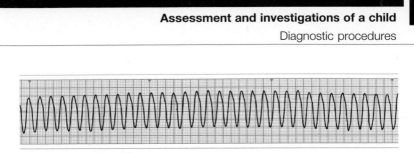

Fig. 2.7 Ventricular tachycardia.

- management: oxygen, antidysrhythmics, possibly lidocaine, possible amiodarone, check potassium levels, if pulseless treat as VF.

Ventricular fibrillation (Fig. 2.8)

Chaotic ventricular rhythm results in quivering ventricular movements and pulselessness. Do not allow sufficient mass of myocardial muscle to fully depolarize and repolarize, so organized ventricular contraction does not take place. Most common presenting rhythm in cardiac arrest:

- aetiology: hypoxia, acidosis, electrical injury, electrolyte imbalance, drugs and toxicity

- clinical significance: a lethal dysrhythmia, with light headedness, followed by loss of consciousness and cessation of circulation and breathing
- management: an emergency, begin BLS, administer oxygen.

Asystole (Fig. 2.9)

This is the absence of all ventricular activity:

- aetiology: may be primary event in cardiac arrest or subsequent to VT, VF, asystolic, PEA arrest. Associated with global myocardial ischaemia and necrosis
- clinical significance: a lethal dysrhythmia, with a poor prognosis,

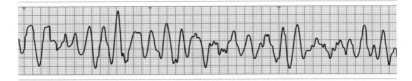

Fig. 2.8 Ventricular fibrillation

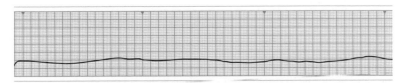

Fig. 2.9 Asystole.

should be confirmed in 3 leads, maximum gain check child and connections!

- management: BLS, administer oxygen, epinephrine (adrenaline), possible pacing.

The 12 lead ECG

It must be remembered that arrhythmias are relatively rare in children. However, after only 30–60 seconds of hypoxia, changes can be observed on an ECG rhythm strip and/or a 12 lead ECG.

Changes to an ECG rhythm can be determined by interpreting changes that occur in time and voltage to the above waveforms (Fig. 2.2) and by using a standardized approach to the diagnosis of arrhythmias detailed previously.

However, it is a 12 lead ECG that a nurse will undertake when cardiovascular changes are suspected. It is more useful when diagnosing cardiac disease, despite the problems with interpretation, than the rhythm strip. It can be performed simply, quickly, and views the heart electrically in a 3D manner. The limb leads are attached to the forearms and calves, with a small amount of conduction gel, and allows three bipolar leads (I, II, III) and three augmented unipolar leads (AVR, AVL, and AVF) to be recorded. Chest precordial unipolar lead placements are secured again by applying a small amount of conduction gel over the six V lead positions (V_1, V_2, V_3, V_4, V_5 and V_6), and allow the heart to be viewed in the horizontal axis from the chest wall.

Thus the 12 lead ECG produces a representation of what is happening directly underneath the electrode, whereby a nurse and/or doctor can determine if the conduction pathway of the heart is normal or damaged. These changes occur if cardiac muscle is damaged (determined in conjunction with cardiac enzymes) the electrical waves within the heart have to travel via an alternative route, and this will alter the pattern of the ECG and identify the affected area.

Cardiac catheterization

This is an advanced skill and used for diagnosis of cardiac conditions and to give detailed information about anatomy, blood flow and pressures within the heart. A radio-opaque catheter is inserted into one of the large arteries or veins, threading the catheter up into the heart. A dye is injected and X-rays are taken. This technique can be used to diagnose and treat abnormal electrical conduction through the heart and relieve symptoms or treat a number of cardiac defects. In some instances cardiac catheterization has replaced the need for invasive cardiac surgical procedures.

The procedure is not without risks:

- arrhythmias
- vascular complications, e.g. haemorrhage, thrombosis
- allergic reactions to the contrast medium.

The children need careful preoperative assessment and preparation and close postoperative monitoring of vital signs and may include the addition of a cardiac catheterization care pathway.

Section 3

Children's nursing interventions

3.1 Interventions

Blood transfusion therapy

The cardiovascular system can compensate for blood loss, which is designed to minimize the effects of blood loss. However, compensation for blood loss depends on a child's age. Blood loss should be treated with blood, especially when blood loss is substantial.

Blood groups

ABO system divides into four main groups:

O – 47% of population compatible with donor O

A – 42% of population compatible with donor A or O

B – 8% of population compatible with donor B or O

AB – 3% of population compatible with donor AB, A, B, or O.

The Rhesus (Rh) system

This blood group system is in addition to the ABO antigen, and expresses a D antigen on red blood cells. This factor is present or absent and termed Rh D positive or negative:

■ Rh D$^+$ comprises approximately 85% of the western population.

■ Rh D$^-$ comprises the rest of the population.

The Rh D factor is significant in both blood transfusions and pregnancy:

■ Blood transfusions:
  – AB blood group with RhD (AB) factor negative is the universal recipient, as they can receive blood *from* any four blood types, but is rare.
  – O blood group with RhD negative (O$^-$) is the universal donor and can donate blood *to* all four blood types.

■ Pregnancy
  – Significant when a woman's blood is RhD$^-$ but is carrying a fetus that is RhD$^+$.
  – The mother carrying the infant builds up antibodies against the RhD$^+$ red blood cells of the fetus; this does not affect the first pregnancy (this includes a miscarriage), but is stored in the immune system memory.
  – In the second pregnancy the antibodies are activated quickly and this can lead to damage to the fetus.
  – Following the birth of a first child Anti-D is administered to the mother to prevent reoccurrences in the second pregnancy.

Blood is collected under strict aseptic technique in a plastic vacuum container, from a donor and then mixed with an appropriate anticoagulant solution, such as: citrate-phosphate-dextrose (CPD) or oxalate salts, which prevent clotting by binding with calcium ions. The blood can then be stored under refrigeration for several weeks at a temperature of 1–4 °C.

Changes in blood begin within 24 hours of storage, and continue throughout the entire 21 days, after which blood is considered outdated (Edwards 1998). Box 3.1 shows the changes that occur in stored blood.

Blood transfusion reactions (TF)

■ When mismatched blood is infused, a transfusion reaction occurs and the

---

Box 3.1 Changes that occur in stored blood

Acid-base changes

Because blood is stored in an air-free container, aerobic metabolism cannot take place, but anaerobic metabolism does occur, yet, the end product is lactic and pyruvic acids. Therefore, the longer a unit of blood is stored, the greater will be the amount of acid end products that it contains. The CPD solution used as an anticoagulant adds another acid component to banked blood and reduces the pH of the blood from a normal body pH of 7.4 to about 7.0.

Alterations in electrolyte concentration

When blood is stored the sodium and potassium concentration undergoes alteration. It can be expected that a unit of stored blood will contain approximately 75–80 mEq of sodium and 5–7 mEq of potassium. There is also a progressive loss of red cell viability and the red blood cells tend to take up water, causing a leftward shift in the oxyhaemoglobin dissociation curve and transfused blood cells to be less capable of releasing oxygen to the tissues than would be normal red blood cells.

The microaggregate load in stored blood

An increased aggregation of platelets and leukocytes occurs in stored blood and blood has been filtered through 170 μm filters to remedy it. However, the formation of microemboli considered smaller than 170 μm, have been identified and microfilters with pore sizes ranging from 20 to 90 μm are required. However, because those conditions which require massive blood transfusions are generally an emergency, it is extremely difficult, if not impossible, to prove that the use of microfilters during massive blood transfusions decreases the development of ARDS.

Depletion of clotting factors

Stored blood is deficient in most of the factors necessary for normal coagulation; it is specifically deficient in factors V, VIII, IX and platelets. However, the depletion of platelets and clotting factors vary from patient to patient and it is recommended that patient's clotting screen and bleeding status be closely monitored during transfusion.

The temperature of stored blood

Blood is stored at a temperature between 1 and 6°C, which is considerably colder than human blood. The normal temperature is generally approximately 37°C. The infusion of large quantities of cold blood can cause patients to become hypothermic. This compromises the patient's heart rate, blood pressure, cardiac output, and coronary blood flow. The consequent hypothermia impairs the metabolism of citrate and lactate, and increases the patient's risk of a metabolic acidosis, it increases the affinity of haemoglobin for oxygen, and may impair clotting, and impairs the possibility of detecting a major transfusion reaction.

donor and recipient's red blood cells are attacked by the recipient's immune system.

- Transfusion reaction can occur with the infusion as little as 10–15 ml.
- The agglutination of the foreign red blood cells blocks small blood vessels throughout the body and is destroyed. This causes a reduction in the capacity of red blood cells to carry oxygen and obstruction to blood flow causing organ damage, both of which are lethal.
- TF can also cause
  - urticaria, itching, discomfort
  - anxiety
  - rash
  - shortness of breath, nausea, collapse
  - tachycardia, hypo/hypertension
  - pain: chest, back, abdomen or loin
  - generally feeling unwell, complains of a feeling of impending doom.

!

If any serious adverse reaction or event occurs during or after a blood transfusion it should be reported on the serious adverse blood reactions and events (SABRE) system, accessed by the serious hazards of transfusion (SHOT) website at http://www.shotuk.org.

- Complications associated with blood transfusion:
  - pulmonary damage
  - metabolic acidosis
  - blood group incompatibilities
  - transfusion reactions
  - hyperkalaemia
  - hypothermia – with infants or large transfusions a blood warmer should be used.

Nurses have to be vigilant in checking:

- The correct blood group and Rh D antigen factor
- Confirming with the parent or child the identity
- Checking the ID band, e.g. date of birth, hospital number (no wristband – no transfusion)
- Donor number matches, CMV negative
- Integrity of the bag, e.g. no damage has occurred
- Expiratory date of blood
- Kell or other antibodies/CMV negative
- Blood been autoclaved
- Observing for any signs of transfusion reactions. If any of signs occur STOP the transfusion! Report the reaction
- Monitoring vital signs:
  - temperature
  - pulse
  - respiratory rate
  - blood pressure.

Other blood product derivatives

- Packed red cells (whole blood from which most of the plasma has been removed) is generally only used to treat anaemia.
- Fresh frozen plasma (FFP) should never be used as a volume expander in this situation. It is better to use FFP for patients with bleeding disorders, whereby there is a deficiency in platelets or clotting factors, e.g. in disseminated intravascular coagulation (DIC), warfarin overdose, trauma or thrombotic thrombocytopenia.

For a more detailed account of blood products see Table 3.1.

Table 3.1 Current blood products

Blood product	Constituents	Uses
Whole blood (510 ± 45 ml)	Use is restricted to circumstances where red blood cells as well as plasma proteins are needed i.e. where large amounts of blood are lost.	Ideal in hypovolaemic shock, since it increases both oxygen carrying capacity and expands circulating volume.
Packed cells (280 ± 60 ml)	This is whole blood, but the majority of the plasma has been removed. It contains half the volume of whole blood, less sodium, potassium, albumin and citrate. Does contain some white blood cells and platelets.	Ideal in chronic anaemia, sickle cell disease, thalassaemia and renal disease. It is not recommended in iron deficiency and vitamin B_{12} or folate deficiency as these should be treated with the appropriate vitamin e.g. iron tablets.
Washed packed cells	These are packed cells with all the white blood cells, platelets and plasma removed.	Indicated for patients who have a long history of transfusion reactions.
Fresh frozen plasma (FFP) (200–300 ml)	This is blood product, which is nearly always frozen and contains all the coagulation factors.	Used for the treatment of coagulation deficits. It is not recommended as a volume expander, except in certain neonatal conditions.
Cryoprecipitate (20 ± 5 ml)	Prepared from FFP and contains mainly clotting factors (factor VIII and fibrinogen).	Used to treat haemophilia or AIDS patients.
Platelets (50 ± 10 ml)	Produced from the residue left over from the production of plasma and leucocyte-depleted red blood cell concentrates.	Indications for use are thrombocytopenia, when platelet content of blood is reduced due to bleeding or diluted following massive transfusion, in acute leukaemia, aplastic anaemia, DIC or sepsis.

AIDS, acquired immune deficiency syndrome; DIC, disseminated intravascular coagulation.

Despite blood products being essential, they are at times scarce, or difficult to source in emergencies and thus other methods have been introduced, namely: autotransfusion, synthetic blood products, or colloid and crystalloid therapies.

Autotransfusion

- Minimizes the need for blood transfusion by a blood donor.
- During surgical procedures blood can be salvaged through an autotransfusion device.
- Blood can be re-infused back into the patient during surgery if blood loss is great, or saved for transfusion at a later date.

Synthetic blood products

- Artificial blood substitutes, or perfluorochemicals, have become available for clinical use.
- Used in cases of severe anaemia when transfusion of blood products is not an option.
- Use of these products to treat blood loss is still under investigation.
- When perfluorochemical microdroplets (which have a high solubility of oxygen) are infused intravenously, oxygen is dissolved in the microdroplets and transported to capillaries for diffusion across capillary walls (Edwards 1998).

Side effects include:

- pulmonary oedema
- arrhythmias
- chest pain
- respiratory distress.

Positive effects of perfluorochemicals do not endure beyond 24 hours after infusion due to their short half life.

- May reduce blood recipient adverse reactions from donor blood.
- Minimizes the use of and improves the cost effectiveness of blood transfusions.

Fluid replacement therapy

Crystalloid therapy

- Crystalloid solutions used are 5% dextrose (not a true crystalloid as it contains no electrolytes), 0.9% sodium chloride; dextrose saline and Hartmann's (see Table 3.2).
- Any solution that contains electrolytes will influence fluid movement; the most powerful is sodium.
- Sodium added to the extracellular fluid compartment as in intravenous infusion will keep sodium at a normal level and have no effect on fluid movement but the infused solution of 0.9% normal saline/Hartmann's solution will stay in the circulation and increase/maintain circulating volume.

Maintenance fluid

- It is extremely important to administer the correct volume.
- Devices should be used to administer the fluids and set at the correct rate over a specific period of time, and documented on a fluid balance chart.

Table 3.2 Crystalloid infusions

Crystalloid	Constituents	Used in	Avoided in
0.9% normal saline	Contains sodium and chloride, no calories, osmolality 308 mOsm/l	Increases mainly extracellular volume with no significant increase in intracellular volume	Dehydration, acidosis, oedema, hypernatraemia, neuro patients, diabetes insipidus, heart failure, increase in chloride
5% Dextrose (not a true crystalloid as it contains no electrolytes)	Contains only 200 calories per litre, adds water to the extracellular compartment and reduced osmolality of extracellular fluid.	The water will pass into the intracellular fluid to reach equilibrium, does not stay in the circulation, good for dehydration.	Hypovolaemia, for feeding purposes, neuro patients with increase in ICP
4% Dextrose 0.18% normal saline	Contains a combination of both of the above.		
Hartmann's solution	Contains sodium, potassium, chloride, bicarbonate, calcium, osmolality 278 mOsm/l	Hypovolaemia, maintenance fluid	Hyperkalaemia, renal patients, acidosis

Some methods of calculating maintenance fluids:

- Body weight and fluid required per day:
  first 10 kg = 100 ml/kg
  second 10 kg = 50 ml/kg
  subsequent 20 kg = 20 ml/kg
- Body weight and fluid required per hour:
  first 10 kg = 4 ml/kg
  second 10 kg = 2 ml/kg
  subsequent 20 kg = 1 ml/kg

Resuscitation fluid

If crystalloids are used as the primary resuscitative agents, for example in hypovolaemia, the volumes required to achieve normal haemodynamic values are from two to four times those required with colloids.

Massive crystalloid fluid resuscitation may predispose the patient to adult respiratory distress syndrome (ARDS) or pulmonary oedema, which is thought to be absent with colloid therapy.

Colloid therapy

- Colloids work as they contain various amounts of large molecules, which draw fluid into the circulation from the intracellular spaces (the largest fluid compartment of the body), increasing circulating volume (volume expanders).

- There are two different types of colloid gelatines and starches (see Table 3.3).

- Colloid supplementation, in the presence of normal kidney function, may aid the excretion of excess extracellular fluid.

- Using colloids in haemorrhage is to restore plasma volume, and improve or maintain oxygen transport.

- Haemodynamic stability is achieved by increasing the blood volume by giving plasma expanders, and thus, providing adequate oxygen and nutrients, which are needed for the maintenance and restoration of cellular function.

- Inadequate circulatory blood volume, owing to haemorrhage, causes pooling of blood in the microcirculation, the major effect being a marked decrease in venous return, and a diminished cardiac output.

- By administering plasma expanders there is an improvement in oxygen availability, oxygen consumption, circulating volume, haemodynamic status and tissue perfusion.

- Colloid is not easily excreted by the kidneys as the renal tubules do not allow protein and other large molecules in the filtrate, thus the effect can increase, giving rise to fluid overload.

- Massive fluid replacement therapy of crystalloid or colloid can lead to the development of pulmonary oedema and haemodilution.

The main argument against using crystalloids or colloid to avoid blood transfusions is that it can lead

Table 3.3 Colloid infusions: gelatins and starches

Colloid	Contents	Used in	Avoided in
Gelatins Volplex, Gelofusine	Large molecules suspended in crystalloid	Hypovolaemia – lasts longer than saline	Should not give too much as protein does not leave the ECF
Starches Voluven, Volulyte	Large molecules: Voluven suspended in solution close to saline Volulyte suspended in solution close to Hartmann's	Hypovolaemia – stays in the system longer	Fluid overload, prone to allergies as can lead to anaphylaxis, clotting disorders

to haemodilution. The blood becomes so dilute that the measured blood haematocrit becomes reduced:

- decreases colloid osmotic pressure
- reduces haemoglobin content
- reduces coagulation factors
- reduces electrolytes
- reduces white blood cells.

There are less of these elements in relation to fluid contained within blood. This increase in fluid in relation to solutes in the blood will serve to dilute body sodium, increases blood osmolarity and via the renin angiotensin aldosterone system stimulates the release of aldosterone, which will reabsorb more sodium (due to reduced body sodium) and water. The renin–angiotensin–aldosterone mechanism stimulates, via osmoreceptors, the release of antidiuretic hormone (ADH) more water reabsorbed from the renal tubules, causing a net increase in extracellular fluid volume and total body weight. Haemodilution is serious and will require the administration of a blood transfusion to replace the reduction in blood solutes. It is imperative that the cardiopulmonary dynamics be monitored.

Cannulation

A cannula is a vascular device inserted into a peripheral or central vessel to provide:

- Diagnostic blood sampling
- Therapeutic administration of medications, fluids and or blood products

- Invasive pressure monitoring:
  - central venous pressure monitoring (CVP)
  - pulmonary artery pressure monitoring (PAP)
  - arterial pressure monitoring.

The cannula for these is attached to a transducer, which converts the pressure to a waveform display.

An intravenous cannula (for the first two bullet points above) inserted into a peripheral vein is a common procedure increasingly performed by nurses; therefore nurses must be aware of:

- relevant anatomy and physiology
- criteria for choosing vein and equipment
- potential problems
- health and safety regulations
- adherence to aseptic technique
- comfort of the patient
- adequate information regarding the procedure and complications.

Veins used are:

- median cubital veins
- cephalic vein
- basilic vein
- metacarpal veins.

Considerations when choosing a vein:

- must be best for the child
- injury, disease or treatment prevent use of a limb
- how the infant/child is positioned
- age and weight
- if the infant/child is in shock or dehydrated poor superficial peripheral access may be present

- temperature will influence venous dilatation e.g. if the child is cold, no veins may be visible.
- medications can influence choice e.g. anticoagulants, steroids, risk of bruising.

  Insertion:

- Consider whether cannula is actually necessary.
- Child will be anxious about the procedure and pain. Thus it is essential to use local anaesthetic prior to procedure.
- Choose a site away from a joint.
- Improve venous access by:
  - Ensuring good lighting
  - A tourniquet above the cannulation – check local policy
  - Opening and closing of the fist, forcing blood into the veins
  - Lowering the arm below heart level to increase blood supply
  - Light tapping of the vein may be useful, but can be painful and lead to haematoma
  - Ointment or patches containing small amounts of glyceryl trinitrate to cause local vasodilatation.
- Prevent infection of skin flora contamination from nurse to child:
  - appropriate personnel protection equipment should be used
  - use aseptic technique and wash hands
  - all wipes should be undertaken in one direction, used for at least 30 seconds, allowed to dry (check local hospital policy).
- Reduce the number of attempts to cannulate as increased number of

puncture sites equates increased entry sites for infection.
- Check patency using normal saline.
- Cover the cannula with a dressing which is transparent and semipermeable, allows the site to be viewed easily.
- Change the cannula site every 48–72 hours – this has been shown to reduce infection rates at the cannula site.

  Insertion site checked regularly for signs of:

- Extravasation/infiltration (see Table 3.4 for infiltration scoring system):
  - inadvertent administration of a drug into the surrounding tissues
  - clinical symptoms of infiltration are coolness, leakage at the site, swelling and tenderness.

Phlebitis

- Acute inflammation of a vein directly linked to the presence of any vascular device.
- Infants may cry or children may report pain.
- If treated early enough often the symptoms will resolve without further intervention required.
- Substances that often cause phlebitis tend to be isotonic solutions, e.g. 0.9% sodium chloride (NaCl) or blood products.
- Phlebitis can be further classified into mechanical, chemical and infective, depending on the cause:
  - mechanical is predominantly due to cannula problems
  - chemical due to the incompatibility of drugs infused

Table 3.4 Infiltration scoring system

Grade	Clinical criteria
0	No symptoms
1	Skin blanched Oedema 2.5 cm in any direction Cool to touch With or without pain
2	Skin blanched Oedema 2.5–15 cm in any direction Cool to touch With or without pain
3	Skin blanched, translucent Gross oedema 15 cm in any direction Cool to touch Mild to moderate pain Possible numbness
4	Skin blanched, translucent Skin tight, leaking Skin discoloured, bruised, swollen Gross oedema 15 cm in any direction Deep pitting tissue oedema Circulatory impairment Moderate to severe pain Infiltration of any amount of blood product, irritant or vesicant

- – infective is where infection is at the tip of the cannula (usually confirmed when blood cultures show the same microbiology as the tip which is sent for culture).
- Treatment is removal of the line and the application of heat to the site and prescribed analgesia.

Flushing of cannula

- Flushing guidance is often overlooked, and is an essential component of good care.
- Flush volume should be equal to at least twice the volume of the catheter, usually 5–10 ml of 0.9% NaCl (RCN 2003).
- An associated hazard is speed shock as a systemic reaction that occurs when a substance foreign to the body is rapidly introduced – occurs most commonly with rapid bolus injection.

Before undertaking cannulation nurses must undergo appropriate training, supervision and assessment by an experienced member of staff and keep updated.

Infections

- Fairly minor irritation at the site (local infection)
- Bacteraemia (bacteria are present in the blood)
- Septicaemia (systemic infection), which is more serious.

Infections are divided into two groups:

- Exogenous – where the microorganisms originate outside the patients' body (this is usually due to cross infection, e.g. hands of health care professionals and equipment).
- Endogenous – this is present due to organisms already present on or in the patients' body.

Anaphylaxis

Anaphylaxis is a systemic immediate hypersensitivity reaction caused by an immunoglobulin (Ig) E-mediated immunological release of mediators of mast cells and basophils, and with potentially life-threatening consequences.

- With increased use of medicines and antibacterials, medicine induced anaphylaxis and anaphylactoid reactions have increased.
- Other causative agents include NSAIDs, anaesthetics, muscle relaxants, latex and radio contrast media.

Anaphylaxis is often unpredictable and so we need to focus on strategies to decrease risks:

- Ensure detailed patient history and full physical examination.

- Consider the route of the medicine and the rate of the medicine and/or fluid.
- Identification of patients with known causes of anaphylaxis.
- Sound knowledge of the medicine, as some cross react and also are contraindicated.
- Greater number of years since the last administration of the offending agent, the less the chance of a recurrence.
- Parenteral route increases the severity and frequency of a reaction, so review the choice of the medicine and route, and if the patient still needs IV route, they remain under medical supervision for 20–30 minutes after medicine administration.

Recommendations for practice

Immediate actions following anaphylaxis depends on the severity of the reaction and these can range from a mild skin reaction to cardiovascular collapse.

- Discontinue suspected medicine.
- Get help, resuscitation call.
- Administer oxygen, epinephrine (adrenaline), IV fluids.
- Start ABCDE.
- Start CPR if no pulse.
- Monitor patient; oxygen saturation, vital signs, ECG.
- Provide reassurance and adequate information and communication.
- At least 2 hours observation if mild and in severe cases at least 24 hours monitoring of the patient.
- Ensure prompt and appropriate reporting and recording in the patient case records and consideration of the Yellow Card Reporting scheme,

which advocates the reporting of adverse medicine reactions.

■ Patient will require advice for the future and this might include: the use of a Medic-Alert (e.g. bracelet) ID system and an Epinephrine kit.

Oxygen therapy

Hypoxia is oxygen deficiency in the body cells caused by:

■ Deficient oxygenation of the blood – due to respiratory disease or chest injuries.

■ Inadequate transport of oxygen by haemoglobin – as in anaemia or haemorrhage.

■ Circulatory inadequacy as in heart disease or emergency situations, e.g. cardiac arrest.

■ Inability of cells to use oxygen – rare – an example is cyanide poisoning.

Oxygen therapy is a specific medical treatment and is given as prescribed by the medical staff who will write the percentage of oxygen and the method of administration on the prescription sheet. However, the premise of the 'prescription only' status of supplemental oxygen is challenged, as delayed oxygen administration because of the need for a medical order may significantly affect an infant or child's outcome (Wong and Elliott 2009).

The concentration given depends upon the condition being treated and an inappropriate concentration may have lethal effects:

■ Oxygen toxicity – may follow prolonged periods (over 24 hours) of administration of high (over 50%) concentrations of oxygen.

■ Atelectasis – alveolar collapse increases with oxygen greater than 50%, as nitrogen is washed out and replaced by oxygen.

■ Retinopathy or prematurity – high concentrations of oxygen obliterates developing retinal vessels leading to blindness.

Although there are risks associated with oxygen administration to infants and children with acute illness the risks of not providing oxygen are far greater and can ultimately be fatal. High concentrations of oxygen (above 50%) are often prescribed in a severe asthma attack and in pneumonia but may also be seen in shock, haemorrhage, and diabetic ketoacidosis. The British Thoracic Society (2008) recommended that oxygen should be given to patients immediately in most emergency situations without a formal prescription.

The effects of oxygen administered can be monitored using pulse oximetry, which records the oxygen saturation using a non-invasive procedure. The aim is to keep the saturation above 90% if possible.

Oxygen may be given by:

■ mask

■ nasal cannulae

■ oxygen tent

■ ventilator

■ endotracheal tube

■ Ambubag in an emergency.

Nasal cannulae are not suitable for all children because they are not accurate when giving low percentages of oxygen and if a higher percentage is needed there is inadequate humidification. They are useful when a child finds the conventional mask claustrophobic as often happens in children.

If high concentrations of oxygen are used, some form of humidification will be needed or the oxygen will have a very drying effect on the mucosa. If the patient's own airways have been bypassed as when oxygen is given via an endotracheal tube, humidification is essential.

Humidified oxygen

Oxygen which is delivered in high concentrations and/or over prolonged periods of time can lead to increased secretions and dried mucous membranes. Thus, humidified oxygen therapy is commonly used in the paediatric patient for the treatment of chronic pulmonary conditions, which require very high concentrations of inspired oxygen.

Indications for the use of heated humidification systems:

- Patients receiving high concentrations of oxygen (where FiO_2 exceeds 40%) for periods of time exceeding 24 hours.

- Patients with conditions causing poor mucociliary transport, sometimes found in patients with severe inflammation of the oropharyngeal mucosa.

- Patients with hypothermia. Heated humidified oxygen therapy may help increase a patient's core body temperature when used in combination with other treatments.

- Humidified oxygen therapy is the process of delivering moisture inspired oxygen to patients receiving mechanical ventilation, non-invasive ventilatory support or who are able to breathe independently but require humidified oxygen.

- Humidified oxygen can be delivered as a heat and moisture exchanger (HME) or in the form of heated humidification.

Heat and moisture exchanger

HMEs operate by capturing the heat and moisture exhaled by the patient and then circulating it back into the patient's inhaled gas. Commonly used during transport or when bagging a patient who is using a humidified breathing circuit.

- HME filters should be changed every 48 hours.
- Be alert to signs of inadequate humidification.
- If the use of HME exceeds 96 hours, patients showing signs of inadequate humidification (e.g. mucous plugging) should receive heated humidification.

Heated humidification

Heated humidifiers increase the heat and water vapour content of a gas before delivering it to the patient. Suitable for patients with excessive:

- secretions (chronic bronchitis, cystic fibrosis, etc.)
- bloody secretions (pulmonary contusion or haemorrhage), very high or very low tidal volumes
- spontaneous minute ventilation which exceeds 10 l/min, during hypothermia (body temperature less than 32°C)
- patients requiring ventilation exceeding 96 hours.
  - Inspired gas temperature should be no greater than 37°C

- Change the 2-litre irrigation flask just prior to it becoming empty
- Tubing and chamber should be replaced once weekly
- Keep the patient's circuit clear of condensation.

Modes of delivery

Humidified oxygen via Headbox is a means of delivering oxygen therapy to infants and neonates by enclosing the head and neck within a transparent shell of circulating gas.

Humidified oxygen via nasal cannulae that are small plastic tubes inserted into each nostril. The advantage of this method is that the child can continue to feed and play without the mask getting in the way. Nasal mucosa can become very dry so it is essential that the oxygen is humidified.

Humidified oxygen via Thermovent/ Hydro Trach T. Children who are able to spontaneously breathe but who require intubation to protect their upper airway may benefit from the Thermovent/Hydro Trach T. This device can be attached onto the Protex connector in order to increase the water vapour content of inspired air. Note that the Thermovent/Hydro Trach T does not provide sufficient humidification to patients with thick or excessive secretions.

Humidified oxygen via Trachy Mask: Tracheostomy is a means of delivering mechanical airway ventilation via a tube inserted into the trachea through an incision in the neck. A Trachy Mask is worn around the neck and attaches to the opening of the tracheostomy tube in order to direct humidified oxygen into the airway.

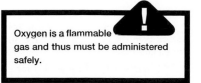

Oxygen is a flammable gas and thus must be administered safely.

Rewarming procedures

As core temperature drops below 35°C treatment becomes imperative, rewarming of the hypothermic child is not the only aspect to be considered in the care (Edwards 2003b). This can occur due to exposure, falling into cold water (drowning). The nurse has a broader role in managing and caring for hypothermic children, s/he should: be vigilant during fluid administration; observe blood results and the ECG; document urine output; and ensure that any drugs administered during rewarming are not toxic, and normal prescribed dosages may need to be reduced.

Passive rewarming

- Once the patient's core temperature is less than 35°C, steps should be taken to prevent them losing further heat to the environment. Remove all wet clothing; gently dry the patient if needed then insulate them with blankets. Patient is allowed to rewarm using just normal metabolic heat production.

- Patient may be covered with polythene sheeting, and placed in a warm room. Space blankets prevent radiant heat loss, but not that lost by conduction or convection. As these may cause sparks, they also present a hazard when oxygen is used, so are best avoided. Remember that heat is lost from the head and the back, so insulate these areas.

- This method is recommended for both mild (32.2–35°C) and moderate (28–32°C) hypothermias that have an onset of less than 12 hours. Passive rewarming treatment will not rewarm an arrested hypothermic patient, and may have limited value for those who are severely hypothermic e.g. a temperature of less than 28°C.

- Close observation, cautious use of fluids and avoidance of vigorous movement to prevent cardiac arrest are essential. Movement contributes to heat loss through convection and may reduce temperature further if not closely monitored. If the temperature fails to rise, and patient becomes persistently hypotensive, active external rewarming should be commenced.

Active external rewarming

- Patient's skin is warmed, using hot baths, hot air blowers or radiant heat. This method can also be used as an adjunct to internal active rewarming. One of the most effective methods is convective warming therapy which forces heated air directly on to the patient's skin through a disposable blanket.

- Method may be used when the hypothermia has occurred slowly, e.g. over a 12-hour period and is mild or moderate in nature. It is not recommended for use alone in the treatment of patients with severe hypothermia.

- Patient's vital signs and peripheral temperature must be monitored, as rewarming shock may occur in the severely hypothermic patient as a consequence of rewarming the peripheries before the core.

- Peripheral rewarming promotes vasodilatation, returning cold, acidotic blood to the heart that has significant effects on myocardial depression. To minimize this effect it is recommended that only truncal rewarming be undertaken. If the patient is persistently hypotensive, or their core temperature continues to fall, active internal rewarming should be started.

Active internal rewarming

This is an invasive procedure, whereby the deep tissues of the body are warmed. It allows the lungs and heart to be rewarmed first. Methods include:

- warm fluid for gastric and peritoneal lavage.
- mediastinal and pleural irrigation.
- continuous arteriovenous or venovenous rewarming.
- extra-corporeal rewarming.
- cardiopulmonary by-pass.
- The advantage of active core rewarming is that it avoids the peripheral vasodilatation associated with surface rewarming, and allows correction of any fluid deficits.
- The disadvantage is that afterdrop may be observed in patients after internal active rewarming is discontinued. A decrease in temperature of as much as 2°C may occur as blood circulates to the peripheries, recools, and returns

to the core. Thus, when more invasive active internal rewarming methods are discontinued, attention is directed to the need for passive and active external rewarming, to prevent afterdrop in temperature.

- the method is best incorporated when the hypothermia has occurred very quickly, e.g. in less than 12 hours, and is moderate or severe in nature. The treatment is to reduce the risk of cardiac arrest, by reducing the time the patient's core temperature is below 32.2°C.

- Process of rewarming should proceed at no faster than a few degrees per hour (Edwards 2003). If a patient is rapidly rewarmed oxygen consumption, myocardial demand and vasodilatation increase faster than the heart's ability to compensate and death can occur.

3.2 Maintaining nutrition in children

Effects of nil by mouth and malnutrition

Absorptive and post-absorptive states:

- Absorptive state – process of eating/digestion
- Post-absorptive state – fasting should be no more than 12 hours as after this time:
  - All glycogen stores in the skeletal and liver is utilized (it is likely this will occur before 12 hours due to stress and to conserve glycogen

stores for the brain), eventually the brain has to use fat as a source of energy.
  - Lipolysis of adipose tissues is being converted by the liver producing ketones, which can effect acid base balance – body building processes do not take place in an acid environment and reduces wound healing, production of white blood cells, energy
  - Finally, catabolism of cellular proteins occurs.

This leads to:

- Anaemia.

- Reduction in the production in white blood cells, immunoglobulins – susceptibility to infection.

- Reduction in adeno-triphosphate (ATP) in skeletal muscle cells leading to weakness, lethargy, reduced mobility – potential deep vein thrombosis and pulmonary embolism.

- Reduction in ATP can also lead to weakened diaphragm and muscles of breathing which can lead to a chest infection or pneumonia.

Some surgeons argue that following bowel or some abdominal surgery the bowel should be rested and fasting is the common practice to allow healing of anastomosis or from handling of the bowel during surgery. However, this practice will lead to a lack of nutrients (utilised due to the stress response) for healing to take place. But the combination of stress and nil by mouth practices can lead the GIT to stop functioning. The GIT lining can be compromised leading to septicaemia from what are normally harmless bacteria living in the bowel, moving into the systemic circulation. Therefore, feeding is essential and should be commenced immediately. The bowel cannot tolerate nil by mouth for very long and even if other forms of feeding are being instigated, e.g. parenteral nutrition, fluid has to be given (minimum 30 ml/hour) to maintain gut integrity, thus if 30 ml can be administered then this can be increased at regular intervals until feeding is resumed.

Enteral feeding (EF)

Enteral feeding (EF) includes any method of delivering nutrients for gastrointestinal tract absorption (Richards and Edwards 2008) and should be initiated at the earliest possible point because it:

■ maintains gut integrity
■ reduces risk of bacterial translocation
■ dampens the inflammatory response
■ reduces complications from sepsis
■ more cost effective in comparison to parental nutrition.

Early enteral feeding (EF) following any type of surgery is possible (i.e. within 6 hours of insult) and only contraindicated in complete gut failure – which is purported to be very rare. EF includes feeding via:

■ nasogastric route
■ nasoenteric route (i.e. placed in the duodenum or jejunum).

Types of tubes

Nasogastric/nasoduodenal are the most commonly used and are suitable for short-term use such as postoperatively or during period of critical care ventilation.

■ *Wide bore tube* is used initially to allow easy assessment of gastric contents and aspiration typically occurs every 4 hours to assess gastric content/absorption and pH.
■ *Narrow bore tube* should replace the wide bore tube to facilitate long-tem feeding. In addition, the narrow bore tube is more comfortable for the patient and less likely to cause oesophageal irritation or interfere with swallowing.

Gastrostomy if long-term feeding is anticipated due to upper gastrointestinal obstruction. Avoids delays in feeding, less discomfort, and is cosmetically acceptable.

■ Percutaneous endoscopically gastrostomy (PEG) – made from polyurethane or silicone and held in place by an inflatable balloon. Disadvantage is that it requires local anaesthetic, sedation and radiological support to ensure tube is positioned correctly.
■ Jejunostomy tube – placed in the jejunum and is the preferable method if the patient has undergone upper gastrointestinal surgery or has severe delayed gastric emptying.

Methods of administration

■ Bolus feeding: if the patient is restless or confused as the patient may dislodge the tube.
■ Intermittent continuous feeding: if feeding needs to be interrupted or discontinued to allow gastric emptying, for example for physiotherapy.

- Gravity drip – allowed to flow through over a given period of time
- Pump assisted feeding – connected to a pump for the majority of the day and typically rested overnight. Most commonly used in the critical care setting, various flow rates per hour from 1 ml to 300 ml.

Complications of enteral feeding (EF)

Complications can be prevented provided the nurse both understands and anticipates the potential problems associated with EF:

- Altered gut motility, that is absent bowel sounds can lead to gastric and colonic stasis.
- Effects of sedation and analgesia can lead to ileus/pseudo obstruction and distension.
- Pulmonary aspiration.
- Nausea and vomiting.
- Diarrhoea, constipation, large aspirates.
- Blockage of tube.
- Trauma to the nose.
- Incomplete calorific delivery due to the above.
- Overfeeding.

Strategies to avoid complications associated with EF:

- Large aspirates – give prokinetic agents, e.g. pantoprazole.
- Early commencement of EF – day 1 of critical care admission, monitor feeding regime, avoid stopping and starting feed, follow feeding regime.

- Care of nasogastric tube to prevent blockages.
- Bowel sounds are not required for enteral feeding to commence.
- Treat diarrhoea, constipation and vomiting to aid enteral feeding.

Overfeeding

The energy requirements of disease have been overestimated to account for:

- high temperature
- increased cost of breathing.

This is inappropriate as a child's resting energy expenditure may represent only 20–30%, rather than 50% as offset by the decrease in physical activity. The energy requirements of patients who are unwell are usually similar to or less than that of healthy subjects. Excess carbohydrate and lipid intake can cause:

- Hepatic steatosis.
- Abnormal liver function.
- Lead to excess carbon dioxide production, which can precipitate respiratory failure.
- Lipids may be deposited in the:
  - lung and impair diffusion of gases
  - produce infusion hyperlipidaemia.

It is recommended that hypocaloric feeding be the current practice in hospital feeding regimes, especially in the early stages of injury (e.g. 1500 kcal/day for up to a week). This would reduce the risk of liver, lung complications and metabolic instability and their consequences. An increase in calorie intake should take place in the recovery phase, when nutrition level is normal and the patient is no longer at risk.

Parenteral nutrition (PN)

Parental nutrition (PN) is the provision of all nutritional requirements intravenously. Instead of food being fed into and absorbed by the gastrointestinal tract, nutrients are infused directly into the venous circulation, thus bypassing the gut. PN contains essential nutrients in quantities to meet the requirements of the individual patient. It is administered via a central venous line. PN is indicated for:

- prolonged ileus
- uncontrolled vomiting
- chronic diarrhoea or malabsorptive states
- severe radiation enteritis
- short bowl syndrome
- gastrointestinal obstruction
- severe pancreatitis with fistula
- critical illness
- hypercatabolic states
- multiple trauma or burns
- hepatic or renal failure
- inflammatory bowel disease.

Routes of administration

- CVP usually subclavian vein:
  - problems with infection
  - all the complications of a CVP line
  - limits mobility.
- Skin-tunnelled catheter for long-term nutrition
  - peripherally inserted central catheter (PICC)
  - can block very easily.

PN solution contains:-

- Amino acids – both essential and non essential 1–2 g/kg/day.
- Glucose – carbohydrate energy source it provides 3.75 kcal/g – 25–50% glucose ↑ in insulin, fatty liver.
- Fat emulsion – fat energy source generates 9 kcal/g – 10 or 20% solutions ↓ insulin and ↑ in ketones.
- If an insufficient energy supply from carbohydrates/fats – encourages the use of protein for energy.
- Electrolytes, e.g. sodium, potassium, magnesium, calcium and phosphorus.
- Vitamins, minerals and trace elements are required.

Nurses' role

- Administration sets need to be changed every 24 hours.
- Feeding line should never be used for the administration of additional medicines – PN is incompatible with numerous other medicines.
- Separate lumen should be used for other medicines, blood products or CVP readings.
- Volumetric infusion pumps should be used.
- Incomplete bags should be discarded.
- Site of the subclavian catheter observed for inflammation/infection.

Monitoring of PN

- Temperature, pulse and respiratory rateand BP.
- Body weight – increases.

- Fluid balance − +ve balance.
- Urine testing – sugar and ketones.
- Blood testing – blood urea nitrogen (BUN), creatinine, urea, glucose, sodium, potassium.
- Mouthcare due to limited oral intake.

Complications of PN

Central line complications

- Pneumothorax
- Arterial puncture
- Air embolism
- Sepsis
- Vein thrombosis
- Catheter blockage and accidental removal.

Metabolic complications:

- Fluid overload
- Hyperglycaemia
- Hypoglycaemia
- Translocation of bacteria/sepsis.

Reduction in trace elements and vitamins

- Metabolic acidosis – chloride/CO_2
- Refeeding syndrome
- Electrolyte disturbances:
  - hyperammonaemia
  - hyponatraemia
  - hypernatraemia
  - hypokalaemia
  - hypocalcaemia
  - hypophosphataemia
  - hypomagnesaemia.

Required nutritional intake

A child's energy requirements is dependent on:

- age
- sex
- weight
- stress activity.

Generally, 25–32 kcal/kg/day is required to maintain an adequate nutritional intake. Nitrogen intake, 0.17–0.3 g N/kg/day (maximum nitrogen intake is 18 g/day). If too much nitrogen is taken (> 0.3 g/kg/day) then this may cause a negative effect on weaning and have an effect on renal biochemistry.

Protein intake should be 1–1.9 g protein/kg/day.

Carbohydrates should not exceed glucose oxidation rate of 3–5 g/kg/day. Carbohydrate overload can cause hyperglycaemia, hypercapnia, possibly fatty liver and elevated tryglycerides. A high-fibre diet is beneficial.

3.3 Peritoneal dialysis (PD)

PD is a slow form of dialysis, utilizing the peritoneum as the dialysis membrane. Typically, a much slower correction of fluid and electrolyte imbalance is preferred in the critically ill and the need for complex equipment is avoided making this a safer option. However, the procedure is labour intensive and does predispose the patient to peritoneal infection. With the advent of haemofiltration, PD is rarely used within critical care.

PD access

A trochar and cannula are inserted through a small, superficial, midline incision under local anaesthetic. However, a lateral approach can also be used. Once inserted the trochar is withdrawn slightly and the cannula advanced to the pouch of Douglas. Its position may be tested by infusing fluid into the peritoneum before the final advancement of the trocar and cannula.

PD technique

Warmed peritoneal dialysate is infused into the peritoneum, 1–2 litres at a time. Fluid is left for periods of 4–6 hours in the peritoneal cavity before draining. Heparin (500 iu) may be added to the initial PD cycles but only required thereafter if the drainage fluid is cloudy or bloody.

Peritoneal dialysate

Dialysate is a sterile balanced electrolyte solution. Standard preparation fluid vary Dianeal glucose 1.36% w/v 13.6 mg/ml to glucose 3.86% w/v 38.6 mg/ml dependent on whether a greater fluid removal is required. Potassium is only added if necessary as it can cause problems due to slow exchange in PD.

Complications

- Fluid leak around the catheter
- Catheter blockage
- Infection
- Hyperglycaemia
- Diaphragmatic splinting.

3.4 Plasmapheresis

Plasmapheresis or plasma exchange is the process of removing autoantibodies from the bloodstream mechanically using a process similar to that used in renal failure treatment. It is performed at many major medical centres and critical care units across the country. In autoimmune diseases, the immune system attacks the body's own tissues and the main attack mechanisms are antibodies and proteins that circulate in the bloodstream until they meet and bind with the target tissue. Once attached, they impair tissue functions, and encourage other immune components to respond.

The function of plasmapheresis is to remove antibodies from the bloodstream, thereby preventing them from attacking tissues. Plasmapheresis does not directly affect the immune system's ability to make more antibodies, and therefore may only offer temporary benefit. It is most beneficial in acute, self-limited disorders such as:

- myasthenia gravis
- Guillain–Barré syndrome
- Lambert–Eaton syndrome
- chronic demyelinating polyneuropathy
- Goodpasture's syndrome
- pemphigus
- rapidly progressive glomerulonephritis

- systemic lupus erythematosus
- thrombotic thrombocytopenia
- immunoproliferative diseases
- multiple myeloma
- Waldenstrom's macroglobulinaemia
- poisoning.

Plasmapheresis process

Plasma, the fluid element of the blood, is removed from blood cells by a device known as a cell separator. The separator works either by spinning the blood at high speed to separate the cells from the fluid or by passing the blood through a membrane with minute pores, that only plasma can pass through. Cells are returned to the person undergoing treatment, while the plasma, which contains the antibodies, is discarded and replaced with other fluids.

Plasmapheresis treatment

- Insertion of a venous catheter, either in a limb or central vein to allow higher flow rates.
- Involves the removal of blood, separation of blood cells from plasma, and return of these blood cells to the body's circulation, diluted with fresh plasma or a substitute.
- Because of concerns over viral infection and allergic reaction, fresh plasma is not routinely used. Instead, the most common substitute is saline solution with sterilized human albumin protein.

- During the course of a single session, 2–3 l of plasma is removed and replaced.
- Takes several hours and can also be undertaken on an outpatient basis, this is dependent on the patients underlying disease and overall condition.
- Can be uncomfortable but normally not painful.
- Number of treatments needed varies depending on the particular disease and patient's general condition.
- Average course of plasma exchanges is six to ten treatments over 2–10 weeks.
- Treatments vary according to clinician's preference, in some centres; treatments are performed once a week, while in others, more than one treatment per week is performed.

Replacement fluid

- This is when replacement fluid is given intravenously post plasmapheresis.
- Some hospitals give a plasma substitute e.g. partial crystalloid replacement or 5% albumin.
- The only indication to replace plasma loss with all fresh frozen plasma is when plasmapheresis has been undertaken to replace missing plasma factors.

Risks associated with plasmapheresis

- Hypotension is the most common problem, which can be connected to episodes of faintness, dizziness, blurred vision, coldness, and sweating or abdominal cramps.

- Circulatory instability in that there are intravascular volume changes and removal of circulating catecholamines and hypocalcaemia during plasmapheresis.

- Plasmapheresis may not be suitable for patients with clotting disorders as anticoagulation therapy is required.

- Bleeding can occur because of the anticoagulant given during the procedure to prevent the blood from clotting.

- Some of these medications can cause other adverse reactions, for example, tingling around the mouth or in the limbs, muscle cramps or a metallic taste in the mouth. If left untreated, these reactions can lead to an irregular heartbeat or seizures.

- Can cause bleeding in that during the exchange there is removal of coagulation factors.

- Allergic reaction to the reinfusion of human plasma solutions used to replace the plasma can prove life threatening. This type of anaphylactic reaction usually begins with itching, fever, chills, wheezing or a rash. If this occurs, plasma exchange must be stopped and person treated with intravenous medications.

- Excessive suppression of the immune system can temporarily occur; since the procedure is not selective about which antibodies it removes. In time, the body can replenish its supply of needed antibodies, but some physicians give these intravenously after each treatment.

- Care must be taken with asepsis and infection control strategies when treating this group of patients so not to increase their susceptibility to infections. Bacterial infection is a real risk, especially when a central venous catheter is used.

- Medication dosages need careful observation and adjustment, because some drugs can be removed from the blood or changed by the procedure.

3.5 Transplantation

Transplants involve the donation of organs from one person to another and enable people to take on a new lease of life in the UK every year. Transplants are the best possible treatment for most people with organ failure with kidney transplants most commonly performed. Transplants of the heart, liver and lungs are also regularly carried out. As medicine advances, other vital organs including the pancreas and small bowel are also being used in transplants. Tissue such as corneas, heart valves, skin and bone can also be donated.

The increasing effectiveness of transplantation means that many more patients can be considered for treatment in this way. However, there is a serious shortage of donors. For some people this means waiting, sometimes for years, and undergoing difficult and stressful treatment. For many it means they may die before a suitable organ becomes available.

Organs that can be transplanted

- Kidneys
- Heart

- Liver
- Lungs
- Pancreas
- Small bowel
- Skin
- Bone
- Corneas
- Heart valves.

3.6 Circulatory support

Intra-aortic balloon pump (IABP)

The IABP is a tool for assisting the failing heart. It does this by lowering the systolic blood pressure and raising the diastolic blood pressure. This technique gives support to the heart by:

- Providing extra oxygen and nutrients in the blood to the heart muscle.
- Reducing the need for oxygen by decreasing the work of the heart.
- Balloon pump allows time for surgical and medical interventions and for the body's own healing powers to restore the heart to life-sustaining function.
- It increases blood flow to the coronary arteries, thereby increasing oxygen supply to the myocardium.
- It decreases the workload of the heart by lowering pressure in the aorta.

  It can be used for:

- Impending myocardial infarction or myocardial infarction.
- Refractory low cardiac output.

- Left ventricular failure or insufficiency
- Inability to be removed from cardiopulmonary bypass following open heart surgery.

Complications

- Vessel damage – trauma of the aorta, iliac and femoral arteries during IABP insertion.
- Peripheral emboli – most frequently encountered problem, any foreign body in the blood stream enhances clot formation around it.
- Problems with the IABP:
  - early inflation of the IABP will interfere with aortic valve closure and possibly regurgitation in the left ventricle
  - late inflation of the IABP will not maximize the effect of IABP
  - late deflation of the IABP will interfere with the onset of the next systole
  - early deflation of the IABP will not maximize the effects of IABP therapy
  - leaking of the balloon – if this is suspected then the pump should be turned off.

Special care considerations

- IABP is an invasive procedure performed by the doctor assisted by the nurse. This can either be performed within a theatre setting, cardiac laboratory or PICU setting.
- The area of skin is prepared and draped with sterile towels and a local anaesthetic is administered.

- Catheter is inserted percutaneously through the femoral artery route after the initial guide wire is inserted. Following predilation, the IABP catheter can be advanced over the guide wire, through the subcutaneous tissue and into the arterial system. Following insertion, an X-ray should be taken to ensure proper positioning in the descending thoracic aorta distal to the left subclavian artery.
- Once the position of the IAB has been confirmed by the medical staff, IABP therapy may commence.
- The inflation and deflation phase settings are set by the medical staff.
  - Regular observations must be carried out to detect early signs of shock, infection.
  - Antithrombotic therapy will commence and regular monitoring of blood coagulopathy must be carried out.
  - Patients will require assistance to move and gain comfortable position and they will also require assistance with hygiene needs.
  - Appropriate pain assessment and analgesia.
  - Appropriate psychological support.

Mechanical circulatory support

Mechanical circulatory support is where a ventricular assist device (VAD) is used to either supplement or to completely replace ventricular function. It can be seen as:

- a bridge to transplantation
- a bridge to recovery
- a permanent basis 'destination therapy'.

Indications for VAD therapy

- Escalating inotropic support
- Myocarditis, when the VAD is used to bridge recovery
- Ischaemic heart disease
- Congenital disorders
- Cardiomyopathy where the treatment is used as a bridge to transplantation
- Post cardiotomy where it is difficult to wean the cardiopulmonary bypass post surgery.

Patient care

- Respiratory management – wean from ventilatory support
- Haemodynamic monitoring – HR, ABP, CVP, PAP, CO
- Monitoring of VAD values/function
- Monitor renal monitoring – urine output, renal function
- Close monitoring of fluid management – input and output
- Monitor abdominal function – risk of reduced gut motility, nutritional problems
- Drug management – weaning of inotropic support, anticoagulation therapy
- Reduced mobilization – passive and active leg exercises, cardiac rehabilitation programme
- Haematological monitoring – coagulation, FBC
- Infection control management – care of IV access, use of antibiotic therapy,

use of appropriate dressing to minimize infection risk, hand washing

- Psychological management – promote rehabilitation and family care.

Complications

- Air emboli intraoperatively
- Haemorrhage
- Neurological damage due to thromboembolic complications
- Impaired renal function
- Right sided heart failure
- Infection from entry site of VAD access
- Reduced gut motility, nausea and vomiting
- Mechanical failure
- Psychosocial issues related to VAD therapy.

Extracorporeal membrane oxygenation (ECMO)

ECMO works on the principle of giving the lungs a chance to rest and heal by taking over the supply of oxygen and the removal of carbon dioxide from the lungs.

- ECMO consists of an extracorporeal venoarterial circulation with high blood flows being circulated via a gas exchange membrane
- ECMO ensures that the majority of the body's gas exchange requirements are achieved and maintained so that there is a preservation of life.
- The main disadvantage of ECMO is that it requires the insertion of large bore cannula and high corporeal

blood flows. This combination predisposes patients to a potentially high risk of cell damage, infection and blood disorders.

Indications and criteria for ECMO

- Failure of improvement and sustained adequate gas exchange, despite maximum critical care support.
- Rapid failure of ventilatory support despite FiO_2 1.0.
- Slow failure of ventilatory support despite a recognized period of critical care management.

Contraindications

- Chronic systematic disease which includes any major organ, e.g. emphysema.
- Lung failure > 7 days.
- Burns $> 40\%$ body surface.
- Four organ failure, including lung failure.

Extracorporeal CO_2 removal (ECCO₂R)

$ECCO_2R$ is an extracorporeal venovenous circulatory device that allows for the clearance of CO_2 via a gas exchange membrane. Low blood flows are adopted so that partial oxygenation support is achieved. Low frequency positive pressure ventilation is typically used with $ECCO_2R$ with the adoption of continuous oxygenation delivery throughout inspiration and expiration. The lungs are helped in expiration with high positive end-expiratory pressure (PEEP) levels (20–25 cm H_2O), limited peak airway pressures (35–40cmH_2O), with a continuous fresh gas supply. Therefore lungs are rested so that recovery of pulmonary problems are reversed.

3.7 Intubation and ventilation of a child

Non-invasive ventilation (NIV)

Non-invasive positive ventilation (NIV) is a form of respiratory support, which increases tidal volume without the use of endotracheal intubation. When used in combination with standard therapeutic treatments, non-invasive mechanical ventilation has been shown to decrease rates of endotracheal intubation and complications which arise from invasive forms of airway management. NIV is an adaptive form of positive pressure ventilation because it can be removed and re-initiated, and it does not depend on taking control of the lower airway.

Non-invasive ventilation is commonly used in children with:

■ Obstruction to upper airway.

■ Acute respiratory infection.

■ Expiratory muscle fatigue.

■ Hypoventilation and hypercapnia resulting from neuromuscular disorders.

■ Conditions and diseases such as skeletal disease, neuromuscular

disease, cystic fibrosis and Prader–Willi syndrome (PWS).

■ NIV can provide effective ventilatory support to children in PICU with immune deficiency, pneumonia and haematological malignancies (Mesiano and Davis 2008).

■ Obstructed sleep apnoea syndrome (OSAS) and respiratory failure as a consequence of neuromuscular disease are most common indications for the long-term use of NIV in children.

■ NIV treats chronic respiratory failure by improving sleep quality, decreasing the work of respiratory muscles, improving respiratory function and increasing ventilatory sensitivity to carbon dioxide (Mesiano and Davis 2008).

Breathing involves muscular work; O_2 consumed at rest is 1–3% of total body O_2 consumption. If more used for respiratory muscles less for heart and brain increases to 25–30% aggravating tissue hypoxia. In respiratory failure management, the goal is to reduce the work of breathing and improve tissue O_2 supply.

Terminology includes:

■ Non-invasive positive pressure ventilation (NIPPV)

■ Trademark names such as Nippy and BiPAP

■ Nasal ventilation

■ BTS (2002) guidelines use NIV to describe all types of non-invasive ventilatory support including continuous positive airway pressure (CPAP)

■ Guidelines refer to bilevel systems as bilevel NIV.

Modes of NIV

NIV is available in two forms: as CPAP or bi-level positive airway pressure (BPAP).

- CPAP is the simplest form of non-invasive ventilation, supplying distending pressure to the airway.
  - CPAP improves the functional residual capacity and pulmonary compliance when used in patients with some level of spontaneous respiration.
  - CPAP reduces the work of breathing by providing active assistance on inspiratory and expiratory phases of the respiratory cycle.
  - Commonly used as long-term treatment for decreasing the work of inspiratory muscles and decreasing airway resistance.
  - CPAP is also of benefit in recently extubated patients who need support in reducing the work of breathing.
- BPAP is a form of non-invasive ventilation which can be used to treat any form of respiratory failure.
  - Increases tidal volume, decreases the work of respiratory muscles and supports alveolar ventilation.
  - BPAP provides support during both inspiratory positive airway pressure (IPAP) and expiratory positive airway pressure (EPAP).
  - Distending pressure provided by BPAP supports lung recruitment and functional residual capacity, while the inspiratory pressure of BPAP increases ventilation, promotes lung recruitment and supports expiratory pressure.
  - Use of BPAP is limited to only patients who can assume control of the airway.

Bilevel NIV gives pressure support and CPAP combined or alone. It is relatively simple and easy to use. Generally uses room air with supplementary oxygen.
Alternates between:

- Inspired positive airway pressure (IPAP)
  - increasing breath size
  - clears CO_2 and reduces patient's work of breathing
  - inspiration higher level airway pressure.
- Expired positive airway pressure (EPAP)
  - expiration low level prevents atelectasis
  - expands collapsed alveoli, improves gas exchange.

Ventilation should work in synchrony with the patient by recognizing:

- Patient breaths in (trigger to IPAP)
- Patient breaths out (trigger to EPAP)
- Triggering and cycling should be recognized automatically as breathing patterns change
- Matched to patient effort to ensure comfort
- Sensitive triggers require smooth bore ventilator tubing to prevent turbulence triggering the ventilator
- Low resistance filter should be used between tubing and the machine.

Administration of NIV

- The relative success of non-invasive mechanical ventilation is contingent upon its practical application in critical care. Factors such as mask choice and ventilator settings can have a substantial impact on a patient's initial reception and overall outcome (Navalesi et al 2000).

- Effective NIV is provided via nasal prongs or a well fitting oral–nasal mask.

- Masks and flow equipment which support this technology may be prone to leaks, and flow-generating devices should compensate for gas loss which occurs around the seal of the patient's mask (Mesiano and Davis 2008).

- Masks which create a reliable seal without producing excessive skin pressure area ideal (Mesiano and Davis 2008).

- Aspiration is the most serious complication that NIV poses, but it is largely confined to the use of full-face masks in infants, young children and disabled children (Navalesi et al 2000).

- Use of heated humidification can resolve minor complications arising from NIV, such as congestion, epistaxis and xerostomia

  Disadvantages of CPAP

- discomfort

- pressure ulcers – tight fitting masks

- hypercapnia – arterial blood gases

- reduced lung compliance – reduced by prolonged CPAP

- Cardiovascular instability – reduces venous return

- Gastric distension – air is swallowed

- Noise – irritating and impairs sleep

- Non-compliance – uncomfortable/stress.

Assessment of patients with CPAP and bilevel NIV

- Chest wall movements

- Co-ordination of respiratory effort with the ventilator

- Accessory muscle recruitment

- General observations/measurements:

- TPR, BP and CVP

- Arterial blood gas analysis

- Samples from an arterial line

- Not safe on a general ward

- Interpretation

- FEV_1 (forced expiratory volume in one second)

- Mental state

- Patient comfort.

Continued evaluation of patient's condition

- Maintenance of airway

- Suctioning forms a significant part in maintaining a patient's airway, indications:
  - Ineffective cough
  - Depressed level of consciousness
  - Thick, tenacious mucus
  - Impaired respiratory function

- Types of suctioning:
  - Suctioning using catheter and gloves
  - Using catheter in sleeve
  - In-line closed suctioning system.

  Areas to consider:

- Suctioning can be a frightening experience for any child, therefore explain the process clearly.

- Use correct size of catheter.

- Pressure used between (80–120 mmHg).

- Too low will be ineffective.

- Too high can cause:
  - atelectasis
  - hypoxaemia
  - airway collapse
  - ulceration.

- Pre-oxygenation and duration of suctioning (no longer than 10–15 seconds).
- Equipment, preparation, procedure, documentation.

CPAP vs bilevel NIV

Due to smaller starting pressures for bilevel NIV (4 cmH$_2$O), CPAP (5 cmH$_2$O) there is less reduction in cardiac output. Bilevel NIV is more comfortable and quieter than CPAP. CPAP reverses pulmonary oedema more rapidly, although bilevel NIV provides better systemic perfusion. Bilevel NIV provides better long-term physiological effects.

A high proportion of hospitals offer NIV as a treatment choice. The BTS (2002) recommends that NIV should ideally be used in high dependency settings, where there are appropriately trained nurses and usually one nurse for every two patients.

Endotracheal intubation

Endotracheal intubation is the insertion of an artificial airway (endotracheal tube) to secure the airway. Intubation can be required for the following reasons:

- protect the patient's airway
- provide positive pressure ventilation to patients with respiratory failure or serious hypoxaemia
- allow tracheal suctioning
- support respiratory function during anaesthesia
- enable patient rest.

Paediatric endotracheal intubation without anaesthesia

- Anaesthesia should not be administered to patients requiring intubation if any of the following indications are met:
  - cardiopulmonary resuscitation
  - loss of respiratory function
  - cases where airway preservation is required
  - unconsciousness or airway obstruction
  - or cases where the aspiration of sputum is required.
- Rapid sequence intubation should be used on conscious, non-fasted patients with unprotected airways in emergency situations.
- In this instance, anaesthesia should be used to induce an unconscious, neuromuscularly blocked condition.
- Due to a greater risk of aspiration, the introduction of a nasogastric tube or the use of positive pressure ventilation should not proceed until a secure airway has been assumed.
- Cricoid pressure should be applied once the patient is fully sedated in order to secure access to the airway (Lutman and Mok 2006).

Paediatric endotracheal intubation under anaesthesia

Airway management can be carried out through the following techniques:

- spontaneous ventilation with face mask or laryngeal mask airway
- controlled ventilation with face mask or laryngeal mask airway

- for brief surgical procedures, the use of tracheal intubation and spontaneous ventilation
- controlled ventilation with tracheal intubation.

Indications for tracheal intubation

- Infants younger than 12 months of age
- Provide airway protection
- Support a clear airway during oral or ENT surgery
- Provide mechanical ventilation during exceptionally long surgery or surgery requiring extensive muscle relaxation
- Allow for reduced breathing work and improved efficiency of mechanical ventilation
- Intubation of burn victims should occur as early as possible because the progressive swelling of the airway may pose difficulties when attempting to gain airway access.

Paediatric airway evaluation

Paediatric endotracheal intubation under anaesthesia should be preceded by an evaluation which seeks to identify patients with difficult airways (Holm-Knudsen and Rasmussen 2009).

- Congenital syndromes which impact upon respiratory anatomy and physiology (e.g. Down's, Klippel–Feil, Pierre Robin, Treacher Collins, Hurler's/Hunter's syndromes)
- Airway problems relating to upper respiratory tract infection
- Past history of difficulty during intubation.

- Conditions such as sleep apnoea, face malformation, excessive snoring, feeding problems should be noted as potential sources of a difficult airway (Patel and Meakin 2000)
- Evaluation should include looking for facial abnormalities, an internal examination of the oral cavity and oropharynx, an identification of any loose teeth in children aged 5–10 years, and any range of motion difficulties in the neck.

Anatomical differences between child and adult airway

- Any health care professional undertaking endotracheal intubation must have a sound knowledge of the anatomical differences between children's and adult's respiratory systems.
- Differences between adult and paediatric respiratory anatomy are significant at ages falling below or above 8–10 years of age.
- After 8–10 years but before the stage at which full development has been reached, differences between children's and adult's respiratory systems are solely attributable to size rather than anatomical function (Patel and Meakin 2000).
- Laryngoscopy tends to be a more difficult procedure to carry out in infants and children than in adults.
- Because of their smaller anatomy, infants and young children present a specific set of difficulties during endotracheal intubation.
- First, desaturation progresses much more quickly in infants and young

children due to their more limited residual lung capacity and higher oxygen consumption.

- Second, tongue displacement is complicated by a shorter jaw and larger tongue relative to the surrounding oral cavity. In infants their large tongue relative to the size of the oropharynx area contributes to an increased risk of airway obstruction.

- Visualizing the laryngeal inlet with conventional laryngoscopy is also made difficult by a long, narrow epiglottis and the cephalad position of the larynx.

- The higher and more anteriorly inclined larynx in children presents added difficulty when trying to bring the vocal cords into view (Patel and Meakin 2000).

Selection of endotracheal tube

- An uncuffed tracheal tube is sometimes used in children because of the funnel shaped larynx with the narrowest aspect of its passage sitting at the cricoid cartilage.

- The cricoid cartilage is a ring of cartilage that is rigid and not distendable.

- Forcing a tube through the cricoid ring will compress and traumatize the mucosa.

- Airway is vulnerable so airway oedema and post-intubation stridor can be easily induced if care is not taken.

- From the age of 8 years the cricoid cartilage becomes wider and a cuffed tube may be used to prevent air leakage. With the advent of modern low-pressure cuffed tubes, the cuffed tube can be used safely without an increased rate of complications.

- Some prefer to use a cuffed tube as it is thought to result in fewer reintubations due to ill-fitting tubes, provided the cuff pressure is carefully monitored and kept as low as possible to prevent causing airway oedema, or scarring and stenosis (Holm-Knudsen and Rasmussen 2009).

- Refer to your hospital policy when choosing the type of endotracheal tube. Box 3.2 details a formula for calculating endotracheal tube size related to age, oral and nasal length.

- Table 3.5 gives measurements that should be used as a guideline when selecting an endotracheal tube for an infant.

Principles of the procedure

- Before beginning intubation, ensure that at least two healthcare professionals are able to assist with the procedure; this may involve an anaesthetist, an experienced critical care nurse and a less experienced nurse who wishes to learn.

- Child should be monitored by appropriate equipment, such as an arterial catheter, oxygen saturation probe or ECG.

- To reduce vomiting and aspiration, patients with a nasogastric tube should have the contents of their stomachs aspirated prior to intubation.

- Prior to the procedure, you must have four essential conditions:
  - a cleared, suctioned airway in which visualization of the vocal cords is possible
  - mask ventilation with oxygen flow
  - laryngoscope for tube insertion
  - correctly sized endotracheal tube.

Box 3.2 Formula for calculating endotracheal tube size

Endotracheal tube size (mm) = [Age (years)/4]) + 4
If cuffed tubes are used, the formula is changed to [Age (years)/4] + 3.5
   (Holm-Knudsen and Rasmussen 2009)
Oral length (cm) = [Age (years)/2] + 12
Nasal length (cm) = [Age (years)/2] + 15
For example: selecting an ET tube for child aged 4 years
Size: 4/4 = 1 + 4 = 5.0 mm
Oral length: 4/2 = 2 + 12 = 14 cm
Nasal length: 4/2 = 2 + 15 = 17 cm
For example: selecting an ET tube for child aged 2 years
Size: 2/4 = 0.5 + 4 = 4.5 mm
Oral length: 2/2 = 0 + 12 = 12 cm
Nasal length: 2/2 = 0 + 15 = 15 cm

Table 3.5 Endotracheal tube size guide for infants

Age	Uncuffed	Cuffed
Newborn weighing less than 3 kg	3.0	0.0
Newborn	3.5	3.0
4 months	4.0	3.5
12–16 months	4.5	4.0

- As patients are unable to respire during intubation, the procedure should take no longer than 30 seconds and should begin only after the patient has received at least 15 seconds of high-concentration ($\geq 85\%$) oxygen ventilation.

- Small infants and neonates should be positioned differently to young children, children, adolescent and adults because of their relatively large head size and occiput.

- Small towel should be placed below the shoulders of the infant, while a pillow under the head suffices for access to the airways of all other age groups.

- A young child should have their head positioned so that the neck is neutral or somewhat extended.

- Mask size is an important consideration: masks should be large enough to cover an open mouth but not so large as to cover the child's eyes.

- Transparent, rather than black, for visualization of possible aspiration.

- Children benefit from seeing and playing with masks prior to induction (such as in a hospital orientation programme), while older children who are anxious may respond well to taking part in holding the mask over their mouths during induction.

- A combination of drugs is administered to the patient as the procedure progresses.

- It is therefore important that a nurse relay the patient's vital signs to the intubator so that the intubator's primary focus is on the procedure itself.

- A laryngoscope provides a pathway along which the endotracheal tube can be passed into the airway.

- When bringing the airway into visualization with a laryngoscope, ensure that the tongue is positioned to the left as the blade is slowly introduced into the midline until the epiglottis comes into view.

- The blade should then be introduced further until it reaches the vallecula.

- The endotracheal tube should then be slowly advanced between the vocal cords through the cricoid cartilage.

- The cuff should be inflated once the tube has been safely secured into place.

- Chest observation and auscultation at the mid-axillary level should be performed in order to ensure that air is flowing into both the right and left bronchus.

- Secure the tube and begin ventilation with high oxygen concentration and appropriate humidification.

- Continuously assess breath sounds, for bilateral chest rise, child's colour, heart rate on the monitor, and pulse oximeter.

- Intubation difficulties can be overcome by adjusting the patient's position, using a differently sized laryngoscope blade, applying cricoids pressure and using external laryngeal manipulation.

- When intubation cannot be performed, tracheostomy by an ENT surgeon may provide an alternative option. However, nasal intubation is a preferable option as these patients tend to have fewer complications and shorter ICU stays.

- Endotracheal extubation may occur once the child is on spontaneous ventilation when they are either awake or anaesthetized.

- However, extubating a conscious patient is less likely to lead to laryngospasm and other airway complications and should therefore be undertaken in patients whose airway posed difficulty during induction.

Psychosocial needs of parents and intubated children

Intubation is particularly stressful for parents of sick children because of its invasive nature and the fact that their child will be sedated:

- Nurses need to communicate information and allay fears and misconceptions about invasive medical procedures.

- It is crucial that nurses support parents' emotional and informational needs throughout the course of a child's treatment.

Mechanical ventilation

Ventilation is the movement of gas between the lungs and ambient air. Patients who show clinical and laboratory signs of the inability to respire with adequate oxygenation and/or ventilation should be considered for mechanical ventilation.

What happens in mechanical ventilation (Gehlbach and Hall 2007):

- Peak airway pressure is the total pressure required to transport gas to the lung and is normally measured and reported by the ventilator.

- It is mathematically defined as being equal to the sum of resistive pressure (the resistance met during inspiratory flow), elastic pressure (the degree to which the chest wall and lung recoil) and PEEP, or pressure within alveoli (which occurs at the start of a breath).

- The mathematical product of airflow and circuit resistance is resistive pressure. This type of pressure is made more pronounced by increases to a patient's airflow, so long as pressure in the patient's airways, endotracheal tube and ventilator circuit is held constant.

- The mathematical product of volume of gas pushed into the lung and the elastic recoil of the lung/chest walls is defined as elastic pressure. This type of pressure increases with restricted diaphragm/chest wall excursion or stiffness in the lung. Elastic pressure is inversely related to physiological compliance with mechanical ventilation.

- End-expiratory pressure, also referred to as intrinsic PEEP or auto PEEP, is usually equal to atmospheric pressure. End-expiratory pressure may be positive in relation to atmospheric pressure if airway obstruction, restricted airflow or decreased expiry time impinge on the ability of the alveoli to fully empty.

There are four phases of the ventilator cycle:

1. Triggers: Change from expiration to inspiration, i.e. what triggers a breath.
2. Breath delivery (inspiration): Determined by control variable.
3. End of a breath: Change from inspiration to expiration or what cycles a breath
4. Expiration: Passive process dependent on time.

Key terms in ventilation:

Tidal volume (Vt)

- Volume of gas delivered to the patient with each breath. Vt is only set for volume controlled modes of ventilation and is usually 6–8 ml/kg of body weight.

- Often the most manipulated variable in response to abnormal levels of CO_2.

- In pressure control modes of ventilation the Vt will be displayed on the ventilator but it is not set by the clinician.

- Excessive tidal volumes have been linked to ventilator induced acute lung injury (volutrauma).

- Acute lung disease produces some areas of the lung that are severely diseased and others that are nearly normal.

- The flow of gas will follow the pathway of least resistance. If large tidal volumes are delivered under positive pressure the delivered gas flows more rapidly and forcefully into the normal areas.

- Rapid forceful introduction of gas causes over distension of the alveoli in these areas leading to parenchymal injury, loss of surfactant and possible alveolar rupture.

Minute volume (MV)

- Quantity of gas expired in one minute (tidal volume × frequency).
- Rate is also determinant of ventilation and adjusted in response to CO_2 levels.
- Minute ventilation is the rate multiplied by the tidal volume ($R \times Tv = MV$).

Oxygen percentage

- Fraction of inspired oxygen (FiO_2) delivered to the patient.
- FiO_2 can be expressed as a decimal fraction or a percentage.
- FiO_2 concentrations of more than 50% for greater than 24 hours increase the risk of oxygen toxicity.

Functional residual capacity

- Amount of gas that remains in the lungs after normal respiration.

Peak airway pressure (PAP)

- Is an indication of global alveolar pressure.
- Monitored continuously usually by a sensor at the Y-connector in the breathing or ventilator circuit.
- Highest pressure is known as the peak airway pressure or peak inspiratory pressure (PIP).
- Excessive pressure can lead to lung damage and barotrauma. Vent will alarm if the PIP exceeds a set value (determined by the vent) and gas entry will stop until the next breath is triggered.

- In pressure controlled modes the PIP will be constant for each breath. In volume controlled modes the PIP will vary from breath to breath.
- Normal PIP on a ventilated patient with normal lungs is 20 cmH_2O. This pressure varies from patient to patient.

Positive end expiratory pressure (PEEP)

- Normal airway pressure at the end of expiration and before inspiration is zero.
- PEEP aids provide a scaffolding for alveoli that would otherwise collapse during the expiratory phase, known as 'recruitment'.
- PEEP enhances oxygenation by maximizing the number of gas exchange units 'alveoli' and is adjusted in response to oxygen concentration.
- Physiologic peep is normally 5 cmH_2O. Therapeutic range from 10–35 cmH_2O depending on patient needs.

Pressure support (PS)

- A support breath is pressure controlled, patient triggered, pressure limited and patient cycled.
- Can be used in combination with other ventilator modes that permit spontaneous breathing.
- Works by responding to the patients' inspiratory effort with a positive pressure breath delivered at a set pressure.
- Pressure support can be used to compensate for airway resistance due to the endotracheal tube and in weaning from mechanical ventilation.

- Pressure support enhances spontaneous Tv and is adjustable in response to CO_2 levels. Ranges from 5–30 cmH$_2$O.

Inspiratory pause

- Determined by the set volume or pressure, peak flow and flow pattern.
- It lengthens the inspiratory time and may exceed the flow duration.
- May be used to increase the time for gas exchange in the alveoli.
- Must ensure that sufficient time is available for expiration, otherwise it may result in air trapping.
- Used to manipulate I:E ratios.

Expiratory time and air trapping

- Expiratory flow is primarily determined by the resistance of the small airways and the resistance of the artificial airway.
- If airway resistance is high flow will be reduced.
- If flow is reduced more expiratory time will be required for the alveoli to empty thus increasing the risk of air trapping.
- Air trapping will increase inspiratory pressure, decrease tidal volumes and can cause significant discomfort for the patient.

Ventilator mode: a description of how breaths are delivered to the child. The mode describes how breaths are controlled.

Mechanical ventilation can be set according to two modes: volume-cycled ventilation and pressure-cycled ventilation (Gehlbach and Hall 2007).

- *Volume-cycled ventilation* provides a predetermined tidal volume and a variable airway pressure. Assist-control (A/C) and synchronized intermittent mandatory ventilation (SIMV) are both forms of volume-cycled ventilation.
  - Assist-control (A/C) ventilation: A breath will be delivered if the patient fails to do so spontaneously within a set frequency; on the other hand, if a patient makes the effort to breathe beyond the set frequency, a fixed tidal volume will be delivered.
  - Synchronized intermittent mandatory ventilation (SIMV): Like A/C, SIMV provides respiratory support at a volume and frequency that is in line with the patient's own respiratory efforts. Any breath taken beyond the set rate is accommodated by an intake valve which opens as a result.

- *Pressure-cycled ventilation* provides a predetermined inspiratory pressure to the lung with a tidal volume which fluctuates according to resistance from the respiration system (Gehlbach and Hall 2007). It is available in non-invasive, mask-based forms as well as in pressure control ventilation (PCV) and pressure support ventilation (PSV).
  - PCV: Full pressure support is provided for a pre-determined time. Continuous flow of gas allows the patient to interbreathe between ventilator breaths.
  - PSV: No minimum inspiration rate is established as all breaths are delivered in response to a patient's own efforts. This helps patients wean from mechanical ventilation by allowing them to do more breathing work. A derivation of

PSV is non-invasive positive pressure ventilation (NIPPV), which uses a mask to provide ventilation to patients who are already able to spontaneously breathe.

Pressure-regulated volume control (PRVC)

PRVC can be thought of as a combined volume control (VC) and pressure control (PC) mode of ventilation which responds to the patient's physiological measures of compliance.

- Specifically, PRVC calibrates inspiratory pressure by comparing a preset tidal volume with a volume/pressure calculation of the patient's previous breath.
- Increasing oxygenation, distributing ventilation evenly throughout the lung, and augmenting collateral ventilation by decelerating the inspiratory flow of ventilation within a pre-defined set of safe parameters.

Airway pressure release ventilation (APRV)

This is a form of mechanical ventilation defined by CPAP and airway pressure release occurring on an intermittent, time-cycled basis (Mesiano and Davis 2008).

- APRV is particularly suited to patients who require ventilation due to ARDS or acute lung injury.
- CPAP cycle of APRV supports improved oxygenation, while its periods of release support the removal of carbon dioxide while providing tidal volume.

- APRV also allows for spontaneous breathing from the patient, which contributes to redistributed ventilation within dependent areas of the lungs.
- Has the effect of synchronizing the child's spontaneous breathing with that provided by APRV

High frequency ventilation

This is used for patients who have not responded to conventional ventilation. High frequency ventilation provides very high respiratory rates and very small tidal volumes. This type of ventilation minimizes airway pressure changes and supports oxygenation through a high mean airway pressure.

High frequency ventilation can be delivered through the following three methods (Mesiano and Davis 2008):

- *High frequency positive pressure ventilation*: increases the set respiratory rates of a conventional ventilator; not commonly used in current clinical practice.
- *High frequency jet ventilation*: directs pressure-driven air into the bronchi through a small tube which feeds into the patient's endotracheal tube.
- *High frequency oscillatory ventilation* (HFOV): generates very low tidal volumes and uses active inspiratory and expiratory phases; delivers and withdraws gas into the lungs at a high frequency (> 2.5 Hz, or 150 bpm).

Table 3.6 details ventilator alarms, their interpretation and nursing interventions.

Table 3.6 Ventilator alarms, interpretation and interventions

Alarms	Cause	Action to be taken
Ventilator inoperative	Ventilator failure	Manually ventilate patient and have someone else trouble shoot or change ventilator
Low pressure Low PEEP/CPAP Low exhaled volume	Patient is losing some or all of his tidal volume	Is the patient disconnected? Is the tubing disconnected? Is airflow adequate? Is the ET tube in the right position? Check heating wire connections **Manually ventilate patient until cause found**
Apnoea or low rate alarm	No spontaneous breaths taken in a preset number of seconds	Encourage patient to breathe or give patient a single breath. Consider whether rate should be increased. Consider sedation/ neurological condition of the patient
Pressure limit alarm	Patient's PIP reached preset limit Tidal volume dumped when limit reached Obstruction in airway Obstruction in circuit	Does the patient need to be suctioned? Is the patient biting the ETT tube? Has water accumulated in the ventilator circuits? Has the patient's compliance decreased? (Lung injury) Is the patient out of synch with the ventilator

Table 3.6 Ventilator alarms, interpretation and interventions—cont'd

Alarms	Cause	Action to be taken
Decreased minute or tidal volume	Leak around ET tube or from the system Leak from chest tube Decreased patient triggered respiratory rate Decreased lung compliance Sensor malfunction	Check all connections for leaks Check respiratory rate Check airway secretions Check patient ventilator system Change sensor
Increased minute or tidal volume	Increase patient triggered respiratory rate Altered settings Hypoxia Increased lung compliance Sensor malfunction	Check respiratory rate Check patient ventilator system Evaluate patient $ETCO_2$ SpO_2 Obtain an ABG Patient improvement Change sensor
Sudden increase in maximal inspiratory pressure	Coughing airway secretions or plugs Ventilator tubing kinked or filled with water Kinked ET tube Patient position ET tube in right main stem Patient ventilator asynchrony Bronchospasm Pneumothorax	Alleviate uncontrolled coughing Clear airway secretions Check for kinks and water Consider repositioning Verify position Identify cause Decompress chest
Gradual increase in maximal pressure	Increased lung stiffness Diffuse obstructive process	Measure static pressure Evaluate for reversible problems: Atelectasis Increased pulmonary oedema Bronchospasm
Sudden decrease in maximal inspiratory pressure	Volume loss from leaks in system	Clearing secretions Relief of bronchospasm Increasing compliance

(Continued)

Table 3.6 Ventilator alarms, interpretation and interventions—cont'd

Alarms	Cause	Action to be taken
FiO$_2$ drift	O$_2$ analyser error Blender piping failure O$_2$ source failure O$_2$ reservoir leak	Calibrate analyser Correct failure Check ventilator reservoir Check circuit and connections
I:E ratio < 1:3 or > 1:1.5 Inspired gas temperature inappropriate	Altered inspiratory flow rate Alteration in sensitivity setting Airway secretions (pressure ventilator) Subtle leaks Altered settings – thermostat failure	Check ration settings Clear airway secretions Measure minute ventilation Correct temperature control setting Replace heater or ventilator
Changes in delivered PEEP	If ventilator control used: Changes in compliance Changes in tidal volume	Correct problem if possible if not increase PEEP setting to deliver desired level of PEEP
Changes in static pressure	Changes in lung compliance	Evaluate patient and correct if possible
Changes in inspiratory flow rate, sigh volume, assist or control mode, alarm status, dead space volume	Changes in these settings resulting from deliberate or accidental adjustment of dials or knobs	Check to determine whether current settings match the child's and modify the parameters accordingly

Ventilatory weaning

Ventilatory weaning is a process which assists a patient in transitioning from mechanical ventilation to independently assuming the work of spontaneous breathing. Usage of this term varies according to medical setting: in the ICUs, weaning is often used to describe extubation, whereas in the post-ICU setting, weaning refers to the gradual process of withdrawal from mechanical ventilation.

■ Endotracheal intubation is the most common means of delivering mechanical ventilation to children in ICU settings.

- Children in post-acute settings often have tracheostomies because of an unsuccessful response to weaning in the ICU.

- Prolonged use of mechanical ventilation is linked to complications, such as recurrent hospitalization, respiratory infection, injury or deterioration from equipment failure, limited mobility, poor feeding and restricted communication (O'Brien et al 2006).

- Prolonged use of mechanical ventilation can lead to the development of a physiological dependence on sedatives and narcotics (Randolph et al 2002).

Principles of weaning

- A successful weaning care plan has an important role to play in avoiding the prolonged use of mechanical ventilation and thus decreasing the likelihood of complications.

- The time period during which weaning occurs is difficult to define due to its patient-specific parameters. Some patients may be able to abruptly resume the work of breathing, while others may require the gradual withdrawal of mechanical ventilation.

- Regardless of the duration or form that weaning takes, it is important to begin weaning at the first sign of a patient's ability to cope with breathing on their own.

Successful weaning from mechanical ventilation is a crucial component of patient wellness:

- An inappropriately weaned child or infant faces increased risk of reintubation, respiratory complications and mortality.

- Inappropriate weaning from mechanical ventilation contributes to poor psychological outcomes in the patient.

- Parents of intubated children need additional support and information to help them cope with a potentially difficult weaning process.

- Deciding upon patient readiness for ventilatory weaning is ultimately the responsibility of the physician, whose decision is often influenced by clinical guidelines and past experience of weaning patients with similar case histories and clinical profiles.

- One drawback to physician-initiated weaning is that physicians are rarely able to provide bedside support on an ongoing basis.

- It is therefore crucial for nurses to be experienced and familiar with various modes of ventilatory weaning.

- Weaning guidelines/protocols should be developed and made available to respiratory and acute care teams looking after mechanically ventilated patients. A detailed prescription of weaning should be provided by the physician.

- While weaning guidelines/protocols tend to prolong the weaning process, they have been shown to decrease rates of reintubation, reduce weaning failure and promote consistency in clinical care (Keogh 2004).

Before weaning can commence for the mechanically ventilated child, these indicators should be assessed to establish patient readiness:

1. Adequate pulmonary functioning and gas exchange:
   a) Evaluating respiratory function consists of measuring minute

volume (along with spontaneous tidal volume and respiratory rate), vital capacity (with regard to millilitres per kg of body mass) and negative inspiratory pressure.

b) Tidal capacity should be 15 ml/kg or greater before weaning can be safely initiated, while negative inspiratory pressure should be -30 mmH$_2$O or less.

c) If any of the following gas exchange parameters are observed, weaning should not commence: abnormal arterial carbon dioxide tension, chest or abdominal dyssynchrony, dyspnea, tachypnoea and vital sign instability.

d) The presence of some of these signs may indicate that the patient is attempting to resume spontaneous breathing *against* or *in addition to* the efforts of the ventilator (Hanneman 2004). Careful judgement must therefore be made in order to differentiate between the root causes of these physiological signs.

e) Ventilation support has not been strengthened or made more frequent in the 48 hours leading up to the decision to wean (O'Brien et al. 2006).

f) Chest radiograph that shows stability in the respiratory system.

g) Supplemental FiO$_2$ level that does not exceed 0.4.

2. Ability to spontaneously breathe:

a) By temporarily stopping ventilation or setting the ventilator's mode to 'flow by', the patient's spontaneous minute volume can be evaluated.

b) Presence of spontaneous minute volume may also be apparent from a patient's attempts at undertaking spontaneous breathing beyond that provided by the ventilator's set rate.

3. Blood levels of nutritional status indicators:

a) Blood PaCO$_2$ level that is no more than 10% above the baseline measurement, and a blood pH that falls within a normal range.

4. Haemodynamic and physiological stability:

a) Assessment of cardiac function is a vital component of evaluating readiness to wean.

b) Haemodynamic parameters should be evaluated closely in patients who are being evaluated for weaning readiness following cardiac surgery.

c) Haemodynamic instability is signposted by lowered arterial blood pressure, tachycardia/ bradycardia dysrhythmias, low peripheral pulses, elevated pulmonary capillary wedge pressure, reduced cardiac output and lowered mixed venous oxygen saturation (Hanneman 2004).

d) Heart rate that does not exceed 95% of the maximal normal according to age.

e) No presence of acute pain, infection or other conditions that may hinder the weaning process.

5. Appropriate level of consciousness:

a) In the postoperative period, alertness is one criterion of readiness to wean because it signifies that anaesthetic agents have been reversed.

b) Reduced consciousness does not always imply a lack of readiness to wean.

c) It is *changes* in the patient's level of consciousness that should prompt further neurological evaluation, as they may signify metabolic instability, residual anaesthesia or cerebral emboli, to name a few (Hanneman 2004).

Weaning methods commonly used for the critically ill child:

- Initiating a spontaneous breathing trial with the option of using CPAP.
- T-piece circuit trials, which allow for intermittent phases of spontaneous breathing.
- Tapering down the level of ventilator support such that a minimal level of pressure support ventilation is met (this may be aided by a mechanical safeguard which ensures that a minimal level of breaths per minute is met).
- Progressively reducing the ventilation rate when using SIMV.
- Gradually decreasing pressure when using PSV.
- Use of BPAP technology.

Process of weaning

- Prior to weaning, sedative drugs need to be managed to ensure patients' comfort without negative effect on ventilatory drive (Randolph et al 2002)
- Weaning begins by reducing the ventilator's respiratory rate and/or level of PIP.
- If these reductions are tolerated well by the patient, additional reductions can be made every 2–3 days.
- Reductions to the ventilator's respiratory rate and/or level of PIP, which occur during the patient's sleep, should only occur during the final stages of the weaning process.
- Previous studies have identified the following conditions as contributing to a child's failure to wean: airway mass or granuloma, pulmonary

atelectasis, aspiration pneumonia, haematological disorders, abnormal cognitive function, sedation, poor nutrition, gastrointestinal illness, metabolic abnormalities or immune conditions (O'Brien et al 2006).

Long-term ventilation

A number of medical conditions affecting the paediatric patient can lead to a long-term reliance on assisted ventilation and these include:

- spinal injury
- neuromuscular disease
- bronchopulmonary dysplasia
- Ondine's curse
- craniofacial abnormality.

The extent of respiratory support a patient requires varies according to their condition and can range from basic mask CPAP to round-the-clock positive pressure support with tracheostomy. Discharge from hospital care to the home environment for children requiring assisted ventilation is suitable when the following conditions are met:

- stable airway
- stable oxygen requirements ($<40\%$)
- pCO_2 levels which can be held within safe limits by equipment within the home nutritional intake which can be viably maintained
- stable remaining medical conditions
- appropriate family support within the home.

Discharge procedure is carried out by a multidisciplinary team, which is headed by a community-based practitioner (responsible for coordinating activities of community and family members) and a case manager (a nurse or social worker who is responsible for liaising with members of the hospital team). There are guidelines on discharge procedures for children in acute care environments who require assisted ventilation in the home.

Key aspects of the discharge procedure are :

- ITUs should not be transferred to a home care environment; instead, parents and caregivers should be trained to use simple equipment which can be easily maintained and transported.

- Children who are unable to stay off a ventilator for 6 hours or more should be given a second ventilator upon discharge.

- Families should be given copies of their child's full medical records as well as 24 hour access to telephone support.

Tracheostomy

Tracheostomy is an artificial surgical opening in the trachea usually between the 3rd and 4th tracheal rings into which a tube is inserted and through which the child breathes. It is required when normal respiration through the mouth or nose is not possible. It may be a permanent or temporary measure.

Reasons for tracheostomy:

1. Congenital abnormalities
   - laryngeal abnormalities: webbing, papilloma, haemangioma
   - vocal cord paralysis
   - subglottic stenosis
   - choanal atresia
   - tracheo-oesophageal anomalies

   - micrognathia (Pierre Robin syndrome).
2. Trauma.
3. Infection.
4. Foreign body airway obstruction.
5. Long-term ventilation of a child.

Tracheostomy tubes

The surgeon usually selects the most suitable tracheostomy tube, which is based on the child's upper airway anatomy, physiological needs, and presenting condition. There are a variety of tubes available and these vary in length and diameter.

- May be rigid or flexible silicone or polyvinyl chloride (PVC) or less frequently, silver.

- Tracheostomy tubes may be cuffed, uncuffed or fenestrated (i.e. with a hole in the cannula to facilitate speech).

- Infants and children are usually fitted with uncuffed tubes as their airway lumen is narrow with soft membranes which may become damaged by a cuffed tube resulting in further airway stenosis (Wilson 2005).

- Tubes are available in sizes 3.0–6.5 (size usually refers to the internal diameter of the tube in millimetres).

- Tubes vary in length to suit the neonate, child and older child.

- Each tube is supplied with a smooth, rounded introducer, which facilitates insertion and reduces trauma to trachea.

- Tube is cut straight rather than slanted to avoid occlusion.

- Tubes are supplied in sterile packaging.

- Tubes are almost always disposable and are inserted for a specified period (often a week) and then changed and discarded.

Parts of the tracheostomy tube

- Cannula – curved part of the tube which is inserted into the stoma and maintains the airway and allows suction to remove secretions.
- Flange – sits against the neck and has securing ties attached to it
- Hub – is a 15 mm connector that enables direct connection to ventilator tubing and other equipment.

Nursing the child with a tracheostomy

- The child must never be left alone.
- Airway patency is essential as the tracheostomy tube is the primary airway.
- Requires competency in all aspects of tracheostomy care and management.
- Competency in the resuscitation of a child with a tracheostomy (mouth to tracheostomy and using an Ambubag) is vital.
- Resuscitation and suction equipment with correct tracheostomy fittings should be kept by the bedside and checked every day.
- When mobilizing the child, essential equipment such as spare tracheostomy tube, oxygen and suction should be included.
- Parents and carers must receive training to be proficient in these skills before the child is discharged from hospital.

- Children with tracheostomies are usually cared for within the community by parents who have received appropriate training in tracheostomy care, changing the tube and resuscitation skills.
- Community nurses link between hospital and home by providing support and advice to families.

Essential aspects of tracheostomy care

- Emergency care – knowing CPR and basic life support (BLS).
- Caring for a newly formed tracheostomy.
- Suctioning.
- Administering oxygen and humidification.
- Cleaning the stoma.
- Changing the tube ties.
- Changing the tracheostomy tube.

Early warning signs of obstruction include:

- increased respiratory rate – tachypnoea
- laboured breathing
- stridor
- tachycardia
- decreased oxygen saturations
- increasing anxiety
- cyanosis, bradycardia and apnoea are late signs of severe respiratory distress.

Potential complications

- Airway obstruction
- Blocked tube
- Aspiration

- Tracheal trauma
- Displaced tube
- Pneumothorax
- Atelectasis
- Infection of stoma or trachea-bronchial fistula
- Granulation tissue
- Tracheal stenosis.

Equipment required for the child with a tracheostomy

When a child has a tracheostomy there is a constant risk that the tube may become dislodged or blocked. Therefore it is essential that equipment is easily accessible at the child's bedside in hospital, in the home and should travel with the child at all times:

- Suction equipment and suction machine
- Oxygen equipment and tracheostomy mask
- Spare tracheostomy tube (child's usual size)
- Spare tracheostomy tube (one size smaller)
- Tracheal dilators (as per local policy)
- Tracheostomy ties and scissors
- Water based lubricant such as KY jelly
- Stoma cleaning equipment
- Dressing pack and non shedding gauze/cotton buds
- Disposable gloves (powder free)
- 2 ml syringes of 0.9% sodium chloride for emergency use (renew every 24 hours)

- Neck roll (roller towel or small blanket)
- Hazardous waste disposal bag.

Caring for a newly formed tracheostomy

In a newly formed tracheostomy, it is customary for the first tube change to be carried out by the ENT surgeon or ANP to ensure that the stoma has healed sufficiently. During the surgery the child will have had sutures inserted on either side of the tracheal opening (stay sutures). If an emergency tube change is required in the first few days postoperatively these sutures can be pulled on to open the stoma and the new tube inserted. These stay sutures are usually removed by the surgeon at the first tube change.

- First tube change is recommended after 1 week, but some hospitals may do it sooner.
- The ENT surgeon or advanced nurse practitioner will perform the first change.
- Vital signs are recorded until the child recovers from the stoma formation.
- Check tube for air entry and observe chest for bilateral chest movement.
- Use a stethoscope to check for equal air entry.
- Tapes' tension should be checked to ensure tension is optimal, not too tight or too loose.
- Observations of the child for signs of complications, e.g. neck swelling, bleeding, surgical emphysema.
- Observe for surgical emphysema, which is swelling caused by air leaking around the tube into the surrounding tissues.

- Secretions may be blood-tinged but should become clear within a few hours.
- Perform hourly suctioning for the first 12–24 hours and then as required.
- Observe for signs of accidental decannulation or tube displacement and take emergency action if either occurs. Tube may be reinserted but force never used.
- Tapes must be checked frequently to ensure that the tapes are secure.
- A newly formed stoma is a surgical wound so will require daily cleaning and dressings according to hospital policy.
- Observe stoma site for signs of inflammation or infection.
- The dressing should be inserted behind the flanges to protect the skin. Never use cotton wool or gauze dressings as loose fibres can be inhaled.
- The dressing should not be bulky as can cause tube displacement.
- Administer humidity via sterile water and elephant tubing.
- Do not use an HME for the first week as child requires extra humidity to prevent occlusion.
- Teach parents how to care for the tracheostomy if it is a long-term intervention.

Suctioning a tracheostomy

Suctioning is a frequent procedure required to remove secretions and maintain a clear airway. The tube can cause irritation resulting in increased mucus production. Second, the tracheostomy prevents the child from increasing intra-abdominal pressure sufficiently to cough and clear secretions normally.

- Suctioning should be dictated by the child's needs rather than being a routine procedure.
- Suctioning is essential if any signs of respiratory distress are observed.
- Some infants and children at risk of hypoxia may require pre-oxygenation prior to suctioning.
- Suctioning is a clean procedure and gloves are usually worn (as per local policy).
- If the tube is fenestrated then an unfenestrated inner tube should be inserted to prevent the catheter going through the fenestration.
- Suction catheters of correct size for the child's tracheostomy (see Table 3.7). Too small a size will not remove secretions efficiently. Too large a size will block the airway, cause bradycardia, and reduced oxygen levels.

Table 3.7 Child suction catheter related to size of tracheostomy

Tracheostomy tube size (mm)	3.0	3.5	4.0	4.5	5.0	6.0	7.0
Recommended suction catheter size (Fr)	7	8	8	10	10	10 12	12

- The catheter should be half the internal diameter of the tracheostomy tube.
- The catheter should only be inserted to 0.5 cm below the length of the tracheostomy tube. Catheters that are too long will cause damage to tracheal mucosa and scarring.
- Suction pressure kept to a minimum as excessive pressure can cause trauma and atelectasis. Generally pressures should be at 60–80 mmHg for newborns and infants and up to 120 mmHg for older children.
- Suction pressure is only applied on withdrawing the catheter to prevent possible mucosal damage.
- If catheters with multiple eyelets are used, rotation is not necessary.
- Suctioning should last for no longer that 5–10 seconds to avoid hypoxia and discomfort.
- Use a clean catheter on each insertion.
- Constantly observe the child during suctioning as there is a risk of causing hypoxia, atelectasis, cardiovascular changes, and pain.
- Observe secretions, e.g. bloodstaining may indicate trauma of the airway.
- Observe secretions for signs of infection, e.g. yellow/green secretions, thicker mucus, and odour.
- Report any changes in secretions and send a specimen for culture and sensitivity.

Methods to loosen secretions

The instillation of 0.9% sodium chloride (NaCl) is potentially hazardous and should not be undertaken routinely with children. Recent evidence suggests that NaCl is unable to mix with mucus and thin the secretions, and it may cause a decrease in oxygen saturations (Ridling et al 2003).Guidelines recommend that greater effort should be made to maintain adequate humidification in order to keep secretions mobile rather than rely on normal saline instillation (American Thoracic Society 2000). Nebulized NaCl is now used in most areas.

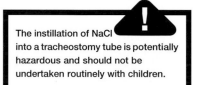

The instillation of NaCl into a tracheostomy tube is potentially hazardous and should not be undertaken routinely with children.

Tracheostomy humidification

During normal respiration air is inhaled through the upper airway (nose, oropharynx and trachea). These normal structures that filter, warm and moisten air are bypassed in the child with a tracheostomy. This results in inadequate humidification and warming of air which can cause thickened secretions, loss of ciliary action and damage to mucous glands. Hence, warming and humidifying the air inspired via a tracheostomy prevents secretions becoming thick and tenacious thus reducing the risk of tube blockage.

- Humidification may be heated, cold or provided via an HME (often termed 'Swedish Nose' or Thermovent) (Edgtton-Winn and Wright 2005)
- Ideally, warm humidification should be used when delivering supplementary oxygen to the child.

- Cold humidification can be used to keep secretions mobile and thus increase tracheobronchial clearance. It may be provided via a nebulizing humidifier.

- The most common method of providing humidity to the child who does not require oxygen is via an HME. This small device is fitted directly to the child's tracheostomy tube and captures exhaled heat and moisture and returns it to the cool, dry air of the next inspiration.

- The HME should be changed every 24 hours or more frequently if it becomes contaminated with secretions or waterlogged.

Stoma site care

The stoma can become soiled by secretions and this can predispose the child to infection and skin irritation. To minimize this risk the stoma site should be cleaned at least daily or more frequently if there are increased secretions. Daily stoma care facilitates inspection of the underlying skin, which is essential as redness or chafing may lead to granulation and unnecessary discomfort.

Depending on local policy either a clean or aseptic technique is used with many healthcare providers favouring a clean technique.

- Clean the stoma site daily and change the ties at least once daily or more frequently if ties become soiled by copious secretions.

- Recommended agent for cleaning the site is 0.9% NaCl and this should be warmed to maintain body temperature at the stoma.

- Cotton wool or dressings that shed fibres should be avoided as these can

be inhaled or trigger an inflammatory response in the stoma (Parker 2000).

- The flange of the tracheostomy tube should also be cleaned.

- Dressings at the tracheostomy site are not used routinely as this may lead to accidental tube displacement. However, this can vary so check your local policy.

- Observe stoma site for signs of inflammation, exudate, and granulation tissue.

- If signs of infection are evident take a swab specimen and send for culture and sensitivity.

Securing the tracheostomy tube

- The tube must be secured in place with suitable ties, e.g. Velcro tapes, cotton ties.

- Velcro tapes are rarely used with infants and children as it is easy for the child to open tapes by tugging which may cause accidental decannulation.

- Cotton ties should be used and tied securely to the side of the neck so that the child is not lying on the knot, and to avoid confusion with other ties such as bibs.

- Only one finger should be able to be placed comfortably under the tapes (to ensure tapes are not too slack or too tight).

Changing the tracheostomy tube

- Regular tube changes are necessary to prevent a build up of secretions, which could block a tube.

- Under normal circumstances tubes can be changed weekly. However, a tube change is not advisable when a child is unwell, tired or irritable.

- Tube change may need to be performed more frequently if secretions are very tenacious and child is showing signs of respiratory distress which is not resolved by suctioning.

- If there are signs of tube obstruction the tube should be changed without delay.

- Once the tube has been changed the child should be closely observed to ensure the problem has been resolved.

  Before the tube change:

- Procedures can be anxiety provoking for the young child and family.

- Need to provide adequate preparation and explanations prior to, during and after this procedure.

- Children will feel less anxious and scared when they know what to expect.

- Explain all aspects of the procedure to the child and parent/carer and gain verbal consent.

- Time a routine tube change appropriately – avoid changing immediately after the child's meal as may cause coughing or vomiting.

- Collect all the equipment required for the procedure.

Procedure for changing a tracheostomy tube

- Two nurses or a nurse assisted by a parent deemed competent in the procedure should perform the procedure.

- Position the child appropriately. A small rolled towel may be placed

under the shoulders to slightly extend the head and improve visibility of the tracheostomy.

- Wash hands.

- Attach the tracheostomy ties to the flange of the new tube.

- Ensure the introducer is properly inserted into the new tracheostomy tube and apply a small amount of lubricant jelly to lubricate the tip (as per local policy).

- Cut the tracheostomy ties and remove the old tube in an outward and downward direction.

- Insert the new tube and immediately remove the introducer.

- Secure the tracheostomy ties on the opposite side of the neck to the old tube.

- If there is difficulty inserting the tube, the smaller tracheostomy tube may be inserted until help is sought.

- If insertion of the smaller tube is unsuccessful, then a suction catheter may be inserted, which will allow some passage of air until help is sought. It is very rare that this happens.

Post tube change principles

- Suction the child if required as tube change may trigger mucus response.

- Observe the child for any respiratory difficulties and reposition child appropriately.

- Document the tube change in the patient notes.

- Dispose of all equipment as per hospital safety and infection control policy.

Communication

A tracheostomy will affect a child's speech and language development. Instead of air passing through the larynx and producing speech it is passed out of the tracheostomy tube which is placed below the level of the larynx. Children with a tracheostomy need to be referred to a speech and language therapist who will identify communication options and methods of developing language skills (Woodnorth 2004). The method of communication should be tailored to the child's preferences and documented so that communication is optimized.

Communication options for the child with a tracheostomy

- Communicating via facial expressions, gestures and body posture.
- Mouth shapes and early sounds (kisses, blowing raspberries).
- Communication aids: pen and paper, alphabet board, laptop, hand held electronic device.
- Sign language.
- Speaking valves (not all children are candidates) – one way valve which is attached to the tracheostomy tube. It closes over as the child exhales and passes air through the larynx and out the mouth.
- 'Pseudovoice' – speech is created by using air trapped in mouth or throat. Can be difficult to understand.
- Electrolarynx – electronic device is held against the neck as the child talks and produces an artificial voice. Can be suitable for older children.

3.8 Acid–base balance

General principles of acid–base balance

- The primary function of the respiratory system is to supply an adequate amount of oxygen (O_2) to tissues and remove carbon dioxide (CO_2).
- The kidneys will excrete any excess acids or alkali.
- The respiratory and renal organs together with the buffering effects of blood maintain hydrogen ion (H^+) concentration. H^+ concentration is one of the most important aspects of acid–base homeostasis.
- When there is an increase or decrease in acid production, blood bicarbonate (HCO_3^-), proteins, and phosphate buffer body fluids (see Table 3.8).
- There comes a point in the disease process when these buffers can no longer maintain appropriate concentrations of H^+.
- Patients in critical care can have life-threatening situations such as diabetic ketoacidosis, asthma, severe vomiting, which alter pH balance and exacerbate their problems.

To maintain homeostasis during stress or illness/diseased states there is generally an increase in depth and rate of breathing due to stimulation of the sympathetic nervous system. High alveolar ventilation brings more O_2 into the alveoli, increasing O_2, and rapidly eliminating CO_2 from the lungs (for chemical abbreviations see Box 3.3).

Table 3.8 The major body buffer systems

Site	Buffer system	Description
Interstitial fluid (ISF)	Bicarbonate Phosphate and protein	For metabolic acids Not important because concentration is too low
Blood	Bicarbonate Haemoglobin Plasma proteins Phosphate	Important for metabolic acids Important for buffering CO_2 and H^+ Minor buffer Concentration too low
Intracellular fluid	Proteins Phosphates	Important buffer of extracellular H^+ Important buffer
Urine	Phosphate Ammonia	Responsible for most of titratable acidity Important – formation of NH_4^+ and hence excretion of H^+
Bone	Calcium carbonate	In prolonged metabolic acidosis

Box 3.3 Chemical abbreviations

Abbreviation	Interpretation
O_2	Oxygen
CO_2	Carbon dioxide
kPa	Kilopascals
pO_2	Partial pressure of oxygen
pCO_2	Partial pressure of carbon dioxide
H^+	Hydrogen ion
HCO_3^-	Bicarbonate ion
H_2CO_3	Carbonic acid
Na^+	Sodium ion
K^+	Potassium ion
Cl^-	Chloride ion
NH_4^+	Ammonium ion

Partial pressure of gases

Dalton's law explains the partial pressure of a gas, which is the pressure exerted by a gas within a mixture of gases independent of each gas in the mixture (Marieb 2004). The partial pressure of each gas is directly proportional to its percentage in the total mixture and in air is determined by atmospheric pressure. Atmospheric pressure is 101 kPa (760 mmHg), 21% of this air is oxygen, and the partial pressure of oxygen (pO_2) in atmospheric air is:

$$\frac{22}{100} \times 101 = 21.2\,kPa$$

Within the alveoli the pO_2 is different to air because of enrichment in the air passages (dead space) with CO_2 and water vapour. Alveolar air contains much more CO_2 and water vapour and much less O_2 and so makes a greater contribution to the near-atmospheric pressure in the lungs, then they do in air. This is due to:

- gas exchanges occurring in the lungs
- humidification of air by the conducting passages
- mixing of gases in the dead space (contains air not involved in gaseous exchange) between the nose and alveoli.

In alveoli pO_2 averages only 13.2 kPa (100 mmHg). Continuous consumption of O_2 and production of CO_2 in the cells means that there is a partial pressure gradient both in the lungs and at the tissue level ensuring diffusion of oxygen into the blood and CO_2 from it.

Changes in partial pressures of carbon dioxide (pCO_2) and H^+ are sensed directly by the respiratory centre central chemoreceptors in the medulla (Guyton and Hall 2000). In contrast, a reduction in pO_2 is monitored by the peripheral chemoreceptors located in the carotid and aortic bodies, which transmit nervous signals to the respiratory centre in the medulla for control of respiration. However, it is the CO_2 'drive' for breathing that dominates in health, although the O_2 'drive' can be significant in some disordered states as an adaptation to chronic evaluations of pCO_2, for example in chronic obstructive lung conditions.

Metabolic generation of acids and alkali

Each day the body produces acids through normal metabolism, and acid or alkali is ingested in diet. The lungs release or strengthen the bond to acids as necessary and the kidneys also effectively eliminate or reabsorb acids, so there is no impact on whole body acid-base status. If there is an increase in production of acids, the body has a number of buffers as outlined in Table 3.8. If there is a reduction in acids or loss of acids the excess bicarbonate (HCO_3^-) is buffered by H^+ to minimize any change in pH.

Normal pH and hydrogen ion concentration of body fluids

The pH is related to actual H^+ concentration (Guyton and Hall 2000). A low pH corresponds to a high H^+ concentration and is evidence of an acidosis, and conversely a high pH corresponds to a low H^+ concentration known as an alkalosis. The interrelationships between O_2, H^+, CO_2 and HCO_3^- are central to the understanding of acid–base balance and reflect the physiological importance of the CO_2/HCO_3^- buffer system (see Box 2.1). The CO_2 / HCO_3^- buffer system largely takes up the majority of the excess H^+. The $H^+ + HCO_3^-$ converts into H_2CO_3 in the presence of carbonic anhydrase (present in red blood cells) and breaks down into CO_2 and water (H_2O) (see Box 2.1). The CO_2/HCO_3^- interaction is slow in plasma, but quicker in red blood cells due to the presence of carbonic anhydrase.

An increase in acids (H^+) in the body is called acidosis.

There are generally two categories of acid accumulation in the body: respiratory acidosis and metabolic acidosis. These are determined if the primary change is either metabolic or respiratory (Table 3.9).

Table 3.9 Acid–base categories and related conditions

Category	The conditions/diseases that lead to acid base abnormalities
Respiratory acidosis – any disorder that interferes with ventilation ($pCO_2 > 5.7$ kPa; pH < 7.35)	Any condition that impairs gas exchange or lung ventilation (chronic bronchitis, cystic fibrosis, emphysema, pulmonary oedema) Rapid, shallow breathing, hypoventilation Narcotic or barbiturate overdose or injury to brain stem Airway obstruction Chest or head injury
Metabolic acidosis ($HCO_3^- < 22$ mmol/l; pH < 7.35)	Severe diarrhoea causing loss of bicarbonate from the intestine Circulatory failure/hypovolaemia Renal disease / failure Untreated diabetes mellitus Starvation Excess alcohol ingestion High ECF potassium concentrations Lactic acid production
Respiratory alkalosis ($pCO_2 < 5.7$ kPa; pH > 7.45)	Direct cause is always hyperventilation (e.g. too much mechanical ventilation, pulmonary lesions) Brain tumour or injury. Acute anxiety Early stages of congestive obstruction airway disease Asthma
Metabolic alkalosis ($HCO_3^- > 26$ mmol/l; pH > 7.40) is the result of excess base bicarbonate ion (HCO_3^-) or decreased hydrogen ion (H^+) concentration, caused by an excessive loss of non-volatile or fixed acids.	Vomiting or gastric suctioning of hydrogen chloride-containing gastric contents: Selected diuretics Ingestion of excessive amount of sodium bicarbonate: Constipation Excess aldosterone (e.g. tumours). Loss of gastrointestinal hydrochloric acid and potassium (e.g. severe vomiting or gastric suctioning) Over-use of potassium wasting diuretics

Respiratory acidosis ($\downarrow$pH $\uparrow$pCO$_2$)

Respiratory acidosis occurs when the respiratory system is unable to eliminate CO_2 produced from cellular metabolism quickly enough (Holmes 1993). An increase in CO_2 increases H^+ ion concentration and the body's pH starts falling below 7.4. However, normally the body is able to particularly maintain acid–base homeostasis, since the increase in pCO$_2$ stimulates central chemoreceptors to increase respiratory rate. When pCO$_2$ can no longer be maintained (for example in COPD), the body can still help to maintain pH by the elimination of excess acid in urine, although this is of a slow onset and will not be so effective in say acute airway obstruction. An individual can live for many years with conditions such as COPD, partly because of the efficiency of renal compensation.

Accumulation of CO$_2$ in respiratory acidosis

It is well known that haemoglobin (Hb) can carry O_2 and CO_2 at the same time, but the presence of one reduces the bonding power of the other, known as the Haldane effect (Carpenter 1991). The Haldane effect is when CO_2 transported in blood is affected by the partial pressure of O_2 in the blood (Marieb 2004). The pO$_2$ in the alveoli normally gives a sufficient pressure (partial pressure) to facilitate CO_2 release from Hb in the alveoli and CO_2 binding in the tissues. The amount of CO_2 transported by Hb in blood is influenced by pO$_2$. When pO$_2$ decreases in conditions such as COPD, the CO_2 is less likely to be released from the Hb; consequently CO_2 levels increase.

In a worsening respiratory acidosis through airway obstruction pO$_2$ decreases in the alveoli and as such cannot sufficiently facilitate the release of CO_2 from Hb. A greater proportion of CO_2 remains attached and will eventually lower pH. The deoxygenated Hb carrying an excess of CO_2 is less likely to bind to O_2, thus exacerbating the problem of poor O_2 uptake. In some conditions administration of oxygen will improve pO$_2$ and facilitate the removal of the accumulated CO_2 from Hb.

Improved release of oxygen in respiratory acidosis

When there is an increase in CO_2 and H^+, as observed in a respiratory acidosis (e.g. COPD), the blood pH will drop. In an acid environment less oxygen can be carried by haemoglobin leading to a reduction of oxygen delivery to cells (Marieb 2004). Conversely, an acid environment in tissues causes haemoglobin (Hb) to release O_2 more readily to cells and facilitates unloading of O_2. This effect is known as the Bohr effect and is an important adaptation to increased acidity in metabolically active tissues. The increased H^+ bind to Hb in red blood cells and alter the structure of the molecules temporarily causing it to release O_2. The Hb molecule therefore gives up its O_2 to tissues under conditions of increased H^+ ion concentration.

Metabolic acidosis ($\downarrow$ pH $\downarrow$ HCO$_3^-$)

Metabolic acidosis occurs when there is excess acid or reduced HCO_3^- in the body (Holmes 1993). Over production or excess H^+ will lead to decreased pH of less than 7.4. This is followed by a reduction in HCO_3^- (used to buffer excess H^+) in an effort to return pH to within the normal range of 7.35–7.45. Body enzymes can only function in a pH range of between 6.80 and 7.80 with reducing pH there is 50% mortality rate at a pH ≤ 6.80.

Compensatory mechanisms for respiratory and metabolic acidosis

When H^+ accumulate in the body chemical buffers in cells and extracellular fluid (ECF) bind with the excess H^+. As H^+ reaches excessive proportions buffers cannot bind with them and blood pH decreases. The compensation for an accumulation of respiratory or metabolic acids occurs in the lungs, and kidneys.

Role of the lungs in compensation

In respiratory acidosis there is a low/normal pO_2 and a high pCO_2 concentration and a low pH. An increase in CO_2 is observed in all tissues and fluids, including cerebrospinal fluid (CSF) and in the medulla oblongata. The CO_2 reacts with H_2O to form H_2CO_3 (quicker in the presence of carbonic anhydrase in red blood cells), that dissociates to H^+ and HCO_3^- (see Box 2.1). When both CO_2 and H^+ are increased in CSF and tissues they have a strong stimulatory effect on central chemoreceptors acting on inspiratory and expiratory muscles leading to an increase in the respiratory rate and depth of breathing (Edwards 2001b).

A reduced pO_2 will also contribute to an increase in ventilation since O_2 saturation will decrease. The role of a reduced O_2 in lung ailments such as pneumonia, asthma or emphysema, plays a major role in increasing respiration via peripheral chemoreceptors and can increase alveolar ventilation as much as five–sevenfold (Guyton and Hall 2000). If the compensation of a deeper and faster respiratory rate is efficient e.g. in asthma it may significantly reduce pCO_2 to maintain O_2 levels (Woodrow 2004). However, the increase in alveolar ventilation may lead to overcompensation and a patient suffering an asthmatic attack may present with a detrimental respiratory alkalosis ($\uparrow$pH $\downarrow pCO_2$) (Figs 3.1 and 3.2).

In metabolic acidosis removal of a proportion of the excess H^+ can occur as CO_2, as the equation presented in Box 2.1 is completely reversible. This allows more H^+ to bind with HCO_3^- to form H_2CO_3 that dissociates to CO_2 and H_2O (see Box 2.1). Respiration is stimulated due to reduction in pH in CSF stimulating central chemoreceptors, leading to hyperventilation. CO_2 is excreted from the body and the arterial pCO_2 therefore reduces.

This explains why patients with a metabolic acidosis have a fast respiratory rate, which further increases as acids continue to rise, and can lead to a reduction in pCO_2 to less than is normal in health (Fletcher and Dhrampal 2003). A complete compensatory respiratory alkalosis through a reduction in CO_2 is unlikely to completely restore normality because, if it were to do so, the compensatory mechanisms would be eradicated. Therefore, in a metabolic acidosis, respiratory compensation is not sufficient alone.

If pCO_2 cannot be reduced and compensation becomes inefficient, in conditions such as a chest infection or asthma pCO_2 may eventually start to rise. This may be an indication to instigate additional interventions such as NIPPV (Butler 2005) or invasive intubation.

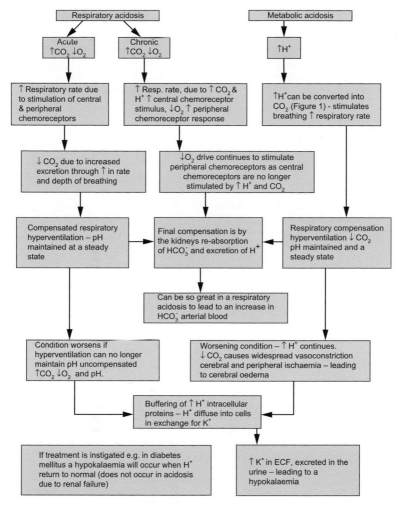

Fig. 3.1 Processes involved in respiratory and metabolic acidosis.

Role of the kidneys in compensation

As blood acidity increases, renal compensatory mechanisms act slowly in maintaining pH (Yucha 2004).

In respiratory acidosis excess CO_2 can be converted through the equation in Box 2.1. The retained CO_2 combines with H_2O to form large amounts of H_2CO_3.

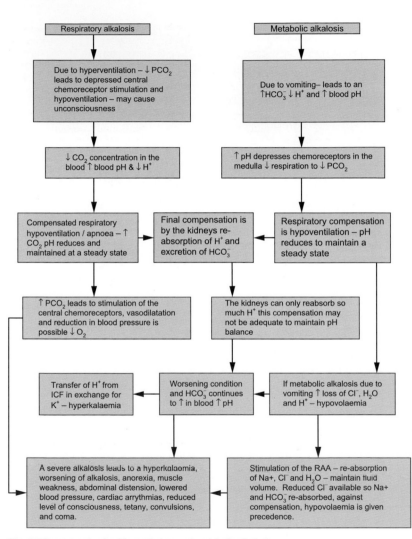

Fig. 3.2 Processes involved in respiratory and metabolic alkalosis.

In the kidneys H_2CO_3 dissociates to release free H^+ and HCO_3^-, and stimulates the kidneys to retain HCO_3^- and sodium ions (Na^+), and excrete H^+. The HCO_3^- retained is recirculated and helps to buffer further free H^+.

Similar effects occur in a metabolic acidosis. After about 30 minutes the kidneys start to compensate for the acidosis by secreting excess H^+ secreted in the renal tubule and excreted in the urine as weak acids (Yucha 2004). For every H^+ ion secreted into the renal tubule, a sodium and bicarbonate ion is reabsorbed and returned to the blood. The pH is unlikely to be completely restored as this would reduce the efficiency of compensatory mechanisms. CO_2 and HCO_3^- will be far from their normal values, as a consequence of altered buffering capacity and respiratory compensation.

It takes around 3 days for a patient to have established a steady state of compensation (e.g. a respiratory hyperventilation) (Guyton and Hall 2000). The kidney can only retain so much HCO_3^- with the consequence that the blood contains a higher concentration of HCO_3^- than produced by the CO_2 retention alone (see Box 2.1), hence an improved base excess (BE).

H^+ buffer by intracellular proteins in exchange for K^+

If the concentration in H^+ in extracellular fluid rises to a level beyond the compensatory mechanism H^+ move into cells by simple diffusion to be buffered by intracellular proteins, in exchange for potassium ions (K^+) (Holmes 1993). As cells need to maintain a balanced membrane charge cells release K^+ into blood in exchange for H^+, this may lead to a high blood K^+ (hyperkalaemia) and characteristic changes in the ECG (peaked T waves and abnormal QRS complexes) may be observed (Richards and Edwards 2008). However, with normal renal functions the majority of excess ECF K^+ will be excreted in urine. If normal ventilation is restored or the acidosis is treated for example in diabetic ketoacidosis is treated with insulin and glucose, the K^+ will return into the intracellular fluid (ICF) in exchange for H^+ and the patient may then develop a hypokalaemia.

Decrease or loss of acids (H^+) in the body (alkalosis)

There are generally two categories of reduced acids in the body: a respiratory alkalosis and a metabolic alkalosis (see Table 3.9). These two conditions stimulate compensatory mechanisms that serve to maintain acid base homeostasis.

Respiratory alkalosis ($\uparrow$ pH $\downarrow$pCO$_2$)

Respiratory alkalosis occurs when the respiratory system eliminates too much CO_2. This reduction of pCO$_2$ below the range of 4.5–5.6 kPa (30–35 mmHg) causes a reduction in H^+ generation. The decreasing H^+ concentration raises the blood pH above the normal range of 7.45. Any condition that causes hyperventilation can cause a respiratory alkalosis.

Processes of carbon dioxide excretion

When ventilation is increased above the normal rate excessive amounts of CO_2 are excreted in expired air. In this situation CO_2 is washed out of the body leading to a hypocapnia the pH rises. A rise in pH is sensed by central chemoreceptors in the medulla and CSF. Both CO_2 and H^+ concentration are reduced resulting in a decrease in ventilation. This reduces the elimination of CO_2 and reduces pH to within the normal range. Arterial blood gas analysis will show a lowered pCO_2 and respiratory rate may be decreased in both depth and rate.

Binding of Hb and O_2 in alkaline states

When there is a decrease in CO_2 and H^+ the pH will rise and consequently more oxygen remains bound to Hb in the tissues (Marieb 2004). Oxygen delivery to cells is therefore reduced as the Hb/O_2 bond is strengthened (the Bohr effect). This will maintain O_2 saturation, but not cellular oxygen delivery. Therefore, the apparent normality of O_2 saturation can be misleading in an alkalosis.

Metabolic alkalosis ($\uparrow$ pH $\uparrow$ HCO_3^-)

Metabolic alkalosis (HCO_3^- > 26 mmol/l; pH > 7.40) is the result of excess HCO_3^- or decreased H^+ concentration, caused by an excessive loss of non-volatile or fixed acids. Metabolic alkalosis over excites central and peripheral nervous systems.

Compensatory mechanisms for respiratory and metabolic alkalosis

When the body HCO_3^- increases in ECF these bind with H^+. As the bicarbonate reaches excessive proportions H^+ cannot bind with them sufficiently to buffer the consequences of pH and blood pH increases. The compensation for a respiratory or metabolic alkalosis occurs in the lungs, kidneys and by the release of H^+ from cells.

Role of the lungs in compensation

In alkaline environments blood H^+ has been lost or there is an excess base HCO_3^-. The unbound excess HCO_3^- elevates blood pH. The arterial blood will show a pH above 7.45, a pCO_2 below 4.5 kPa (35 mmHg) and HCO_3^- above 26 mmol/l. In an alkalosis blood and tissues give up more H^+ as a compensatory response (Edwards 2008). So as HCO_3^- starts to accumulate in the body H^+ combines with it to form H_2CO_3; this chemical reaction buffers excess HCO_3^-.

An increase in blood pH is sensed in the CSF and depresses respiratory centre central chemoreceptors in the medulla. This reduces respiration, CO_2 is retained in an attempt to increase blood pCO_2 and decrease pH. However, this is limited since as the reduction in respiratory rate and depth lowers O_2 levels. The reduced CO_2 and H^+ observed in a metabolic alkalosis combine to form two powerful respiratory inhibitory effects on the peripheral chemoreceptors opposing the excitatory effects of a diminished oxygen concentration (Guyton and Hall 2000). A blood sample taken now will show decreasing HCO_3^- and pH as the body attempts to compensate (Woodrow 2004).

Role of the kidneys in compensation

After approximately six hours the kidneys start to increase excretion of HCO_3^- and reduce the excretion of H^+. This renal compensation returns the plasma H^+ concentration towards normal and urine will be very alkaline with a high pH. To maintain electrochemical balance, excess sodium ions (Na^+) and chloride ions (Cl^-) are excreted along with HCO_3^-. This can lead to hyponatraemia.

The decreasing pH may in turn cause the respiratory centre chemoreceptors to increase respiratory rate and consequently a compensatory hyperventilation may ensue. If the pCO_2 becomes too low, due to the hyperventilation, this imposes a respiratory alkalosis on top of the metabolic alkalosis and hence metabolic compensation may not be adequate (Yucha 2004). At this stage the patient could have bradypnoea or Cheyne–Stokes respiration.

A prolonged alkaline environment leads to vasoconstriction, which increases cerebral and peripheral hypoxia (Fig. 3.2). As alkalosis becomes more severe calcium ions increasingly bind to proteins and so hypocalcaemia develops. This increases nerve excitability and muscle contractions. If left untreated an alkalosis can put excess strain on the heart and central nervous system.

Alkalosis in severe vomiting

An alkalosis can be seriously exacerbated if there is a severe drop in circulating volume, for example in vomiting. In persistent vomiting of gastric contents, electrolytes are no longer available to the body from the alimentary canal to replace those lost in the vomit and in urine (Na^+, Cl^-, HCO_3^-). The principal electrolytes, in addition to water lost as a result of vomiting gastric contents, are:

- hydrochloric acid (hydrogen and chloride ions)
- sodium chloride (sodium and chloride ions).

The single electrolyte lost in greatest amounts is Cl^-, as a result the plasma Cl^- concentration falls. A loss of fluid and plasma volume due to vomiting can lead to a hypovolaemic state, which can affect acid–base balance.

Compensation for a hypovolaemia will impose powerful compensatory mechanisms stimulating the kidney to release renin from the juxtaglomerular apparatus stimulating the adrenal gland to release aldosterone. The effect of aldosterone promotes sodium (Na^+) and chloride (Cl^-) reabsorption (and hence water) in the renal tubules to maintain circulating volume in exchange for K^+ and H^+.

The low concentration of chloride in the plasma results in a relatively small filtered load of Cl^- by comparison with Na^+. There are less chloride ions to balance the reabsorption of sodium. The body cannot respond by reducing Na^+ reabsorption, which is required to restore circulating volume. The only mechanism available to the kidney is to increase the re-absorption of Na^+ and HCO_3^- and consequently increase the excretion of K^+ and H^+. Vomiting therefore leads to processes of Na^+ and HCO_3^- re-absorption, K^+ and H^+ loss due to excess Cl^- depletion because of vomiting. This triggers mechanisms that are inappropriate in an existing alkalosis (Fig. 3.1). The retention of electrolytes and fluid during a hypovolaemia takes precedence over acid–base homeostasis.

A cautious intravenous infusion of isotonic sodium chloride solution at this stage may improve the patient's hypovolaemia. The replacement of the principal ECF electrolytes necessary (e.g. Na^+ and Cl^- will return fluid volume towards normal). It switches the drive from retention of Na^+ and HCO_3^- and excretion of K^+ and H^+, to those of correction of metabolic alkalosis (e.g. the retention of H^+, Na^+ and Cl^- and excretion of K^+ and HCO_3), putting the acid–base problem in order.

H^+ release from cells in exchange for ECF K^+

A decreased H^+ level in ECF causes H^+ to diffuse passively out of cells to buffer excess HCO_3^-. To maintain balance of charge across the cell membrane, ECF K^+ moves into cells. When K^+ cannot be replaced by absorption in the alimentary tract there is a severe depletion of the body's total ECF K^+ content (hypokalaemia), which can ultimately lead to confusion and arrhythmias (Richards and Edwards 2008).

The primary function of the respiratory system is to supply an adequate amount of oxygen to tissues and remove carbon dioxide. The kidneys will excrete any excess acids or alkali. The respiratory and renal organs, together with the blood, maintain hydrogen ion concentration. Hydrogen ion concentration is one of the most important aspects of acid–base homeostasis. When there is an increase or decrease in acid production by body tissues, the blood bicarbonate, proteins, and phosphate buffer body fluids or both. There comes a point in the disease process when these buffers can no longer maintain adequate concentrations of hydrogen ions. Patients admitted to hospital can have life-threatening situations, which alter pH balance.

3.9 Caring for a child in a variety of settings

Acutely/critically ill child

Critical illness has a major impact on the child and family. The diagnostic groups include:

- prematurity/dysmaturity
- respiratory illness
- surgical conditions, e.g. gastroschisis, tracheo-oesphageal fistula, imperforate anus
- congenital anomalies, e.g. congenital heart disease
- postnatal problems
- postoperative monitoring
- medical conditions, e.g. meningitis, sepsis.

Children may be classified by age:

- preterm neonates (gestational age < 37 weeks)
- newborn (= 40 weeks)
- neonates (0–30 days).

Early warning systems

Early identification and management of a deteriorating child is a crucial aspect of paediatric critical care. Clinical deterioration is impossible to reliably predict and can lead to life-threatening conditions, such as cardiopulmonary failure. The use of paediatric early warning systems therefore has a vital role to play in the management of acutely or critically ill children. Nurses must be trained to implement and interpret early warning assessment tools, as serious complications can arise if the results of such tools are misunderstood or improperly acted upon.

Severity of illness may be measured at admission by either of two validated scores: the Pediatric Risk Mortality Score (PRISM) (Pollack et al 1988) for neonates and children; the Clinical Risk Index for Babies (CRIB) (International Neonatal Network 1993) for the preterm neonates.

Assessment

■ Temperature, heart and respiratory rate, respiratory effort and blood pressure should be recorded initially and then recorded again at varying intervals. Good record keeping allows trends in vital signs to be spotted and can prevent or halt deterioration.

■ Increased work of breathing is an indicator of respiratory distress and should be noted during intake and observation.

■ Signs of increased breathing work include nasal flare, see-saw breathing, and recession of the supraclavicular region, sternal and substernal regions, and subintercostal and intercostal regions.

■ Fatigue may develop as a consequence of increased work of breathing. Infants and young children are more susceptible to respiratory fatigue because their breathing relies heavily on the diaphragm, and the diaphragm's low muscular twitch fibres make it prone to fatigue.

■ Muscle fatigue can either suddenly or progressively lead to respiratory failure

and therefore must be closely monitored and treated.

■ Cardiovascular assessment in the acutely ill child is a cornerstone of paediatric clinical care.

■ To carry out cardiovascular assessment effectively, the physiological and anatomical differences between the cardiovascular systems of infants, children and adults must be properly understood.

■ To begin, the heart's cardiac output (volume of blood pumped through the body over the course of one minute) is related to heart rate and stroke volume, whereby an increase in either one or both leads to an increase in cardiac output. In adults, cardiac output is influenced by stroke volume (quantity of blood pushed into the ventricles by each contraction); in infants and children, cardiac output is influenced by heart rate (beats per minute). This is an important distinction to be made, because respiratory distress, exercise and fever all increase the cardiac output of infants and children, making heart rate an important signpost during evaluation.

■ Evaluation of cardiac function requires a complete physical examination of the child: respiratory function, body/extremity temperature, skin colour, capillary refill time and abdominal distension should all be noted.

■ Particular signs to watch out for include
 – pyrexia (may signify infection)
 – lower temperatures in extremities (compromised peripheral perfusion if the environmental temperature is comfortable)

- depression in the chest wall (indicative of accessory muscle use during respiratory distress)
- abnormal neck vein pulsation/ appearance (sometimes occurs in congestive heart failure)
- abdominal distension (may signify right-sided heart failure and hepatomegaly).

■ Areas for palpating pulse are the same in both children and adults, and include points along the dorsal pedis, brachial, radial and femoral arteries.

■ It is recommended that the peripheral pulse of a child or infant be taken from the brachial artery, with the femoral or carotid arteries providing good central pulse measurements.

■ Auscultation is used to measure the apical pulse rate and identify heart characteristics and abnormalities. The apical pulse should mirror the brachial and radial pulse rates.

■ Raised heart rate can indicate septic shock or other serious illness. Other early warning indicators include abnormal respiration, dehydration, delayed capillary refill, cool extremities, poor skin turgor and low heart rate.

■ The following signs may indicate an intermediate risk for serious illness: abnormal communication and response;
- flared nasal passages
- reduced passing of urine
- oxygen saturation equal to or less than 95% in air
- fever which persists for five days or longer.

Children presenting with respiratory disease should be admitted for critical care if any of the following conditions are present:

■ requiring endotracheal intubation
■ children with chronic respiratory problems requiring mechanical ventilation with tracheostomy
■ progressive pulmonary disease at risk of progressing to respiratory obstruction or failure
■ requiring supplemental oxygen
■ patients with tracheostomy
■ requiring apnoea evaluation or cardiorespiratory supervision.

Children presenting with cardiovascular disease should be admitted for critical care if any of the following conditions are present:

■ non-life-threatening dysrhythmias that do not require cardioversion
■ non-life-threatening cardiac disease that necessitates low-dose intravenous inotropic or vasodilator therapy
■ undergoing cardiac procedures requiring post-surgical monitoring, and where haemodynamic/respiratory compromise is absent
■ undergoing closed-heart cardiovascular and intrathoracic procedures.

Children presenting with neurological disease should be admitted for critical care if any of the following conditions are present:

■ seizures that respond to treatment but which require cardiorespiratory monitoring, and where haemodynamic compromise is present
■ requiring neurological evaluation due to altered sensorium, and where neurological deterioration is likely

- having undergone neurosurgery which requires postoperative cardiorespiratory monitoring
- presenting with CNS inflammation/infection where neurological problems are present
- progressive neuromuscular dysfunction which requires cardiorespiratory monitoring and where altered sensorium is present.

Children presenting with haematological/oncological disease should be admitted for critical care if any of the following conditions are present:

- severe anaemia where haemodynamic/respiratory problems are present
- sickle cell crisis complications where acute chest syndrome is present
- neutropenia, thrombocytopenia, anaemia or solid tumour where a risk of cardiopulmonary problems is present.

Children presenting with endocrine/metabolic disease should be admitted for critical care if any of the following conditions are present:

- diabetic ketoacidosis (blood glucose < 500 mg/dl) that necessitates insulin infusion, and where altered sensorium is present
- metabolic/electrolyte abnormalities that necessitate cardiac monitoring, such as hypokalaemia, hyponatraemia and hypernatraemia, hypocalcaemia/hypercalcaemia, hypoglycaemia/hyperglycaemia, and metabolic acidosis
- other inborn metabolic problems that may require cardiorespiratory monitoring.

Children presenting with gastrointestinal disease should be admitted for critical care if any of the following conditions are present:

- acute gastrointestinal bleeding and where haemodynamic or respiratory instability is present
- emergency endoscopy where cardiorespiratory compromise is present
- chronic gastrointestinal insufficiency and where coma or haemodynamic or respiratory instability is present.

Children who have undergone surgery and show signs of haemodynamic or respiratory instability should be admitted for critical care if any of the following conditions are present:

- requiring postoperative care after cardiovascular, thoracic, neurosurgical, upper/lower airway or craniofacial surgery
- thoracic or abdominal trauma
- requiring treatment for numerous traumatic injuries.

Children with renal disease should be admitted for critical care if any of the following conditions are present:

- hypertension which necessitates oral/intravenous medication on a frequent intermittent basis and where seizures and encephalopathy are present
- nephrotic syndrome and chronic hypertension
- renal failure at any age
- requiring chronic haemodialysis or peritoneal dialysis.

Discharge of a child from high dependency care to general care

This should occur when the following conditions are met:

- stable haemodynamic measurements which span for no fewer than 6–12 hours prior to discharge
- extubation and stable respiratory status which spans for more than four hours prior to discharge
- reduced oxygen requirements (< 0.4 of fraction of inspired oxygen)
- reduced or no further doses of intravenous inotropic support, vasodilators and antiarrhythmic medication
- cardiac arrhythmias which are managed for no fewer than 24 hours prior to discharge
- neurological stability and an absence of seizures
- removal of haemodynamic monitoring such as arterial lines
- return to baseline status amongst patients given mechanical ventilation.

Critical illness and malnutrition

Critical illness has a major impact on the nutritional status of the child. Research has found that the nutritional status of patients admitted to the PICU was poorer than that of the general population (Hulst et al 2003). Protein-energy malnutrition that develops during an ICU stay is associated with an increase in morbidity and mortality.

- Duration of the patient's stay in PICU is associated with negative nutritional status after discharge.
- Malnutrition is associated with poor growth and reduced or delayed mental and psychomotor development.
- Malnourishment that emerges during the course of a child's PICU stay is most likely the result of poor nutritional intake, interrupted feeding or under-prescribing.
- Nutritional assessment upon admission should help to identify children at higher risk of malnutrition and optimize their nutritional support.

The unconscious child

Unconsciousness – also referred to as coma – is caused by severe impairment of both cerebral hemispheres of the brain or a loss of function to the reticular activating system. Arousal and consciousness are regulated by the reticular activating system, an area of the brain comprised of neuronal circuits connecting the cortex to the brainstem. The unconscious person is unable to respond to stimuli, and unlike someone in deep sleep, the unconscious person cannot be roused or made aware of their self and their surroundings. Unconsciousness can be short in duration (such as that brought about by acute illness), long-term or indefinite in length (Peate and McGrory 2009).

Brain injury, acute illness or intoxication can cause dysfunction in the reticular activating system. In cases where the cause of unconsciousness cannot be treated, a child will continue to pass into decreasing levels of consciousness.

Consciousness can be categorized into the following six levels of altered arousal:

- *Confusion*: slowed cognition, impaired judgement.

- *Disorientation*: inability to think clearly about time or place, compromised memory and poor recognition of self.

- *Lethargy*: impaired speech and motion but can be aroused into wakefulness.

- *Obtundation*: very limited responsiveness to external stimuli, passes into sleep easily and give only minimal responses to questions.

- *Stupor*: deep unresponsiveness which can be broken only through extensive physical or verbal stimulation.

- *Coma*: complete lack of responsiveness to all external stimuli.

Unconsciousness may be brought about by:

- *Seizure*: changes in the brain and the chemical overstimulation of the brain can cause unconsciousness.

- *Heart/lung disease*: hypoxaemia and, in consequence, inadequate levels of oxygen-rich blood flowing to the brain can induce unconsciousness as a result of poor heart and lung function.

- *Tumour or haematoma*: pressure exerted between the brain and skull from a tumour or haematoma can cause brain malfunction and unconsciousness.

- *Traumatic brain injury*.

- *Cardiac arrest*: oxygen-rich blood ceases to reach the brain, leading to malfunction.

- *Infection*: damage to, or malfunction of, the brain can be caused by meningitis or pyrexia from septicaemia.

- *Asphyxiation*: leading to deprivation of oxygen and brain malfunction.

- *Alcohol misuse/recreational drugs*: may cause slowed brain function and low blood oxygen levels, resulting in coma and death if untreated.

- *Carbon monoxide poisoning*: commonly resulting from household poisoning or attempted suicide; carbon monoxide in blood deprives the brain of oxygen, inducing malfunction and unconsciousness.

Vegetative state

Vegetative state (VS) can be described as a condition of sleep–wake cycles in which patients experience wakefulness but lack awareness of their self and their surroundings (Ashwal 2004). This owes to the fact that with VS, the autonomic functions of the hypothalamus and brain stem are either entirely or partially preserved. VS in children is most commonly the result of either:

- acute traumatic brain injury caused by, for instance, motor vehicle accident

- hypoxic ischaemic encephalopathy resulting from oxygen deprivation to the brain caused by, for instance, near-drowning or sudden infant death syndrome

- some metabolic or degenerative diseases in children that progress to a permanent VS with unexpected recovery

- severe congenital CNS disorders (e.g. anencephaly, hydranencephaly) cause VS in infants, with the likelihood of significant neurological improvement being very improbable.

Following acute brain injury, most children fall into a coma and then progress into sleep–wake cycles after a few days to a few weeks.

The signs of VS are:

- interpersonal communication is not possible
- no awareness of one's self or one's surroundings
- no language comprehension/ construction
- no voluntary responses to external stimuli
- erratic periods of wakefulness caused by sleep–wake cycles
- fully or partially functioning cranial nerve and spinal reflexes
- incontinence of bowel and bladder.

Vegetative state and related conditions

- *Persistent VS*: no awareness of self or surroundings; does not perceive pain; sleep-wake cycles are intact; no intentional motor function; normal or somewhat depressed respiration; EEG reveals polymorphic delta/theta; variable prognosis for neurological recovery.
- *Coma*: no awareness of self or surroundings; does not perceive pain; no sleep–wake cycles; no intentional motor function; depressed or somewhat depressed respiration; EEG reveals polymorphic delta/theta; neurologic recovery, VS or death ordinarily occurs within 2–4 weeks.
- *Brain death*: no awareness of self or surroundings; does not perceive pain; no sleep–wake cycles; no intentional motor function; no respiration; EEG reveals electrocerebral silence; no

possible outcome of neurological recovery.

- *Minimally conscious state*: awareness of self exists; perceives pain; sleep–wake cycles are intact; intentional but limited motor function present; normal or somewhat depressed respiration; EEG reveals polymorphic delta/theta; variable prognosis for neurological recovery (Ashwal 2004).

Assessment scales:

- Glasgow Coma Scale (GCS) has widespread application amongst health care practitioners for scoring a patient's level of consciousness and determining a course of treatment. The GCS is most suited for long-term monitoring and sets parameters for the evaluation of body temperature, pulse, blood pressure, respiratory rate, motor response, degree of eye opening and level of verbal responsiveness (see Section 2 for full discussion of this scale).
- Alert, Voice, Pain, Unresponsive (AVPU) scale is a less detailed assessment tool, which is most suited for the early assessment of a patient's level of unconsciousness. The AVPU scale is comprised of alertness, verbal/ motor response, pain response, and level of unresponsiveness (see Section 2 for full discussion of this scale).

Management of the unconscious child

Unconsciousness causes a person's normal protective reflexes to be inoperative, placing huge responsibility on the health care team to provide ongoing care that supports basic functioning (Peate and McGrory 2009). The skills required are:

- Medical and nursing care that has the potential to support the autonomic function of the hypothalamus and brain stem.

- Keep the airway clear – may require ventilatory support or tracheostomy.

- Closely monitor respiratory and cardiac function.

- Evaluate neurological status frequently.

- Appropriate patient positioning to minimize airway obstruction.

- Regular respiratory care and monitoring is necessary to reduce aspiration pneumonia.

- Enteral or parental nutrition – may require gastrostomies for nutritional support.

- Interchanging urinary catheterization with diapers may reduce the risk of urinary tract infections, which are common amongst patients in VS.

- Pressure area care and skin care should occur on a daily basis.

- Medical procedures required to care for intensive care patients – such as mechanical ventilation, cannula and airway suctioning – are unpleasant and painful, making it particularly important to monitor and discern the pain experienced by uncommunicative, sedated or unconscious patients.

- Physiological changes, such as rapid heart rate or rising blood pressure, can serve as indicators of pain.

- Directly observable physiological changes are important signposts of pain, such as changes in facial expression, tears and grimacing.

- When assessing pain in the unconscious patient, one should bear in mind that while behavioural response does not necessarily depend on a particular level of arousal, sedation in patients may mute physiological signs which would otherwise present themselves as strong indicators of pain.

- Certain drugs may alter vital signs, rendering physiological evidence (such as heart rate, blood pressure, sweating, shaking, etc.) less valid measures.

- It is important to conduct pain assessments regularly and ensure adequate analgesia.

Communication with the unconscious child

- The emotional needs of the unconscious patient are easily overlooked in critical care nursing, but it is important to remember that not all non-responsive patients are unable to hear or feel someone's presence (Endean 2006).

- Research has found that some unconscious and unresponsive patients are aware of their surroundings and the people who visit and care for them (Woodward 2008).

- It is essential to communicate with patients diagnosed as in a fully vegetative state, as misdiagnosis abounds and 'vegetative' patients may in fact have some level of awareness.

- Although awareness of one's surroundings is quite rare amongst fully unresponsive patients, the use of functional MRI for fully unconscious patients has emerged in recent years as a diagnostic indicator for awareness of one's surroundings (Woodward 2008).

- Nurses should educate family members and other carers about the importance of addressing the patient's psychological needs by comforting the person through physical touch and verbal communication.

- The patient's privacy and dignity should be upheld at all times regardless of their level of consciousness or communicative ability.

Positioning of an unconscious child

Repositioning of the unconscious and conscious child is a fundamental and essential care element that nurses undertake on a regular basis. It is important to stress the need to correctly position and reposition children frequently and/or as their physical condition allows.

With decreased movement an unconscious patient becomes vulnerable to skin breakdown due to problems associated with pressure, moisture, shearing forces and diminished sensation.

- The child should be turned from side to side in the lateral or semiprone position at least every 2 hours, unless contraindicated.

- The reason for regular repositioning is so that there is a change to the distribution of ventilation and blood flow through the lungs and mobilization of secretions.

- This will also have an enhanced effect on the cardiopulmonary system in that changing ventilation and perfusion of the lungs through gravitational effects enhances oxygen transportation.

- Despite the advent of pressure relieving aids and specialist mattresses and beds, it remains the case that an immobile patient who is not regularly turned will develop pressure sores.

The 'log roll' technique

The *'log roll'* technique is used when there are concerns about the stability of the spinal column and that there may be damage caused by adopting the traditional turning manoeuvre. This technique is a labour intensive process and requires numerous individuals: one to support the head, and two on either side of the patient. A modified 'log rolling' technique is also used when nursing the child prone; like log rolling it is a labour intensive process and requires experienced staff to prevent further complications (e.g. extubation).

Procedure

- The individual at the head end of the bed should be a qualified nurse or doctor experienced in log rolling and airway management.

- The other four individuals will manage the torso, arms and legs.

- When everyone is in position and ready for the manoeuvre, the leader will indicate when turning is to take place.

Children's hygiene requirements

Children are sometimes unable to care for their personal hygiene due to the very nature of their often sedated or unconscious state.

General hygiene

There is some evidence that washing/bathing children before they go to bed rather than in the morning is beneficial. Whatever time is chosen to wash, it must be remembered that regular mouth care, eye care and pressure area care must be performed.

- Washing or bathing may be influenced by factors such as whether the child is sedated.
- If the child is not sedated then the nurse should negotiate with the patient/parent or guardian when the best time may be.
- Night-time washes are often encouraged because it ensures the child's energy is conserved for morning activities.
- Early night-time washes are beneficial as they facilitate long periods of uninterrupted rest to counteract the effects of sleep deprivation and sensory overload.

Mouth care

Drug therapies such as steroids may increase the pathogenicity of these organisms, leading to local and systemic infections. Oral complications can lead to pain, ulcers, infection, bone and dentition changes and bleeding and functional disorders affecting verbal and non-verbal communication, chewing and swallowing, taste and respiration. Therefore, mouth care is an important element of nursing care. See the assessment and scoring tool for mouth care (Box 3.4).

The aim of oral care is to:

- keep the mucosa clean, soft, moist and intact and in doing so prevent infection
- keep lips clean, soft, moist and intact

- remove food debris as well as dental plaque without damaging the gingiva
- alleviate pain and discomfort and enhance oral intake
- prevent dental plaque formation and bacterial colonization
- reduce problems associated with dry mouth and identify early any problems that may require medical treatment
- prevent halitosis and freshen the mouth.

Mouth care involves:

1. Cleaning the teeth with toothpaste and toothbrush after meals.
2. Chlorhexidine gluconate 0.2% 5 ml, four times a day diluted in 100 ml of water which should be retained in the mouth for at least 1 minute before discarding.

Eye care

Eye care of unconscious children is paramount in preventing eye damage, infection and promoting comfort. Normal protective mechanisms like blinking and tear production are often impaired in patients who are receiving sedative drugs or are unconscious. In an unconscious child the blink reflex is lost and the eyes are not flushed or cleaned. Eye infections can result in permanent damage to the eye (e.g. loss of vision). Red, inflamed or oedematous eyes will result in patients becoming distressed, agitated and experiencing pain.

Eye care involves:

- Examining patient's eyes regularly. If the child is conscious and able to interact make sure that you get their permission and explain what you are doing.

Box 3.4 Assessment tool for the mouth

	1 (Low)	2 (Medium)	3 (High)
Lips	Mouth, pink and moist	Dry or cracked	Ulcerated, inflamed or bleeding
Teeth/ dentures	Clean and no debris	Plaque or debris in localized areas	Plaque and covered with debris
Gingiva (gums)	Pink and moist	Dry, oedematous in localized areas	Red, shiny, oedematous with ulceration. Bleeding spontaneously or with pressure
Mucous membranes	Pink and moist	Red, inflamed. May have a white coating	Very red, blistered and/or ulcerated, with or without bleeding
Tongue	Pink, moist and papillae present	Slightly coated, loss of papillae with or without reddened areas, slightly dry	Heavily coated, blistered or cracked, very dry
Saliva	Thin, watery	Thick and tenacious	Little or absent
Swallow	Normal gag reflex, swallows without difficulty	Diminished gag reflex, difficulty in swallowing	No gag reflex an/or unable to swallow
Breathing	Self ventilating	Ventilatory support via CPAP or BPAP, with or without tracheostomy	Fully ventilated via oral ET tube or tracheostomy

Score	**Recommendations**
8 (low risk)	3 hourly moistening of mouth with foam sticks and water. Brush teeth × 1 per shift using toothbrush and toothpaste
9–18 (medium risk)	2 hourly moistening of mouth with foam sticks and water. Brush teeth × 1 per shift using toothbrush and toothpaste
>19 (high risk)	1–2 hourly moistening of mouth with foam stick. Brush teeth × 2 per shift using toothbrush and toothpaste
	Discuss with Consultant and treat with Chlorhexidine mouth gel applied topically to teeth and gums 4–6 hourly after brushing
	Obtain oral swab, if candida present treat appropriately, e.g. Difflam Oral rinse. If patient has herpes zoster/simplex consider antifungal cream applied topically every 4 hours

- If the child's eyes are clean and they have an intact blink reflex then it is acceptable to leave them and reassess every few hours.

- Look for any discharge or cloudiness, ulceration or scratching of the cornea and assess the blink reflex (this may be absent in sedated patients).

- Note any differences between the eyes or changes from any previous documented assessments.

- If there is evidence of red eye, cloudiness, ulceration or discharge report this immediately so that an appropriate medical referral can be made.

- If the eyes appear to need cleaning (they may be 'crusty' or have a discharge) clean the eye with sterile water.

- Wipe from the inner part of the eye (closest to the nose) to the outer part to remove any discharge or 'crust'.

- Use a new piece of gauze for each pass and treat the upper lid before the lower. Always wash your hands before beginning this procedure and when moving from cleaning one eye to the other.

- Always treat a clean eye before one that appears to have a problem.

- If the patient's eyes appear dry speak to the doctors about the use of appropriate drops or ointment.

Eye care procedure

- Equipment required: 2 gallipots (one for the left and one for the right eye), sterile gauze and water.

- Cleaning – use each piece of gauze one only, clean from the inside out.

- Should be undertaken at least 4 times daily for patients without any problem.

- Observation – every 2 hourly, look for redness, discharge or corneal clouding, in these instances eye care should be increased.

- Eye drops – artificial tears (hypromellose, viscotears), these are not routinely used, but prescribed if corneal wetting is inadequate. There should be two bottles of eye drops one for each eye and clearly labelled L and R.

- Antibiotics – may be needed if the eye(s) are red or discharge is present, a conjunctiva swab may be required and sent for microscopy, culture and sensitivity (MC&S).

- Geliperm – may be used to keep the eye closed as it will not cause trauma or irritation, it reduces tear evaporation, prevents infection, keeps eyelids closed and its transparency allows constant observation.

Risk factors for unconscious children

- Exposure to keratopathy – caused by incomplete lid closure

- Dry eyes – drugs or exposure induced

- Infection – mostly pathogens from the respiratory tract (*Pseudomonas* and *Pneumococcus*)

- Ventilator eye – conjunctival chemosis (oedema) caused by IPPV and PEEP.

Pre- and postoperative care

There has been a considerable increase in the use of day surgery for children who require surgical procedures. Day surgery is seen as optimal as children encounter fewer strangers and remain united with their parents throughout most or all of their hospitalization. However, the fast throughput of patients can result in children feeling unprepared and anxious.

Children experience a range of stressors and fears about:

- admission process
- meeting unfamiliar healthcare professionals
- being transported to the theatre
- being separated from parents
- induction of anaesthesia
- undergoing blood tests
- injections and needle sticks
- operation
- receiving medications
- recovery after surgery
- staying in hospital.

Anxiety is a stress response that can suppress the immune system and hence increase pain response, delay wound healing and recovery. Research on postoperative outcomes in children has shown an association between preoperative anxiety and increased frequency of emergence delirium, increased levels of pain and increased frequency of maladaptive postoperative behaviours (Kain et al 2007). Therefore the reduction of anxiety for the child and parents is an important aspect of pre- and postoperative care. When children are adequately prepared for surgery, their coping ability is enhanced and anxiety is lessened (Brewer et al 2006).

Techniques aimed at reducing children's pre- and postoperative anxiety fall into two categories:

- non-medical interventions (e.g. preadmission programmes, supervised play, distraction, parental presence at induction, parental participation, and teaching sessions)
- sedative premedication (e.g. oral midazolam).

A review of studies which measure either form of intervention concluded that families and health care professionals should select techniques that are appropriate for and address the needs of the child as an individual, taking into consideration the child's age, temperament, previous hospital experience and level of involvement that parents are willing to have (Watson and Visram 2003).

Preadmission programme

Research has shown that preadmission programmes which teach coping methods and promote play with hospital equipment are associated with decreased anxiety and increased knowledge amongst children facing surgical procedures (Justus et al 2006, Ellerton and Merriam 1994). Parents of children who did not attend a preadmission programme reported higher instances of postoperative stress-related behaviour – a finding that is corroborated by a number of similar studies (Rossen and McKeever 1996).

Benefits of a preadmission programme:

- Can help reduce preoperative anxiety and should be offered to children and families.

- Equips parents and children with new knowledge and coping skills that can be beneficial to future medical procedures.

- Preadmission programmes for preschoolers aim to familiarize children with the hospital environment by encouraging supervised play that introduces children to medical equipment and procedures.

- Decreases anxiety by addressing the child's emotional concerns and reduce postoperative behavioural changes.

- Helps familiarize parents and children with the hospital layout, ward facilities, and theatre area.

- Helps to encourage children to acknowledge fears or concerns that would otherwise remain hidden or unexpressed.

Additional strategies to reduce anxiety and prepare parents and children:

- Caring for children undergoing surgery requires a family-centred approach.

- Parents should receive information about their child's postoperative behaviour, information about eating and drinking, use of analgesics, and coping behaviour.

- Parents should receive repeated verbal and written information so that they are prepared and can support their child.

- Information sessions that address parents' emotional concerns have the added effect of decreasing preoperative anxiety in the child.

- Give parents a phone call before the scheduled date of surgery in order to gather information, answer questions and provide instructions.

- Information about hospital should be provided directly to children in the most accessible and flexible form.

- Provide information on the pre- and postoperative care according to the child's preferences. Some children prefer information whilst others cope by having less information.

- Prepare children by asking what they know or want to know about the impending surgery and associated procedures and tailoring the information to their needs.

- Assessing preoperative anxiety requires a nurse to pay attention to the nature of the child's questions and coping strategies.

- Where appropriate, parents and healthcare providers should consider the views of children when making decisions about the child's care.

- Nurses need to take an individualized approach to caring for children and their families, and should negotiate care with families by considering their views, experiences and prior knowledge before attempting to provide information or instruction

Interventions to decrease pre- and postoperative anxiety amongst infants and toddlers aged from birth to 3 years. Separation anxiety can feature in infants' pre- and postoperative hospital experiences. To reduce separation anxiety, nurses should ensure that:

- parents are not separated from their child

- the child keeps a special toy for comfort and reassurance

- what is planned is explained in simple words, using the assistance of the play therapist

- parents and child stay together during induction or reduce the time between separation and induction
- painful procedures are only performed after induction
- parents can join their child in the recovery area as soon as possible.

Interventions to decrease pre- and postoperative anxiety amongst children aged 3–6 years:

- Respect the child's privacy by, for instance, closing curtains or doors before asking a child to disrobe.
- Use information provided by parents about the child's likes, dislikes, strengths and weaknesses to aid communication with the child.
- Allow child time to ask questions and respond to his/her requests for information and explanations.
- Explain what is planned in simple words avoiding jargon.
- Seek help from play therapist to allay child's expressed fears or concerns.

Interventions to decrease pre- and postoperative anxiety amongst children aged 6–13 years:

- Engage with the child through open-ended questions about their life at home and school.
- Build on past learning by determining what is already known about the procedure.
- Speak directly with the child rather than relaying information through a parent.
- Explain to the child in simple terms what to expect preoperatively, during surgery and postoperatively.

- Encourage the child's participation and independence by eliciting their preferences and including them in discussions about their care.

Interventions to decrease pre- and postoperative anxiety amongst adolescents aged 14 years and older:

- Involve the adolescent in teaching and information-giving sessions by answering questions and explaining all relevant aspects of their surgery and postoperative care.
- Provide reassurance and support to the adolescent, while bearing in mind the patient's increasing need for autonomy and independence.
- Encourage the child's participation and independence by eliciting their preferences and including them in discussions about their care.

Physical care preoperatively

- Clear and consistent communication between all healthcare professionals is essential to prevent errors occurring.
- Ensure that the procedure has been explained clearly to both child and parents and informed consent obtained for the procedure.
- Ensure child has name band with name, date of birth, age, ward are clearly written.
- Ensure that allergies are clearly documented in the case notes and written in bold letters on the front of the child's case notes.

- Ensure that all investigations and results are included with the case notes.
- Record baseline observations of vital signs, weight and height.
- Check if the child has any loose teeth, document if any, and inform the anaesthetist.
- Ensure child is clean and that nail varnish, jewellery, facial piercings are removed. Tie long hair back with an elastic band.
- If child has a hearing aid or glasses, do not remove these until child is about to undergo the anaesthetic.
- Children are usually allowed to wear their own clothes to the theatre but this policy can vary among hospitals so check your local policy.
- Ensure that the child has been fasting for required duration according to hospital policy.
- Ensure child has had opportunity to empty his/her bladder and ensure that infants have a clean nappy.
- Administer premedication as prescribed. Anxiolytic medications may be administered to help reduce anxiety and promote haemodynamic stability while allowing for verbal response. Anxiolytics administered orally require 15–30 minutes to take full effect.
- The process of administering anxiolytic medication – IV, intramuscular, rectal, intranasal, oral – may counteract its intended purpose of decreasing patient anxiety by actually increasing anxiety or resistance. So for some procedures, premedication may not be prescribed.

- Premedication with sedatives is associated with reduced preoperative anxiety but contributes to increased cost, increased risk of recovery delay, and delayed discharge from hospital.
- Complete the preoperative checklist prior to departure for theatre.

Journey to theatre and anaesthetic room

- Provide age-appropriate toys and allow a child to bring a special item (e.g. teddy bear, blanket) for comfort to the theatre.
- Allow the child to walk to theatre if they have not had a premedication and desire to walk. Some children may prefer to cycle or go on a mobile toy device to theatre. The important issue is to allow choice so the child feels they have some control.
- Parents are encouraged to accompany their child to the theatre.
- Check child into theatre with theatre staff and inform them of any allergies and particular requirements a child may have.
- Successful procedures require teamwork, careful planning and clear communication. All staff are important so if you have any concerns do not hesitate to inform the theatre staff.
- Parents should be allowed to stay with their child in the anaesthetic room until the child is anaesthetized if this is their preference. This policy can vary among hospitals.

Physical care postoperatively

Care will depend on the nature of the procedure but there are standard steps involved in all postoperative care:

- The surgeon should communicate the outcome of the operation, any problems encountered, and the expected postoperative course.

- Parents should be allowed to be present when their child is awakening in the recovery room to prevent distress.

- Once the child has recovered safely from the anaesthetic, accompany the child back to the ward.

- Monitor the child for possible complications associated with the surgery and anaesthetic (e.g. respiratory depression, hypovolaemia, hypoglycaemia, pain, urinary retention, nausea and vomiting, bleeding, and wound complications).

- Monitor vital signs and report abnormal vital signs.

- Monitor wound site for bleeding or any discharge.

- Administer IV fluids as prescribed.

- Monitor and record all inputs and outputs (IV fluids, nasogastric aspirate, urine, vomit and bowel movement).

- Assess the degree and severity of pain using a pain assessment tool (as outlined in Section 1) that is appropriate for their developmental age and level of understanding.

- Children have an increased chance of having moderate to severe postoperative pain because they often receive less analgesia than adults.

- Administer appropriate analgesia so that the child does not experience any pain.

> **!** Many surgical conditions increase caloric needs or prevent adequate nutritional intake. Pay close attention to the child's nutritional intake as poor nutrition will delay wound healing and recovery from the procedure.

Pain management

Early experiences of pain have been shown to have long-term consequences for children's behavioural reactions to pain, rendering pain management to be a crucial aspect of paediatric and neonatal care. The relief of pain is a basic human right and human dignity and respect requires that treatable pain is relieved. Unrelieved pain has adverse physical and psychological consequences such as increased stress response, reduced movement and increased anxieties. The quality of pain management may influence length of hospital stay and incidence of complications.

Acute pain

Acute pain is the most commonly experienced type of pain in children and arises from illness, injury, surgery and other medical procedures. The management of acute pain is best achieved through non-opioids and, for moderate to severe cases, a combination of non-opioids and opioids.

Chronic pain

Chronic pain tends to go untreated in children until changes in the child's normal behaviours and routines are observed. While acute pain serves an important role of red-flagging bodily injury or disease, chronic pain has no useful function and, when left untreated, causes significant suffering and distress. Chronic pain in children often results from underlying disease such as rheumatoid arthritis, sickle cell disease, fibromyalgia and human immunodeficiency virus infection.

Chronic pain can be classified into four broad categories (Chambliss et al 2002):

- pain that spans beyond the expected duration of an injury or disease
- persistent or re-emergent pain without a known cause
- pain resulting from degenerative or neurological disease
- pain resulting from cancer or cancer treatment.

Procedural pain

Procedural pain arising from medical procedures is a form of acute pain that causes both psychological distress and physical discomfort. Procedural pain should be managed with a multimodal approach using a combination of Ametop or Entonox and distraction or coping strategies.

Key points to remember

- Managing pain in children depends upon an accurate and appropriate assessment. So assess pain regularly using a pain assessment tool (see detailed information on pain assessment tools in Section 1).

- Evaluation and management of pain in children should be prioritized upon admission, as failure to do so may result in delayed or inadequate treatment for the patient.
- Plan ahead for pain.
- Never ignore the child's complaints.
- Be aware that children may under report pain if they are afraid of injections so reassure children about different routes for receiving pain medication.
- Record the severity of pain.
- Administer adequate doses of analgesia.
- Common methods of pain management in children include intramuscular analgesia, intravenous opiates, patient-controlled analgesia (PCA), and constructive play or distraction.
- Use infusion pumps when available – PCA/nurse controlled analgesia.
- Monitor for adverse side effects.

Non-pharmacological interventions for pain relief

Non-pharmacological interventions should be used in addition to analgesics as careful attention to factors that promote comfort can reduce the amount of analgesics required.

- Involve parents/carer in assessing the child's pain and in providing comfort measures that the child prefers.
- Use comfort measures such as touch, hugging, holding, rocking, and singing.

- Distraction therapy can help decrease anxiety and promote relaxation, e.g. music, relaxation techniques, bubble tubes, bubbles and fibre-optic lights.
- Use complementary therapies such as massage, aromatherapy and relaxation therapy.
- Electronic games and board games could help provide distraction from pain.

Management of procedural pain

- Provide age-appropriate information to the child about the procedure and the type of pain relief planned.
- Pharmacological interventions depend on the procedure.
- Use non-nutritive sucking for infants.
- Use non-pharmacological alongside analgesic interventions.
- Ensure that the child is aware that something is going to hurt; they will cope more effectively when prepared.
- Ensure that you have the child's cooperation and agreement prior to beginning the procedure.
- Involve the play specialist's expertise to help explain the procedure beforehand.
- Reduce adverse environmental factors, e.g. noise, cold, and cover frightening equipment.
- Allow choices so that the child feels that they have some control over the procedure.
- For unsuccessful venepunctures, use time out periods.
- Limit the number of venepuncture attempts as children find this procedure very distressing and frightening.

- Guided imagery and relaxation techniques can help reduce anxieties during uncomfortable procedures.
- Provide praise and reassurance after the procedure.

Pharmacological pain management

Experience and perception of pain is comprised of physiological and emotional components, both of which must be considered when choosing an appropriate treatment option and route of administration. Aim is to anticipate and prevent pain whenever possible (pre-emptive analgesia) and to target drugs at several parts of the pain pathways at the same time (balanced analgesia). This ensures that:

- lower doses of analgesics used
- produces better analgesia with fewer side effects
- may reduce morbidity and hospital stay.

Recommended analgesic agents

- Mild pain is best treated with paracetamol.
- Mild to moderate pain is best treated with non-steroidal anti-inflammatory drugs (NSAIDs) or a combination of NSAIDs and opioids.
- Moderate to severe nociceptive pain, as well as neuropathic pain, is best managed with opioid analgesics.
- Pain resulting from burn, surgery, postoperative stress responses and opioid withdrawal is best treated with Clonidine.

- Titrated oral opioids are commonly administered to children with advanced stages of cancer; however, epidural or subarachnoid opioid infusions are appropriate for high-dose opioid-resistant patients (such as those with solid spinal/CNS tumours). For more information see Section 6.

Routes of administration

- Oral administration is suitable for mild pain.
- Intramuscular injections are painful and commonly arouse anxiety in children and, where possible, should be avoided as routes of administration.
- Local anaesthetics by subcutaneous or topical administration should be used for short-term relief of painful procedures.
- Regional techniques should be used to provide epidural anaesthesia and peripheral nerve blocks.
- Continuous or patient-controlled intravenous drip which has already been established is a suitable method of administration for moderate to severe pain
- PCA. Children as young as 5 years and older can learn how to use a PCA device in order to provide pain relief without serious toxicity or side effects.

Patient-controlled analgesia (PCA)

- The PCA pump uses an intravenous line and a syringe with ordered medication which is locked inside the pump.

- The pump is programmed so that when the child pushes a button, an analgesic dose is administered.
- If it is too soon, the pump will not deliver the dose because a lockout interval is programmed into the pump by the nurse.
- The child's level of pain needs to be carefully assessed so that the programmed pump dose alleviates the child's pain effectively.
- Advantages of the PCA is that it allows the child some measure of control over his/her pain relief.
- The pump can also be set to administer an analgesic dose at designated time intervals without the child needing to push the button.

Repeated needle procedures in neonates have been shown to cause reduced pain tolerance and adverse behavioural effects in later life, while severe injury may induce lasting changes in an individual's sensory processing (Howard 2003). Many of these effects can be reduced in the clinical setting through the use of analgesia.

Wound care

Caring for a child with wound(s) can be both challenging and time consuming as their treatments can be both complex and diverse.

Structure of the skin

The skin is one of the largest organs of the body and it occupies a surface area of approximately 2 m^2 (Guyton and Hall 2000). It can be divided into two main parts:

- *The epidermis* – composed of mainly stratified squamous epithelial tissue and four major cell types:
  - keratinocytes
  - melanocytes
  - Langerhans cells
  - Granstein cells.

- *The dermis* – composed of primarily connective tissue containing collagenous and elastic fibres. Other structures found in the surrounding regions are:
  - blood supply
  - lymph vessels
  - sensory nerve endings
  - sweat glands and ducts
  - hair, root and follicles
  - sebaceous glands
  - arrectores pilorum.

Functions of the skin

- *Protection* – against invasion by foreign and bacterial matter.

- *Perception of stimuli* – enables constant monitoring of the external environment.

- *Absorption* – allows certain tropical compounds, such as drugs to be absorbed.

- *Synthesis of vitamin D* – synthesized by the body as a result of direct exposure to ultraviolet radiation.

- *Maintenance of body temperature* – through metabolic processes, the body is continuously producing heat. This is primarily dissipated via the skin, facilitated by three processes:
  - *radiation* – ability of the body to give off its heat to another object of lower temperature
  - *conduction* – transfer of heat from the body to a cooler object in contact with it
  - *convection* – movement of warm air molecules away from the body.

- *Water balance* – approximately 500 ml of fluid is lost each day as *'insensible loss'* through evaporation.

Healing process

There are three classifications of healing:

- Healing by *primary intention* – the skin edges are brought together with the aid of suture or skin staples (surgical wounds) or Steri-Strips (minor trauma).

- Healing by *secondary intention* – the skin edges are deliberately not brought together. This is done in order to promote granulation tissue from the base of the wound. Common practice in chronic wounds.

- Healing by *tertiary intention* - a previously sutured wound that has dehisced and has been resutured.

Phases of healing

There are three phases of wound healing, which are all linked:

- *Inflammatory phase* – formation of a blood clot, loosely uniting the wound edges and stimulating the inflammatory response and leading to the characteristic appearance of a wound, e.g. swelling, heat, redness and pain, facilitating healing and repair (0–3 days).

- *Regenerative phase* – tissue starts to fill and granulation tissue starts the process of wound contraction. Signs of inflammation start to subside but the wound may be raised in relation to surrounding tissues (0–24 days).

- *Maturation phase* – process of re-epithelialization begins. Scab should now drop off, as the epidermis is restored to its natural thickness (1–2 years).

Wound drainage

A drain is an abnormal opening in the skin that produces exudates or drainage, which may be caused by disease, trauma or surgery. All drainage should be accurately measured and recorded on the fluid balance chart. Colour, consistency as well as odour and drug therapy must also be noted in the nursing care plan.

Common types of wound or surgical drains are:

- *Corrugated strips of rubber* (e.g. Yeats drain) are used primarily to drain exudates from fat layers, subcutaneous tissues, and occasionally the peritoneal cavity. They guide exudates onto a surface dressing, can be messy and affect normal skin. Application of stoma bag to collect drainage is often used to prevent skin irritation and minimize mess.

- *Tubes and catheter type drains* (e.g. Robinson drain) are most effective type of drain and can be connected to a closed drainage bag system.

- *Suction drainage systems* may involve a closed suction system; ideal for removal of blood and serous fluid (e.g. Redivac drains or under water sealed drains for thoracic surgery).

Wound dressing materials

To undertake appropriate and effective wound drainage requires knowledge and understanding of the skin structure and the normal wound healing process. Factors taken into account when choosing a wound dressing are:

- *Best dressing* – the ideal dressing should ensure that the wound remains:
  - moist with exudates but not saturated
  - free from clinical infection and excessive slough
  - free from toxic chemical particles or fibres released from dressing
  - kept at an optimum temperature for healing to take place
  - not exposed to unnecessary disturbance or wound dressing changes
  - kept at an optimum pH level.

Classification of wound dressings

Wound dressings are classified by their primary functions.

Film membranes

- Permeable to water vapour and oxygen.

- Impermeable to water and micro organisms.

- Provide a warm and moist environment.

- Comfortable and convenient as they provide a direct observation.

Alginates

- Used to fill cavities and sinuses.
- Useful around drainage sites as they absorb exudates and serous fluid and can easily be removed by irrigation methods.

Foams

- Absorb exudate, which then evaporates into the cells of the dressing and is lost as water vapour.
- Non-adherent.

Hydrogels

- Swell when wet and can retain significant proportions of water within their structure.
- Their role is to:
  - rehydrate wounds
  - debride and clean
  - be painless when applying and removing
  - be soothing.

Hydrocolloids

- Withdraw warm fluid to form a gel that produces a moist environment on the wound surface in order to facilitate healing.

Additional therapies

Not all wound dressing materials are suited to all wound types, in particular wounds that are non-healing or copiously draining wounds. However, an alternative method is available in such wounds, the vacuum assisted wound closure system (VAC). This system is often considered when conventional methods have been ineffective.

The VAC system offers:

- a closed, non-invasive, active therapy system
- negative pressure, which increases the effectiveness of the local wound circulation
- active removal of excessive exudates, reducing oedema and haematoma formation
- assists with the control of wound leakage
- promotes angiogenesis.

Specialist support surfaces

Pressure sore complications are a real concern and using specialist beds problems can be reduced or avoided. Specialist beds can help reduce the pressure exerted on pressure points and thus decrease capillary occlusion pressures. In the majority of critical care patients the frequent turning and repositioning alone may suffice.

Factors influencing decision for a specialist bed:

- cardiovascular instability, e.g. extreme episodes of hypotension on turning
- respiratory instability, e.g. extreme episodes of desaturation on turning
- decreased skin integrity, e.g. severe burns
- malnourished
- receiving vasconstrictive drug therapy
- extreme weight, e.g. too thin or obese
- invasive equipment preventing adequate turning, e.g. ECMO, LVAD, RVAD.

Indications for kinetic therapy or continuous lateral rotational therapy

Kinetic or lateral to lateral rotational therapy (rotational therapy) treatment is generally indicated for high-risk patients within a critical care setting who are vulnerable to respiratory associated complications due to immobility and or prolonged ventilation.

Furthermore, rotational therapy should be considered in all mechanically ventilated patients who are at a high risk of developing pulmonary related complications. These are:

- increased pulmonary shunt
- atelectasis
- pneumonia or lower respiratory pneumonia
- ARDS.

Criteria to discontinue rotational therapy/lateral to lateral rotation:

- stable and satisfactory improvement in oxygenation
- patient extubated
- patient is able to sit out of bed
- do not resuscitate order

Sleep

The unfamiliar environment of a hospital may affect the child's ability to sleep. Lack of sleep has the potential to slow recovery (Freeman et al 2001). It is important to allow children to sleep for periods of at least 2 hours to complete all sleep cycles before nursing interventions are carried out. Other factors that can lead to sleep deprivation are sedation and analgesia, stress and technology.

Sedation and analgesia is often administered to children as part of treatment (Milner and Gunning 2000). This is because many interventions are uncomfortable, distressing, frequently painful, and lying in a fixed position for prolonged periods of time may lead to backache and muscular discomfort. Using sedation and various analgesic preparations can also lead to sleep deprivation (Milner and Gunning 2000) and efforts should be made to promote natural sleep.

Promoting rest and sleep

Sleep can be defined as an altered state of consciousness from which a person can be aroused by stimuli of sufficient magnitude. The function of sleep is:

- Considered as restorative and energy conserving, as protein synthesis and cell division occurs for the renewal of tissues, which takes place predominantly during the time devoted to rest and sleep.
- Sleep is needed to avoid the psychological problems resulting from inadequate sleep, which might hinder recovery.
- Sleep deprivation could be considered as an added stressor, over and above those physical and emotional traumas already suffered.

During an average night's sleep, individuals pass through four or five sleep cycles, each cycle lasting about 90–100 minutes. Within the sleep cycle, five successive stages have been defined by their distinctive characteristics. The first four stages of sleep are collectively named non-rapid eye movement sleep (NREM) and demonstrate a progressive increase in the depth of sleep. Final stage is called rapid eye movement sleep (REM), or paradoxical sleep, and is associated with dreaming, learning and memory.

Perpetual awakening and sleep interruption has been associated with increased anxiety, irritability and disorientation, which may have a negative influence on recovery. In addition, total sleep deprivation, for 48 hours, can result in changes such as:

- behavioural irritability
- suspiciousness
- speech slurring
- minor visual misperceptions
- reduction in motivation and willingness to perform tasks which could include mobilization and other aspects of self-care
- lethargy, irritability and disorientation and confusion
- later, delusions and paranoia manifestations.

Strategies that minimize sleep interruptions:

- Turning off/down number of lights, especially at night.
- Keeping noise levels to minimum, e.g. switch off suction equipment.
- Offering cotton wall balls to awake patients.
- Reassessing the need and value of continually interrupting patient's sleep to perform observations and care.
- Centralizing of nursing duties so to minimize touch and stimuli.
- Charting amount of uninterrupted sleep time per shift as evidence of stages of sleep.
- Communicating the patients need to sleep to other health care professionals.

Children's nurses should use their knowledge of:

- the patient's normal sleeping patterns
- supportive family relationships to optimize environment for sleep
- analgesic and sedative administration, according to the patient's felt need and monitor events thereafter to promote sleep and rest.

Early mobilization

Early and progressive mobilization is an important aspect of caring for children. Mobilization is an extension of the physiological principles of turning and repositioning of patients confined to bed.

Reasons for early mobilization:

- encourages ventilation
- increases perfusion
- promotes mobilization of secretions
- promotes oxygenation
- decreases venous pooling
- improves functional residual capacity
- improves patient's psychological state.

When and how patients are mobilized is decided on an individual basis in conjunction with the nurse, doctor, physiotherapist and patient.

Discharge procedure

Compared to adults with similar conditions, children are discharged to the home environment at an earlier stage of their recovery. In the UK, many children may receive specialist nursing care in the home environment with the support of children's community nursing teams.

Discharge procedure should fall within a predetermined framework, which is understood by anyone involved in sending the child home and providing post-hospitalization support (Smith and Daughtrey 2000).

The key principles are:

- Parents should be given information about their child's medical condition as soon as a diagnosis is made in order to allow time for parents to digest the information and approach members of staff with any questions or concerns.

- Parents should be given clear instruction on whom to contact in the event of a complication or concern after discharge.

- Procedures for dealing with post-discharge concerns should be streamlined such that all members of a child's health care team understand their roles and responsibilities.

Managing a sick child in the community

Children should only be admitted to hospital if the care they require cannot be given at home. It is now well accepted that sick children are better cared for by their families within the home, rather than spending lengthy periods in the hospital setting. Meeting the child's healthcare needs within the community promotes family centred care as it avoids the disruption of hospital admissions

- Caring for children in the community setting has expanded over the last decade to meet the needs of a growing number of children who, through

increased survival rates, require complex and technology-based treatments.

- Children with complex needs are children who have significant physical and psychosocial needs that require healthcare services beyond that required for children generally.

- Typical caseload profiles of community children's nurses (CCN) include referrals for children with gastric and dermatological problems to those with cystic fibrosis, tracheostomy, neuromuscular disorders and childhood cancer.

- Referral practitioners include GPs, paediatricians, district nurses, and other allied health care professionals.

Many models of community care exist and these are generally based on two organizational models:

1. Community-based team supplying a service to a defined geographical area. Community care provision involves the general practitioner along with a team of qualified support staff, providing emotional support, medical treatments and individualized instruction to the families of children receiving care in the home.
2. Specialist team as in a hospital outreach service usually focused on a specific client group such as oncology, renal, or neonatal, with the care administered by staff employed by the hospital.

Range of professionals

Smooth coordination of multiple practitioners is essential to ensure that the child's needs are met appropriately and that families are supported in their care giving role. Professionals involved are (Kirk and Glendinning 2002):

- community children's nurse
- specialist paediatric nurse (with specialist qualification but without community nursing qualification)
- generalist paediatric nurse (without community nursing qualification)
- general practitioner
- health visitor or public health nurse
- district nurses
- home care assistants
- practice nurse
- physiotherapist
- occupational therapist
- social worker.

Community services are often configured differently within the country and between countries. Upon discharge from hospital, the clinical responsibility for the management of a child's care usually lies with the child's GP; however, in some cases care will remain with a hospital consultant within community outreach schemes.

Coordination of a child's treatment plan should aim to:

- provide post-hospitalization care planning
- assessing the home environment prior to discharge
- ensure parents are willing and able to cope with continuing the care in the home with the support of community services
- coordinate the involvement of practitioners
- promote information-sharing and communication
- organise services to avoid duplication

- facilitate access to services required by the family
- ensure appropriate training of staff
- monitor outcomes and resource use
- ongoing assessment of outcomes and evaluation of the child's treatment plan.

Parents caring for sick children in the home have been shown to experience difficulty with negotiating their role as carers when an individualized assessment of their needs and expectations has not been carried out (Kirk 2001). Additionally, because lay knowledge has not kept up with the rapid expansion of medical technologies and treatments, support services in the community tend to be underdeveloped and inadequate for families' needs. At times there may be ambiguity regarding the professional roles and boundaries of community services and tertiary services, therefore clear communication is essential.

Strategies to avoid problems with communication

- GP and health visitor/public health nurse should be informed as soon as to when the child will be discharged from the hospital.
- Community practitioners should be involved in the discharge planning if at all possible as they will know the family situation.
- One person in the hospital sector should be responsible for the liaison role between the tertiary and primary services.
- All relevant personnel must be kept informed.

- All visits to the home should be coordinated so duplication is avoided.
- Families can be provided with home-held records to facilitate communication between all members of the team who visit.
- Communication between professionals should be documented so that a clear decision trail is available.

Community children's nurses

Within the UK, CCN services have become recognized as an important component in the care of sick children (Eaton 2000). CCNs work in local communities within multidisciplinary health care teams. Care is often delivered within GP surgeries, local clinics, school nurses or hospital-at-home schemes supported by state programmes. In an ideal situation all nurses working within the community should have both a community and children's nursing qualification. CCN services operate effectively when they are supported by appropriate staff training, patient/practitioner communication, adequate support for hospital readmission and health education resources and activities.

Providing support and information to families in the community

Providing support and information to parents of a sick child in the home is a primary role of the CCN. Participation in caring for a child in the home originally entailed involving parents in everyday

childcare tasks; this later expanded to include medical procedures ordinarily performed in a clinical setting, such as changing tracheostomy tubes, giving injections and placing central venous lines. CCNs should be able to:

- Give instruction on the use of medical equipment and carrying out procedures required for the delivery of treatment and medication
- Demonstrate skills in self-management and hold specialized knowledge relevant to patients in their care
- Aware of relevant sources of information and support within the community
- Know of sources of government funding and assistance which lighten the load for parents of undertaking and coordinating home-based care on a full-time basis.

The education of parents on the aspects of a child's care is a primary responsibility of the CCN as it empowers parents to make informed decisions and take an active role in their child's care. Teaching and education can be carried out in the home and commonly includes:

- educating parents on the medical care, e.g. nature of illness, medical equipment and technologies, carrying out procedures, and safety measures
- ensuring that parents are competent in the performance of nursing procedures
- ensuring that parents are willing to accept responsibility for carrying out the necessary tasks
- provision of equipment and supplies, e.g. tubes, catheters, feeding pumps
- helping parents replace tubes, e.g. nasogastric

- providing skin care and doing dressings
- providing support and advice
- educating parents on non-medical care, e.g. social support, coping strategies, psychosocial needs of the child
- respecting parents' expertise and prepared to learn from parents, offering reassurance where needed.

> **!**
>
> It is important to not assume that parents will want to accept the full responsibility for their child's care. Parents are more willing to take an active role when they know that they will continue to be supported by community care staff when needed.

Caring for a sick child in the home presents a mixture of drawbacks and benefits to family carers. Advantages to the family include:

- reduced travel between hospital and home
- being more involved in child's care
- child not being separated from the family
- frequent contact between family and child.

Families caring for a sick child in the home can experience the following difficulties:

- social isolation
- demands placed upon carers' time and energy associated with taking on increased responsibilities in the home

- increased anxiety/stress due to increased responsibilities for care
- need to schedule and coordinate home visits by external care staff and the resulting lack of privacy in the home
- less time for self-care, lack of sleep, financial burdens and reduced work hours
- lack of time for siblings and other family members.

Transfer of a child

Transfer of a child does not only involve moving the patient within the hospital (for example to imaging department or theatres) but also externally to other hospitals. This may be due to bed shortage within the admitting hospital or need for specialist care and treatment. Prior to transfer of the child there are a number of factors to take into consideration:

- Patient accompanied by experienced nursing and medical staff /and parent or guardian.
- Appropriate equipment and vehicle are sought and utilized.
- Patient fully assessed, stabilized and staff prepared prior to transfer.
- All investigations accompany child on transfer.
- All drugs and delivery systems are readily available and prepared for immediate use.
- Monitoring systems and battery back up are familiar to accompanying staff.
- Continuous monitoring and assessment during transfer.

- Knowledge of area transferring patient to. If another hospital, phone ahead and ensure a member of staff waiting at agreed point. For example, a porter waiting in A&E dept.
- Accurate and concise oral and documental handover.

Organizational and transfer decision-making factors

A designated Consultant is responsible for the decision to transfer a child. They should ensure that:

- transfer is appropriate
- patient can be transferred, risk versus benefits of transfer
- referring hospital is informed
- coordination of transfer runs smoothly
- appropriate staff have been allocated for transfer
- local policies are adhered to
- child is accompanied by a family member.

Specification of transfer vehicle

- Ensure good trolley access with appropriate fixing devices.
- Good lighting, power points and temperature control.
- Sufficient space for attending medical and nursing team.
- Sufficient medical gases, electricity and storage space.
- Robust surfaces to take into account urgency of transfer, mobilization time, geographical distance of transfer, weather and traffic conditions.

Specification of equipment

- Robust
- Lightweight
- Battery powered
- User friendly
- Audible alarms due to unrelated noises during transfer, e.g. sirens
- Illuminated displays
- Emergency equipment available
- Mobile phone for communication.

Accompanying staff

- Experienced doctor, experienced in resuscitation, airway management, ventilation and organ support with previous transfer experience.
- Experienced nurse, operating department practitioner or paramedic experienced in transfer of a child.
- Current staffing levels in many hospitals mean that this level of assistant is not always available.
- Transferring hospital should provide medical indemnity and personal medical defence cover is also recommended.

Importance of patient preparation

- Stabilization of the child prior to transfer is key to minimize the destabilization of the patient on transfer
- Is the child's oxygenation stable?
- Is the cardiovascular system stable?
- Is intravenous access adequate?

- Accompaniment of all relevant investigations
- Full monitoring of patient's vital signs should be in progress prior to transfer
- Securing airway and intravenous line management.

Departure checklist

- Are appropriate equipment and drugs available?
- Sufficient oxygen?
- Suction available?
- Trolley available?
- Ambulance service notified of transfer and patient's condition, nature of transfer?
- Bed confirmed at receiving hospital?
- Receiving hospital notified?
- Medical notes, X-rays and investigations available?
- Transfer letter prepared?
- Return arrangements known?
- Next of kin informed of impending transfer?

Transfer of critically ill child

- Standard of care delivered should be maintained at same level as ICU care.
- Continuous monitoring of patient is necessary.
- Smooth transfer is vital.
- Accurate record keeping is vital.
- In event of emergency, ambulance to be stopped and/or transport patient to nearest A&E department.

Medical and nursing handover

- Direct communication between referring hospital team and receiving hospital team.
- Full handover of patient's hospital stay alongside and treatments, investigations and results.
- Disclosure of next of kin members and contact numbers.

Audit and training

- Completion of audit documentation.
- Completion of any local documentation regarding transfer.
- Attend i – house and external training courses regarding safe transfer of critically ill patient.

Review of all transfers by an allocated Consultant

The clinical conditions possibly eliciting inter-hospital transfer are:

- coma/head injury
- renal/metabolic failure
- requirement for computerized tomography scan (CT)
- plastic surgery
- burns
- cardiac problems
- respiratory failure
- spinal injury
- major sepsis
- recipients of transplantation
- premature babies.

Generally the majority of patients requiring inter-hospital transfer have neurological or respiratory problems requiring further management in a specialist critical care unit. There is an increasing need for inter-hospital transfer of patients requiring liver and cardiac transplant units.

The issue that has led to a decrease in the need for inter-hospital transfer is the development of systems to transmit the images of a CT scan from one hospital to another. This allows the hospital to send the CT images via a phone line to the specialist neuro-centre where the images can be assessed. The specialist neurologist can then decide whether transport of the patient to the specialist centre is indicated.

When to transfer?

The importance of the 'golden hour' and the resulting importance has been debated. Transfer should occur:

- When the staff of the referring centre feel uncomfortable with the course of the illness/injury.
- When it is first realized that the patient requires care in a specialist centre.

Risks to the patient

- Endotracheal tube, intravenous line dislodgement.
- Lack of appropriate equipment in the transfer vehicle if an unforeseen incident occurs en route.
- Breakdown of the transfer vehicle whilst transferring patients – and lives have been lost.
- Vibration of the transport vehicle can cause either hypertension or cardiovascular depression.

- Acceleration forces in an ambulance can lead to transient hypertension and arrhythmias.

The risks of changes in blood pressure can be reduced if the patient is adequately sedated prior to transfer. However, a patient is only ready for transfer after effective resuscitation, after physiological status is stabilized and after mechanical aspects are secured and appropriate equipment is available for transfer.

How should a child be transferred?

- Ground vehicle transport is most often used.
- Boats are sometimes used to transfer critically ill patients from islands to the mainland.
- The use of aircraft is becoming more widely available in this country.
- Helicopters are more frequently being used in the transfer of patients over long distances or where traffic would slow the process of ground transport. The helicopter has the benefit of getting to places not accessible to road vehicles and also does not have to contend with the problems of traffic delaying the transfer.

Staff involved in transfer

Different areas use different disciplines of staff to accompany patients on transfer:

- paramedics – ambulance personnel who have undergone further training
- specially trained flight nurses – mainly in the USA
- specially trained physicians and nurses, facilitated by ambulance personnel.

There is a pretransfer checklist, which identifies the need for:

- assessment
- evaluation
- stabilization
- having equipment available for:
  - airway and breathing
  - cervical spine
  - circulation
  - neurological
  - procedures (catheterization, reintubation)
  - laboratory work (blood gases)
  - continued medication
  - safe delivery and documentation.

The main focus must be on the infant/child's safety during the transport.

Section 4

Common conditions in children and reasons for admission

This section commences by outlining some of the physiological processes of injury and repair that are common to all medical and surgical conditions. In addition, the section details some common conditions that may be observed in infants and children and may be the reason for admission; others may be complications of interventions / treatment that occurred elsewhere.

4.1 General conditions in children: a systems approach

Principles of cellular death, injury and repair

Cellular death/hypoxic damage

When blood flow falls below a certain critical level that is required to maintain tissue viability swelling of the area affected will occur. When the occlusion becomes too great blood supply is cut off. Eventually the loss of blood flow reaches a level where tissue viability can no longer be maintained (Edwards 2002b). This damage can occur due to:

■ generalized ischaemia (hypovolaemia, hypoxaemia or conditions such as disseminated intravascular coagulation (DIC))

■ ischaemia of an organ (acute tubular necrosis of the kidney)

■ ischaemia of the skin or limb (compression bandages or constrictive

devices, such as a tight cast that has been improperly left in place for extended periods of time, crush or pressure injuries, pressure ulcers, swelling of a foot, leg or arm due to fractures or compartment syndrome.

All of these and others can lead to hypoxic injury (Table 4.1), which can affect viability of tissue and its surrounding area. The hypoxic damage may either occur inside the body and is invisible to the naked eye or appear on the surface of skin and be visible. Those areas of hypoxic damage that are invisible are generally due to acute tubular necrosis. Hypoxic injury that is visible is due to occlusions of limbs or pressure ulcers, which may lead to the appearance of offensive unsightly necrotic wounds, which do not heal.

The interrupted supply of oxygenated blood to cells can result in cellular changes, which in turn can stimulate the inflammatory response (IR) (see later). The interrupted supply of oxygenated blood to cells results in anaerobic metabolism and cellular membrane disruption (Fig. 4.1).

Tissue injury: the formation of oedema

Oedema is an abnormal collection of fluid in tissues, which can either collect in interstitial or intracellular spaces (Edwards 2003c). Oedema is a problem of fluid distribution and does not necessarily indicate fluid excess. The causes of oedema are varied (Table 4.1) and include hypoxia (leads to intracellular oedema) (see previous) and the inflammatory response (leads to interstitial oedema) (see later).

Table 4.1 The conditions that lead to cell death, injury and repair

Inflammatory response	Hypoxic damage	Oedema
Trauma	Hypovolaemia/hypotension	Cancer
Head injury (cerebral	Tight compression	Malnutrition
oedema)	bandages/casts	Congestive cardiac
Surgery/anaesthetic	Compartment syndrome	failure
Renal/liver disease	Myocardial infarction/cardiac	Fluid overload
Pancreatitis	arrest	Left ventricular failure
Burns	Shock	
Gastro-intestinal	Heart failure	
disorders:	Deep vein thrombosis	
ulcers	Pulmonary embolism	
hernia	Acute tubular necrosis	
irritable bowel syndrome	Pressure ulcers	
inflammatory bowel	Cerebral thrombosis or bleed	
disease	Peripheral vascular disease	
ulcerative colitis	Neoplasms	
Infection / sepsis		
Pulmonary oedema		
Drugs		
Hypertension		
Heart failure		
Malnutrition		
Anaphylaxis		
Neoplasms		
Leg ulcers		

These processes are not mutually exclusive. The inflammatory response can lead to interstitial oedema causing swelling which can cut off blood supply, leading to hypoxic damage and intracellular oedema. Hypoxic damage leading to intracellular oedema can lead to cellular damage and stimulation of the inflammatory response, which will stimulate the release of mediators. In addition, oedema can lead to hypoxia and stimulation of the inflammatory response.
Modified from Edwards 2003c.

Interstitial oedema is usually associated with weight gain, swelling and puffiness, tight-fitting clothes and shoes, limited movement of an effected area, and symptoms associated with an underlying pathological condition. There are generally many different types of interstitial oedema, named due to the mechanisms that cause it and may be localized or generalized.

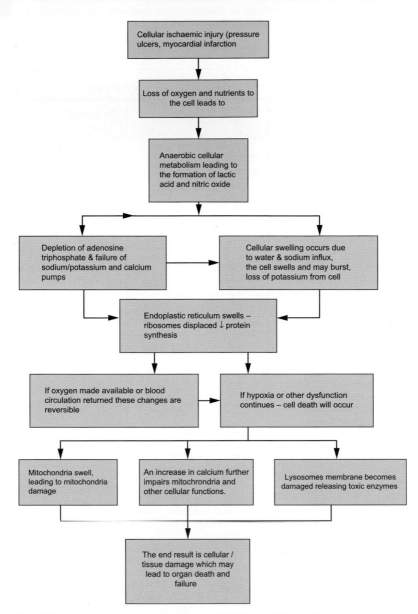

Fig. 4.1 The processes of cellular hypoxia and cell death. Intracellular oedema occurs due to a reduction in ATP, the cell membrane can no longer maintain ionic gradients and sodium and water moves into the cell.

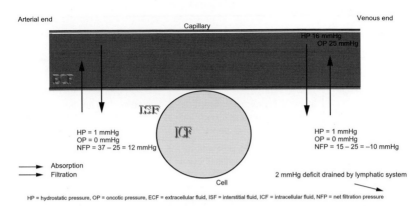

HP = hydrostatic pressure, OP = oncotic pressure, ECF = extracellular fluid, ISF = interstitial fluid, ICF = intracellular fluid, NFP = net filtration pressure

Fig. 4.2 Normal capillary dynamics and pressures allow the normal movement of fluid across a semi-permeable membrane (filtration) to nourish the cell. The majority of the fluid is absorbed (absorption) back into the circulation. The remaining excess is drained by the lymphatic system.

Interstitial oedema is formed in three different ways:

1. Stimulation of the inflammatory immune response (see later).
2. Changes in capillary dynamics (Fig. 4.2) due to increase or decrease in hydrostatic pressure is seen in conditions when the hydrostatic pressure is high (Table 4.2). Decreases in plasma oncotic pressure occurs in a number of conditions leading to poor healing and tissue viability may be affected (Table 4.3).
3. Lymphatic system obstruction.

Tissue repair: activation of the inflammatory response

Cellular damage e.g. leg ulcers, surgical procedures, and trauma (Table 4.1) causes stimulation of the IR that ends with repair to damaged cells and tissues (Edwards 2006). Activation of the IR is

part of the innate immune system, and represents a major physiological event in the body (Fig. 4.3). Following the damage tissues release mediators, the most important are:

- histamine
- kinins
- prostaglandins
- complement
- cytokines (monokines and lymphokines).

The list of these chemical mediators is immense and rapidly growing. The mediators are released at the site of injury and will enhance the activity of the body's own immune and non-specific responses. Release of these mediators is to:

- protect the body from invading microorganisms
- limit the extent of blood loss and injury
- promote rapid healing of involved tissues.

Table 4.2 The conditions that lead to changes in hydrostatic pressure and oedema formation

Condition	Principles	Progression
Liver failure	In liver failure there is a general increase in pressure in the portal venous system and raised pressure in the portal vessels.	This may eventually lead to the formation of an ascites.
Heart failure	In heart failure the pressure can rise in either the systemic veins or the pulmonary veins, depending on which side of the heart is affected. Failure of the left ventricle causes pressure to rise in the pulmonary veins and can lead to oedema formation in the lungs as pulmonary oedema.	In right sided heart failure (complete heart failure) there is an increase in HP in the vena cava and other systemic veins. This tends to cause oedema in systemic tissues and oedema will form in the parts of the body that hang down, such as the wrists, ankles and sacrum.
Renal failure	Certain forms of damage to the kidneys interfere with their ability to eliminate excess water and solutes into the urine, which results in the accumulation of excess fluid in the body.	As a consequence, blood volume increases and blood pressure rises throughout the cardiovascular system. The increase in pressure raises capillary HP, which will increase filtration and reduce absorption processes and lead to the formation of oedema.

The mediators act as a signalling system (chemotaxis) to attract nutrients, fluids, clotting factors, neutrophils and macrophages to damaged sites. The arrival of macrophages to an area of damaged tissue is central to acute inflammation control, but macrophages can remain at sites of prolonged or chronic inflammation. The mediators cause a localized increase in:

- capillary permeability
- vasodilatation to increase blood supply.

The endothelium is a major contributor to activation of the IR. It is not just an inert barrier between flowing blood and the substructure of blood vessels and tissue, but an active metabolic organ responsible for anticoagulation. Coagulation always accompanies injury, to prevent excessive blood loss and to isolate the injured site. A victim of an acute tissue injury or a patient with a wound that will not heal or is infected, varicose or pressure ulcers could potentially release inflammatory

Table 4.3 The conditions that lead to changes in colloid osmotic pressure and oedema formation

Condition	Principles	Progression
Renal disease	Damage to the kidneys can cause increased elimination of plasma proteins in the urine (nephritic syndrome)	This loss of protein triggers a reduction in capillary absorption because of the drop in colloid osmotic pressure
Malnutrition	Starvation will reduce the amount of protein available to form plasma proteins. During malnutrition insufficient amounts of proteins are digested through the gastrointestinal tract.	If the malnourished state is allowed to continue, the proteins stored in the body are broken down and used as a source of energy by the liver to maintain cellular and organ function. This leads to a reduction in plasma proteins which are unable to produce effective colloid osmotic pressure.

mediators that circulate in the blood stream and could alter endothelial integrity elsewhere. This may incite coagulation abnormalities whereby there is a concomitant activation of coagulation or alterations in the haemostatic balance causing systemic thrombosis or gross haemorrhage known as DIC.

A lack of regulation of the IR can lead to an uncontrolled intravascular inflammation that ultimately harms the body. The mediators become toxic to other cells, damaging tissues, vessels, and organs far away from the initial injury. There are currently no conclusive indicators why some inflammatory processes proceed smoothly to healing while others lead to increase tissue damage. If there were such signs then the serious systemic conditions such as multi-system organ failure (MSOF) and systemic inflammatory response

syndrome (SIRS) thought to be caused by over stimulation of the IR could be prevented.

The effect of treatments on the physiological processes

The interventions used to treat the insult/injury can lead to further stimulation of the physiological processes identified above. Some of the interventions used may prevent the physiological processes identified above from causing serious damage and/or complications, treatments such as:

■ The nurses' role is to administer the prescribed fluid regimes for the immediate restoration of an effective circulating blood volume. This may

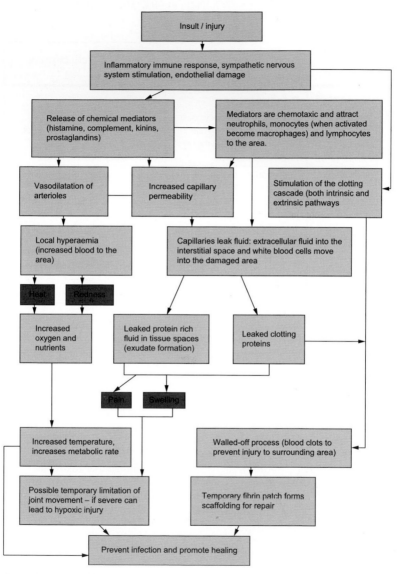

Fig. 4.3 The Inflammatory immune response. An increase in permeability allows protein rich fluid to move out of the extracellular fluid compartment reducing colloidal osmotic pressure, this increases interstitial fluid colloidal osmotic pressure and oedema formation. (Modified from Marieb 2010)

require the use of blood, blood products, a balanced salt and/or water solution, colloid solution or a combination of all solutions.

- Following injury a balance between oxygen supply and tissue demands is fundamental. Oxygen supply and demand is maintained in equilibrium as long as supplies of oxygen are available and carbon dioxide is eliminated through ventilation, perfusion, diffusion and cell metabolism. Any alteration of any part of these processes cause impaired gas exchange. The nurse, therefore, is responsible for administrating humidified oxygen, the continuous frequent monitoring of respiratory rate, depth and pattern of breathing and any signs of change.

- The use of all energy sources following an insult/injury causes an exhaustion of energy stores, deprives cells and tissues of nutrients to support organ function. The loss of energy stores especially protein depletion will contribute to morbidity and mortality of patients following an insult. It is therefore imperative to initiate feeding early in children.

Instigation of these treatments early may stem the IR and neuroendocrine activation and prevent further endothelial damage.

Neurological

Epilepsy

Epilepsy is a neurological condition when the child has recurrent or unprovoked seizures. A child is usually diagnosed as having epilepsy if they have had two or more seizures that started in the brain. Seizures are caused by abnormal electrical discharges in the brain. In the UK, there are an estimated 58 000 children under 18 with epilepsy. Epilepsy usually begins in childhood and affects 1 out of every 100 children. If seizures are 'mini' (petit mal) instead of 'grand mal', it may not be obvious that the child is having a seizure.

Types of seizures

- *Generalized* – where both sides of brain are involved:
  - absence (petit mal) – loss of awareness
  - tonic – sudden stiffening of the limbs or whole body
  - clonic – jerking or twitching of the limbs or whole body
  - atonic – sudden loss of muscle tone
  - tonic–clonic – tonic stage followed by clonic stage (grand mal seizure)
  - myoclonic – shock like contractions of different muscles.

- *Partial (focal)* – where seizure starts in one part of the brain:
  - simple – where no loss of consciousness occurs
  - complex – where loss of consciousness occurs.

The signs and symptoms can vary depending on the type of seizure. Some of the symptoms are outlined below:

- tingling sensation
- unusual smell or taste
- brief staring
- twitching muscle
- convulsive movements
- shallow breathing
- bluish tinge of skin and lips
- drooling of saliva
- loss of bladder or bowel control

- fear and anxiety
- confusion
- change in awareness
- may have no memory of the event
- loss of consciousness.

  Some causes of epilepsy:

- genetically inherited
- brain injury from trauma, surgery, brain tumours
- brain infection (meningitis)
- brain abnormalities
- brain injury at birth
- cerebral palsy
- autism
- intellectual disabilities.

Investigations

- Obtain medical history and duration of seizure.
- Obtain details of antiepileptic medication.
- Apply electroencephalogram (EEG) to record electrical activity.
- Blood tests to exclude possible causes of seizures.
- CT scan, which will show abnormalities in the brain.
- MRI scan, which will show cerebral malformations.

Care and management

- Time the length of the convulsion.
- Stay with the child and lie them on their side.
- Cushion their head with something soft if they have collapsed to the ground.

- Do not put anything in child's mouth or try to restrain the child.
- Loosen tight clothing.
- Remove any objects that could cause injury.
- When the seizure does not subside, this is known as status epilepticus (please read details in Section 1).
- Anticonvulsant drugs are used for long-term treatment. Examples are: sodium valproate, carbamazepine, clonazepam, phenobarbital and phenytoin.
- The type of medication will depend on the type of seizure.
- Children with epilepsy are usually controlled through the use of one anticonvulsant drug.

Long-term care of epilepsy

- Child should wear a medical alert bracelet or carry a card that identifies their condition.
- Medication must be taken as prescribed.
- Blood levels need to be checked periodically.
- Anticonvulsant medication can cause drowsiness and interfere with other medication so it is important that health professionals know all medications the child is taking.
- Seizures can be controlled by medication, surgery or a combination of both.
- Surgery may block the area where seizure begins, remove brain tissue or use vagal nerve stimulation (VNS).
- A ketogenic diet high in fat, low in carbohydrates and low in calories can reduce the number and severity of seizures for some children.

- Avoid or limit known triggers, e.g. flickering lights, lack of sleep, fatigue, noise, exercise, stress and non-compliance with medication.
- Some children can outgrow their seizures by their mid to late teens.
- Children are not allowed to swim alone.
- Children must always wear helmets when cycling, roller blades, or using scooters.
- Young girls may experience seizures prior to menstrual periods, thus medication may need to be adjusted when child reaches puberty.
- Alcohol can affect epilepsy, thus children need to be strongly advised against using alcohol or recreational drugs.
- Young people (18 years) are not allowed to drive until they have been seizure free for 3 months or more depending on the countries driving regulations.

High temperatures

For in an emergency see Section 1. There are four general states of increased body temperature (Edwards 1998b, 2003b):

- *Pyrexia (fever)* – involves a condition whereby the thermoregulatory mechanisms remain intact, but the body temperature is maintained at a high level. It generally has an infective aetiology, but there are other non-infectious causes of a hyperpyrexia. These include haemolysis (seen in reactions to blood transfusions) and thyrotoxicosis.
- *Hyperpyrexia* – the hypothalamus set point temperature is generally very

high e.g. above $40°C$, generally observed in conditions such as septicaemia and meningitis. A temperature between $41°C$ and $43°C$ produces nerve damage, coagulation, convulsions and death.

- *Hyperthermia* - occurs when there is hypothalamic injury, due to neoplasms, surgery, central nervous system problems, and when overheating overwhelms the heat loss mechanisms – causes cerebral metabolism to increase and the brain has great difficulty keeping up with the increase in carbon dioxide production, does not respond to antipyretic therapy.
- *Malignant hyperthermia* – caused by certain drugs commonly used in patients, e.g. diuretics, antiseizure therapy, analgesics, some common anaesthetics, anti-arrhythmics and antibiotics. A malignant hyperthermia also presents in five other conditions:
  - heat cramps;
  - heat exhaustion
  - heat stroke
  - malignant hyperthermia
  - neuroleptic malignant syndrome (NMS).

Heat cramps, heat exhaustion are generally not life threatening. However, heat stroke, malignant hyperthermia and NMS must be recognized quickly, as, untreated, they may be fatal.

During a high temperature due to an infection the treatment by cooling methods such as tepid sponging or fanning has been criticized. Cooling methods are of no use, as they result in:

- A compensatory response by the hypothalamus, which will produce heat-generating activities like chills and shivering.

- Information sent to the hypothalamus that the body temperature is decreasing.
- Compromising an unstable patient by depleting their metabolic reserve and can create a new temperature spike, which is as high or higher than the original one, and may even increase the patient's temperature.
- The patient feeling weak, especially during the early stages when the temperature is still rising.

The best way to treat a high temperature is by the use of antipyrexial drug therapy, in preference to cooling methods.

Hyperpyrexia due to damage of the hypothalamus results in the body failing to activate compensatory cooling mechanisms. This tends to increase cellular metabolism, oxygen consumption and carbon dioxide production.

Unless the temperature is monitored carefully and cooling methods such as fanning and tepid sponging are instituted, irreversible brain damage and death occur.

Hypothermia

A drastic decrease in body temperature is known as hypothermia, and is characterized by a marked cooling of core temperature, and is defined as a core temperature below 35°C (Edwards 1999). Progressive temperature reduction below this level will result in reduced metabolism and risk of cardiac arrest. At 28–30°C, loss of consciousness will ensue. Low temperatures cause compensatory shivering and vasoconstriction, to shunt the blood to vital organs, and prevent excess heat loss

from skin surfaces, causing metabolic and cardio-respiratory stress to ill patients. Hypothermia can be accidental of therapeutic:

- *Accidental hypothermia* is a temperature below 35°C and is a result of sudden immersion in cold water or prolonged exposure to cold environments. Healthy subjects who experience hypothermia often survive profound hypothermia with medical support.

- *Therapeutic hypothermia* is used to slow metabolism and preserve ischaemic tissue during surgery. It can also occur through exposure of body cavities to the relatively cool operating room environment, irrigation of body cavities with room temperature solutions, infusion of room temperature intravenous solutions, and inhalation of unwarmed anaesthetic agents. These types of therapeutic hypothermia can extend into the postoperative period.

The nurse needs to be aware of any patients at risk of hypothermia and take notice of how long the patient has been exposed for in theatre. Rewarming methods are divided into three groups:

- passive external rewarming (removal of wet clothes, blankets, warm room)

- active external rewarming (radiant lights, convection air blankets)

- active internal rewarming (warmed gases to respiratory tract, warmed intravenous fluids).

The process of re-warming should proceed at no faster than a few degrees per hour. If a patient is rapidly re-warmed oxygen consumption, myocardial demand and vasodilatation increase faster than the heart's ability to compensate and death can occur.

Endocrine disorders

The endocrine system along with the nervous system is responsible for control and communication within the body. The glands are ductless and secrete their products directly into the blood stream to act upon a target organ that may be far away from the gland itself (Richards and Edwards 2008).

Diabetes insipidus

This is a disease of the posterior pituitary gland, which is the size of a pea and secretes many vital hormones, important in the control of other endocrine glands, known at the 'leader' or 'master' endocrine gland.

Types of diabetes insipidus

- Central or neurogenic diabetes insipidus – lack of antidiuretic hormone (ADH) being released into the circulation in response to an osmotic stimulus, e.g. osmoreceptors.
  - Most often due to a lesion in the hypothalamus or posterior pituitary gland including:
    - tumours
    - aneurysms
    - thrombosis
    - infections.
  - There is a total or partial inability to concentrate the urine.
  - Total urine output varies between 4 and 12 l per day.
  - Acute onset and dehydration may develop rapidly.

- Transient usually incomplete central diabetes insipidus is noticed frequently in patients with head injury.
- Dipsogenic or psychogenic diabetes insipidus – precipitated by excessive intake of water very rare.
- Nephrogenic diabetes insipidus – deficient action of ADH
- Pregnancy-related diabetes insipidus is also known to occur.

Clinical presentation

- Polyuria
- Nocturia
- Thirst – generally the desire for cold drinks
- Inability to replace water may result in signs of hypovolaemia
- Low urine osmolality – SG 1.001–1.005
- High plasma osmolality due to dehydration
- The essential feature is that urine osmolality is inappropriately low compared to plasma osmolality.
- Urine volumes over 4–6 l/day or 3 ml/kg over 2 consecutive hours (in neurosurgical patients may point toward diabetes insipidus).

Investigations

- Random plasma and urine osmolality.
- Plasma and urine osmolality relationships.
- Blood chemistry – blood glucose, 24 hour urine osmolality an electrolytes, blood and urine electrolytes, urea and creatinine.
- ADH test – if tests above are positive then ADH (usually as DDAVP nasally) is given.

- Hypertonic saline – used to evaluate osmoreceptor mechanism.
- MRI scan – assessment of pituitary function.

Treatment

Replacement therapy with a synthetic ADH:

- Aqueous vasopressin (arginine) – short-acting agent can be given intramuscularly or subcutaneously.
- DDAVP (desmopressin) – long-acting agent, given intranasally.
- Oral hydration is often sufficient.

Diabetes mellitus

This is a common condition characterized by a persistently raised blood glucose level due to a deficiency or lack of insulin. An estimated 1.4 million people in the UK have diabetes (Richards and Edwards 2003).

The pancreas

The pancreas releases glucagon, which is synthesized by alpha cells of the pancreas. When stimulated they lower blood glucose levels and when inhibited blood glucose levels will rise. The target/effect of glucagon is the:

- liver
  - glycogenolysis (glycogen to glucose)
  - glyconeogenesis (synthesis of glucose)
  - release of glucose into blood.
- adipose (fat) tissue
  - fat catabolism, release of fatty acids into blood.

A hyposecretion of glucagon leads to hypoglycaemia, hypersecretion leads to hyperglycaemia.

The pancreas also releases insulin synthesized by the beta cells of the pancreas. Release of insulin is stimulated by high blood glucose levels and inhibited release is by a low blood glucose levels. The target/effect of insulin is:

- all cells except liver, kidney, brain:
  - increased glucose uptake into cells
  - promotes protein synthesis and fat storage
  - encourages glucose storage as glycogen in the liver and skeletal muscles
  - lowers blood glucose levels.

A hyposecretion of insulin leads to insulin-dependent diabetes mellitus as glucose is not absorbed into cells and therefore the body cannot utilize its glucose, which accumulates in the blood and the kidneys attempt to excrete any excess in urine. A hypersecretion of insulin is generally due to an overdose of insulin.

Type 1 diabetes mellitus

This used to be called insulin-dependent diabetes mellitus (IDDM).

- Dependent on insulin without it the patient would die.
- Less than 25% of people with diabetes are insulin dependent.
- Thought to be an autoimmune disorder – beta cells in the pancreas are targeted by antibodies and eventually totally destroyed.
- Some individuals have a genetic predisposition – trigger factor is needed; this is generally a virus.
- Highest incidence around 11–12 years but can occur at any age, uncommon over the age of 40 years.

Clinical features:

- Polyuria
- Thirst
- Polydipsia
- Weight loss – breakdown of protein and fats as source of energy, emaciation
- Production of excessive ketones – acid and appear in urine
- Lack of energy – cells are starving, loss of muscle mass, weakness.

Treatment:

- Insulin therapy – cannot be given orally as gastrointestinal enzymes render it ineffective. May require up to four injections per day (see Section 6).

Type 2 diabetes mellitus

Type 2 diabetes used to be called non-insulin dependent diabetes mellitus (NIDDM).

- There is either insufficient production of insulin or an inability of the body to use the insulin adequately (insulin resistance).
- Patients not dependent on insulin may receive some insulin to help control their diabetes, but can live without it.
- Different from type 1 and does not happen in the young, may have the disorder for years and not know it.
- Symptoms develop much more insidiously, incidence increases with age and as people are living longer, so the disease is getting more common.
- Disorder is linked to obesity, and can run in families.
- Can be controlled by diet alone or by medication such as oral hypoglycaemic agents, to bring down blood glucose.

Respiratory

Asthma

The most common diagnosis for children admitted to hospital is asthma and its related disorders. In the last 20 years, hospitals have dealt with a dramatic increase in both asthma-related admissions and readmissions in the paediatric population. Asthma admission rates are more frequent amongst girls, and the likelihood of readmission is higher amongst children under five years of age. Asthma is an inflammatory condition of the airways mediated by a wide range of stimuli usually the immunoglobulin IgE, the release of chemical mediators, leading to bronchospasm (Fig. 4.4), which is due to an imbalance between:

- cholinergic (parasympathetic) nervous system
- adrenergic (sympathetic) nervous system.

These actions contributes to plugging mucus and oedema (Fig. 4.5).

Extrinsic asthma

This is associated with the following:

- childhood
- identifiable factors provoking it such as wheezing
- hayfever and eczema
- nocturnal cough (only a symptom).

Intrinsic asthma

This is associated with the following:

- begins in adult life and obstruction is more persistent
- there are obvious stimuli other than respiratory tract infection (RTI).

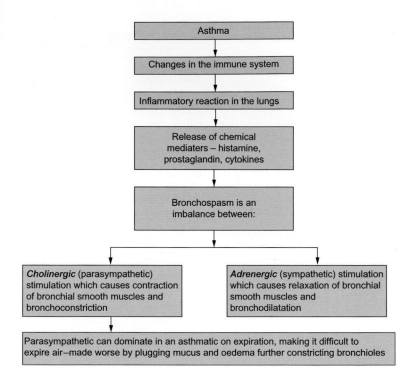

Fig. 4.4 Sequence of events that lead to asthma.

Acid–base changes occur

- respiratory alkalosis – normal physiological process of homeostasis is maintained:
- dyspnoea ↑ respiratory rate
- $ETCO_2$ normal or low
- cough/wheezing
- respiratory acidosis – indicates homeostasis is not maintained and intubation required
- worsening wheeze
- respiratory rate > 30/min
- cyanosis/tachycardia > 110/min
- peak flow < 33%.

Drug therapy:

- Salbutamol inhaler on demand
- Inhaled short-acting steroid (beclomethasone, budesonide, fluticasone)
- Longer acting beta agonist (salmeterol)
- Theophylline, cromoglycate or ipratropium

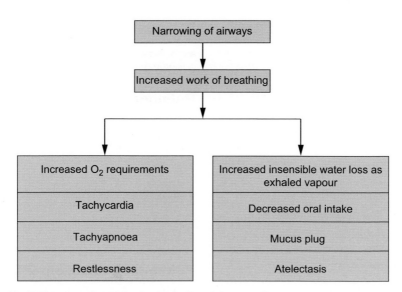

Fig. 4.5 Sequence of events leading from asthma to hypoxaemia.

- Prednisolone
- Antibiotics.

- *Legionella pneumophila*
- *Myobacterium tuberculosis.*

Pneumonia

Pneumonia is an acute inflammation of the substance of the lungs due to:

- bacteria
- chemical causes
- aspiration of vomit
- radiotherapy
- allergic mechanism (asthma).

Common bacteria

- *Streptococcus pneumoniae*
- *Mycoplasma pneumoniae*
- *Haemophilus influenzae*
- *Staphylococcus aureus*

Aspiration pneumonia

Aspiration of gastric contents, either solids or liquids, can lead to severe illness; this can be fatal as gastric acid contents in the lungs is very destructive. Material enters the right lung more readily because of the wider right bronchus. Infection usually caused by an anaerobic organism.

Predisposing factors

- Recent extubation
- Metabolic coma
- Altered consciousness
- Drug overdose, anaesthesia, epilepsy, CVA, alcoholism

- Dysphagia, oesophageal disease
- Stricture, fistula, hiatus hernia, reflux
- Neurological disorders
- Myasthenia gravis, motor neurone disease
- Nasal gastric tubes
- Terminal illness.

Management

- Oxygen therapy
- Mechanical ventilation
- Bronchodilator therapy
- Cardiovascular support
- Bronchoscopy
- Antibiotics
- Corticosteroids.

Prevention

- Posture
- Suction
- Cricoid pressure
- Airway protection
- Nasograstric tube
- Antacid therapy, H_2 receptor antagonists and sucralfate.
- Metoclopramide.

Pneumonia in the immunocompromised patient:

- More common with the emergence of human immunodeficiency virus (HIV)
- Opportunistic infections
- Rapid pneumonias extensive and life threatening

- Viral, fungal, protozoal or bacterial in origin
- *Pneumocystis carinii* pneumonia is the commonest.

Pulmonary oedema

Fluid in the interstitial and alveolar spaces of the lungs. The general cause is by an increase in hydrostatic pressure within the pulmonary circulation due to:

- left ventricular failure
- fluid overload, increased infusions of:
  - crystalloids
  - colloids
- pulmonary hypertension.

Pulmonary embolism (PE)

A PE is an occlusion of pulmonary vascular bed by an embolus or a thrombus, tissue fragments, lipids, fats or an air bubble:

- 90% of PE is the consequence of clots that are initially in the leg veins and the pelvis.
- Half the people diagnosed with pulmonary embolism die within 2 hours of the diagnosis.
- PE is responsible for 10% of hospital death and 80% of the time PE go undetected.
- PE causes hypoxia, vasoconstriction, pulmonary oedema or decrease in surfactant.

The effect of the embolism depends on the extent of the pulmonary blood flow obstructed, the size of the affected vessels, nature of the embolism and the secondary effect. The size of the pulmonary artery in which the blood clot is logged determines the severity of symptoms and prognosis. If the embolus blocks the pulmonary artery and one of its main branches, immediate death may occur. Patient may complain of:

- chest pain
- sudden pain or shock
- a sudden sharp or abdominal pain if embolism blocks smaller vessels.

The pathophysiology of PE

PE is more common in patients who have had surgery of the lower limbs and trauma patients. Permanent lung injury does not occur if the infarction is not severe, patient may present symptoms similar to those of pneumonia dyspnoea, chest pain, VQ imbalances, pulmonary infarction and decreased cardiac output.

Diagnosis of PE

- Bloods are taken to examine leukocyte count and sedimentation rate, which is usually elevated in cases of infarction.
- Impairment in gas exchange that is to say partial pressure of oxygen was low, partial pressure of carbon dioxide was normal and the pH was normal.
- Use of a VQ scan but results can be sometimes inconclusive. Angiography and echocardiography could then be used but they are not easily available in most hospitals.
- PE should be suspected in patients who collapse suddenly 1–2 weeks following surgery.
- If large PE is a medical emergency – leading to death
- Clinical features depends on size of embolus:
  - sharp, knife like pain in the chest, well localized in a small embolus

- if large the pain is more central
- shortness of breath
- anxiety and distress
- haemoptysis
- hypotension, tachycardia, pallor
- cyanosis (suggests a large embolism)
- collapse, cardiac arrest or shock.

Treatment of PE

The aim of the therapy is to prevent further thrombus formation and embolization.

- The administration of oxygen is required to relieve shortness of breath and to supply oxygen to the affected areas of the lungs.
- Morphine 10 mg may be given to relieve chest pain.
- A bolus of heparin is used as a fast-acting drug and then proceed with warfarin.
  - 5000 iu followed by 1400 iu/hour to 2.8 ml/hour of 0.9% saline in a syringe pump
  - a fast acting anticoagulant
  - high molecular weight heparin (LMWH) has a high affinity for anti-thrombin obviously inhibiting blood coagulation
  - heparin is generally used for the treatment of acute PE.

Care of a patient with a PE

- Involves supportive measures and prevention of further emboli formation.
- The primary excessive usage of heparin is bleeding of the gums when brushing teeth, excessive or easy skin brushing and unexplained nose bleeds.

- The vital signs the nurse has to look for include when a child appears to be in shock or having difficulty in breathing and pain.

Pneumothorax

An accumulation of air in the pleural space due to:

- spontaneous formation in young tall thin males
- trauma
- asthma, COAD, TB, pneumonia, lung carcinoma
- cystic fibrosis and any diffuse lung disease
- IPPV, aggressive bagging following intubation
- insertion of a CVP line.

Clinical features

- No symptoms if small and in a fit young person
- Dyspnoea depends on size, mild to very severe
- Pleuritic pain – sometimes transient
- The patient may suggest they felt something 'snap' before the onset of pain and dyspnoea
- Decreased breath sounds, respiratory distress
- Agitation, cyanosis, tachycardia
- Reduced respiratory movement on affected side
- Increase or decrease in BP.

A tension pneumothorax is a medical emergency. A flap develops and acts as a one way valve, air is trapped following inspiration. Mediastinal shift is when the medial structures become misplaced towards unaffected side:

- reduces venous return and cardiac output
- death may occur very quickly

16–18 gauge needle 3rd–4th intercostal space at the midclavicular line will relieve pressure.
Flail chest

- A reduced rigid structure of the rib cage.
- The segment loses continuity with the rest of the chest wall and paradoxical movement occurs.
- When chest expands the flail segment is depressed.
- Limits the negative intrathoracic pressure needed to move air into lungs.

On expiration:

- the flail segment bulges outwards, interfering with exhalation
- the negative pressure on the unaffected side is less than the affected side – the mediastinum shifts towards the affected side
- ventilation impairment depends on injury or presence of pneumothorax or haemothorax.

On inspiration:

- the intrapleural pressures on the unaffected side are greater displacing the mediastinum towards it.

This is known as mediastinal flutter, which:

- impairs ventilation

- reduces cardiac output and venous return
- reduces intrapleural pressure during inspiration
- impairs circulating dynamics and venous filling
- can be observed by visual inspection of movement of both posterior and anterior breathing patterns
- is worsened by pain
- may require ventilator support.

Cardiovascular

Hypovolaemia

For hypovolaemic shock see Section 1. Hypovolaemia is a decline in blood volume produced by continued bleeding, plasma loss, water or fluid shifts, decreases venous return and cardiac output (Edwards 2005c). Numerous compensatory mechanisms are activated when the circulating volume is reduced and the venous return is decreased.

Following blood loss homeostatic mechanisms are activated:

- The baroreceptors (in the aorta and carotid sinus) become stretched to a lesser degree, decreasing their rate of discharge, resulting in vasoconstriction. The vasoconstriction will greatly increase the peripheral resistance, maintain arterial blood pressure and return more blood to the heart.
- A decreased renal blood flow will result in release of renin which stimulates the production of aldosterone, which restores extracellular volume, by conserving sodium and water. Angiotensin II

stimulates the release of norepinephrine (noradrenaline) and when circulating in the blood will cause widespread peripheral vasoconstriction, to improve blood pressure and renal blood flow. However, the continued vasoconstriction in the kidneys may cause the glomerular filtration rate (GFR) to become depressed, as a result, minimal urine is produced. If hypovolaemia is prolonged, severe renal tubular damage results, known as an acute tubular necrosis (ATN).

These protective mechanisms will eventually cease to function and circulatory failure ensues. If the metabolic acidosis, circulatory failure or volume is not corrected or treatment instigated, death will occur in a short period of time.

The principal aetiologies of hypovolaemic states can be classified as haemorrhage, plasma loss, third-space shifts, bleeding disorders, dehydration and high temperatures.

Haemorrhage Hypovolaemia caused by haemorrhage (the loss of whole blood) is the most common cause of shock. The greater the duration and severity of haemorrhage, the more pronounced is the state of shock. The loss of red cells seen in haemorrhage decreases the oxygen carrying capacity of the blood, and contributes to hypoxia.

Plasma loss Hypovolaemia caused by plasma loss is the result of an increase in permeability leading to a shift of plasma fluid from the vascular space into the interstitial space. This type of hypovolaemia occurs most often in individuals with large partial-thickness burns, full thickness burns, or burns over more than 20–25% of the total body surface area.

Third space shifts

Hypovolaemia caused by third space fluid shifts – any type of trauma or cell damage (e.g. surgical, myocardial infarction, head injury) whether it is external and visible or internal and invisible – will automatically trigger an inflammatory response. This normal body response will be to send nutrients, fluids, white blood cells, and clotting factors to the damaged site to repair tissue, prevent infection and if necessary stem blood loss (see trauma section later).

Bleeding disorders

Hypovolaemia caused by bleeding disorders – which involves platelet and coagulation disorders, which can cause or fail to prevent an internal or external haemorrhage. Disorders of platelets include thrombocytopenia and thrombocytosis and can be caused by drugs, such as anti-inflammatory agents, antimicrobials, antidepressants, and adrenergic blocking agents. Coagulation disorders tend to result in more serious bleeding and are usually caused by a deficiency of one or several clotting factors, for example vitamin K, liver disease or DIC.

Dehydration

Hypovolaemia caused by dehydration is more commonly seen in the elderly, but if prolonged can induce hypovolaemic shock. It may be a consequence of a primary deficit of water, a primary deficit of salt or both. A primary deficit of water leads to cellular dehydration and circulatory failure, a primary deficit of salt leads to a reduced extracellular fluid volume, a reduced blood volume, and increasing difficulty in maintaining an adequate circulating volume. For the different types of hypovolaemia due to dehydration see Box 4.1.

High temperature

Hypovolaemia due to a high temperature is due to the vasodilatation observed during a high temperature and can make a patient appear hypovolaemic. As fluid space has increased there is still the same amount of circulating volume. The vasodilatation causes a reduction in BP, peripheral vascular resistance and an increase in heart rate and electrolyte imbalance. Dehydration may result due to fluid loss during sweating and from the lungs due to increased respiratory rate. Dehydration, together with the profuse vasodilatation of blood vessels may serve to add to the 'appearance' of a hypovolaemic state.

Hypovolaemic shock caused by any of the six aetiologies described is indeed a critical state that begins with an adaptive response to illness or injury and if not treated may progress to multiple system organ failure.

Assessment of a child with hypovolaemia

Nurses can collect data to determine the circulatory status of a patient, and every nurse is aware of the crucial importance of astute and accurate observation. This starts from the very moment the patient is admitted, as the nurse automatically observes details such as:

- facial colour
- pallor
- flushed or cyanosed
- any respiratory difficulty
- rapid or shallow breathing
- cool moist or dehydrated skin
- ischaemia of the eyelids, lips, gums and tongue

Box 4.1 The different types of dehydration

Isotonic dehydration

This is where there are alterations in both the total body water (TBW) and electrolyte balance. It generally results from reduced fluid intake rather than increased loss, but can occur from haemorrhage, severe wound drainage, and excessive diaphoresis. The most common cause of reduced fluid intake in clinical practice is the inability of the individual to acquire an adequate amount of fluids. Water dehydration causes weight loss, dryness of skin and mucous membranes, decreased urine output, and symptoms of hypovolaemia, such as, a rapid heart rate, flattened neck veins, and a decrease in blood pressure. In severe causes hypovolaemic shock can occur. The individuals at risk of dehydration related to water deficit include infants, the elderly, or immobilized individuals.

Hypertonic dehydration

This is where there is an increased concentration of extracellular sodium (hypernatraemia) in relation to water. This is associated with fever or respiratory infections, which increase the respiratory rate and enhance water loss from the lungs. Also severe diarrhoea causes water loss in relation to sodium. Insufficient water intake also can cause hypernatraemia, particularly in individuals who are comatose, confused, or immobilized. In hypertonic volume depletion the urine specific gravity will be greater than 1.030, the haematocrit, plasma proteins and plasma osmolality will be elevated above normal.

Hypotonic dehydration

This is where there is a reduction in sodium (hyponatraemia) and an increase in water. This is associated with a reduced intake of sodium, continued diuretic therapy and vomiting. Sodium deficits usually cause a reduction in the plasma osmolarity with movement of water into the cells. This movement will reduce the overall circulating volume and thus give the impression of dehydration.

Dehydration – a deficiency of both salt and water

This is the most appropriate term to indicate both sodium loss and water loss. A deficiency of both salt and water occurs when fluid is lost from the gastrointestinal tract.

- facial expressions
- oedema
- increased or decreased body weight
- pulsating neck veins
- posture and dry mucous membranes

- observations are made for signs of:
  - anxiety or distress
  - evidence of confusion, disorientation, apprehension, restlessness, agitation or calm.

These observations will direct the nurse's subsequent, more systematic objective approach to data collection such as: mental state; central venous pressure; pulses; electrocardiograph; skin temperature; blood pressure; urine output and testing; oxygen saturation and blood analysis.

Mental state

A reduced oxygen supply caused by the loss of red blood cells observed in haemorrhage will stimulate the adrenal medulla to secrete norepinephrine (noradrenaline), which causes vasoconstriction of the systemic circulation. The reduction in blood flow leads to a reduction in blood supply to the brain's reticular formation (located in the brain stem), whose function it is to modulate sensory awareness and input. These changes may account for the deterioration in mental state often observed in hypovolaemic states, and can present themselves in different ways (e.g. apathy, confusion, restlessness and apprehension).

Restlessness in hypovolaemic patients may serve to increase their depth of respiratory movements and may improve venous return by increasing the intrathoracic pressure, helping to compensate for the continued reduction in cardiac output from continuous bleeding. However, other patients are quiet and apathetic, and their senses become dulled, probably as a result of cerebral ischaemia and acidosis. In addition, a reduction in perfusion to the brain stem will affect respiration, blood pressure and heart rate.

A general assessment of the patient's mental state can alert the nurse to impending neurological deterioration. The Glasgow Coma Scale (see neurological assessment) is an example of a specific tool designed to produce a uniform method of determining and recording the activity of the ANS or mental state. It focuses on the evaluation of three parameters: eye opening, motor response and verbal response.

Supporting the patient with hypovolaemia

When considering support for the circulation, there needs to be effective clinical management of bleeding, to ensure the rapid establishment and maintenance of fluid volume replacement and the control of haemorrhage. The immediate restoration of an effective circulating blood volume through the use of blood, blood products, a balanced salt solution, colloid solution, or all four, is needed to minimize, prevent or reverse hypovolaemic states.

The current concepts of fluid resuscitation are complex, full of controversy and there are constant discussions about whether whole blood, colloid or crystalloid therapy should be given (Table 4.4). It might be easy to just propose that blood be given for haemorrhage, colloids be given for plasma loss, clotting factors for bleeding disorders and crystalloid for dehydration, and third-space fluid shifts. However, this argument, even though rationale and logical, is much too simplistic. Please consult up-to-date literature and individual hospital policies for current practices.

Table 4.4 Constituents of crystalloids and colloids used for fluid resuscitation

Fluid	pH/ mOsm	Contents	Normal levels	Uses	Avoid in	Benefits	Problems
0.9% Normal saline	pH: 5.5 mOsm: 308	Na: 154 mmol/L Cl: 154 mmol/L	pH: 7.35–7.45 mOsm: 274–300 Na: 35–45 K: 3.5–5.5 Cl: Cal: Bic: Lactate:	Hypovolaemia Maintenance fluid (not recommended) Dilution of drugs	Dehydration Acidosis Oedema Hypernatraemia Neuro patients Diabetes insipidus Increased chloride Heart failure	Stays in the extracellular fluid space and so can be given for hypovolaemia	Is slightly hypertonic and if too much given can lead to fluid overload.
5% Dextrose	pH: 4.2 mOsm: 278	Glucose: 5 g/100 ml 840 kJ/l (Yorkie bar 1500)		Cellular dehydration Insulin infusion Dilution of drugs	Hypovolaemia Feeding Neuro patients increased ICP	Good for intracellular dehydration and as maintenance fluid	Should not be used for emergency or for hypovolaemia
Hartmann's solution	pH: 5–7 mOsm: 278	Na: 131 Cl: 111 K: 5.1 Cal: 2 Bic: 29 Lactate:		Hypovolaemia Maintenance during surgery	Hyperkalaemia Renal patients Acidosis	Stays in the extracellular fluid space and so can be used for hypovolaemic stages	Is slightly hypertonic and so can lead to fluid overload, some patients may not be able to take the potassium load, so not good for all patients.

(Continued)

Table 4.4 Constituents of crystalloids and colloids used for fluid resuscitation—cont'd

Fluid	pH/mOsm	Contents	Normal levels	Uses	Avoid in	Benefits	Problems
Gelatins (Volplex, Gelofusine)	pH: 7.4 mOsm: 274	Na: 135 Cl: 110 K: Cal: Bic:		Hypovolaemia	Hypervolaemia	Requires less volume than normal saline	Effects of protein can have lasting effects and not excreted by diuretics
Starches (Voluven, Volulyte)	pH: 4-5.5 mOsm:308	Voluven (starch in saline) Na: Volulyte (starch in water) Na: 137 K: 4 Cl: 110 Cal:		Hypovolaemia	Voluven Hypervolaemia Anaphylaxis Volulyte Clotting disorders	Requires less volume than normal saline	Hyponatraemia Hypernatraemia

Renal

Renal function can be affected by a variety of disorders, the common cause is infection. The urinary tract can be obstructed by stones or a tumour. Renal function can be impaired by disorders of the kidney itself or by many other systemic diseases.

- Inflammation (Fig. 4.3) – infection, obstruction, tumours.
- Reduced blood supply to the kidneys (Fig. 4.1) – hypoxic damage, acute tubular necrosis (ATN), hypovolaemia.

Urinary tract obstruction

- Can occur anywhere in the urinary tract.
- Renal stones formed from calcium loading in the urethra.
- Trauma.
- Tumours.
- Neural lesions interrupt innervation of the bladder.
- Renal cell carcinoma common neoplasm.
- Metatastasis to the liver, lung, bone.
- Bladder tumours high rate of recurrence.

Causes a collection of urine behind the obstruction, affecting surrounding organs leading to inflammation and ischaemic atrophy, which is dependent on:

- location within the urinary tract
- unilateral or bilateral
- partial or complete – GFR reduced or zero

- acute or chronic duration – chronic partial obstruction causes compression of kidney structures reducing renal ability
- the underlying cause.

The relief of a renal obstruction followed by a variable period of diuresis, with losses of large amounts of urine lasts for a few days without symptoms of volume depletion

Urinary tract infection (UTI) usually caused by:

- bacteria from retrograde movement into urethra and bladder
- diagnosed by culture of specific organisms
- counts of 100 000 bacteria/ml of freshly voided urine
- can occur anywhere along the urinary tract
- cystitis – inflammation of the bladder, which is the most common site, generally more common in women, common organisms:
  - *Escherichia coli*
  - *Klebsiella*
  - *Proteus*
  - *Pseudomonas*
  - *Staphylococcus*.

Pyelonephritis

- Infection of the renal pelvis acute or chronic (persistent or recurrent).
- Cause is usually bacterial, but can be fungi or viruses.
- Generally spread by ascending organism along the ureters, but may occur via the blood stream.
- Acute responds well to 2 weeks organism-specific antibiotics.

Gastrointestinal tract (GIT)

Patients admitted may have undergone GIT surgery for a number of the conditions identified here or develop bleeding. Some conditions are severe (e.g. peritonitis, pancreatitis) and may require additional interventions. In addition, feeding is a priority and these conditions will inhibit the digestion and absorption of nutrients. It is therefore, imperative that a nurse has understanding of these conditions.

Symptoms of gastrointestinal disease could include the following:

- dysphagia
- dyspepsia
- heartburn
- flatulence
- haematemesis
- abdominal pain/acute abdomen
- GI bleeding
- malaena
- steatorrhoea
- loss of weight
- abdominal pain
- anorexia
- diarrhoea and vomiting
- constipation.

Helicobacter pylori

This organism is a spirochaete and appears in patients with gastric ulcers or cancer and has been known to occur in children.

- It is the commonest cause of gastritis.
- Its mode of transmission is thought to be through kissing or water, otherwise it is uncertain.

- Diagnosis is by C urea breath tests, endoscopic mucosal biopsy and culture of the organism.
- Treatment is by triple regimens:
  - amoxyicillin
  - metronidazole
  - omeprazole.

Inflammatory bowel disorders

Any condition of the GIT can lead to stimulation of the inflammatory response (Fig. 4.2).

These conditions include:

- ulcerative colitis
- Crohn's disease
- diverticular disease
- peritonitis
- appendicitis.

Ulcerative colitis

- Chronic inflammatory disease – inflammation and ulceration of rectum and sigmoid colon.
- Oedema forms and narrows the lumen of the involved colon.
- Mucosal destruction causes bleeding, cramping pain, urge to defecate, diarrhoea.
- Dehydration, malnutrition, steroids/analgesia.
- Periods of remission, with possible surgical resection if therapy unsuccessful.

Crohn's disease

- Difficult to distinguish from ulcerative colitis.
- The rectum is seldom involved and the formation of cancer rare.

- Few symptoms other than IBS, then inflammation, tenderness, weight loss.
- Child may develop pernicious anaemia, deficiencies in folic acid and vitamin D absorption, hypoalbuminaemia.
- Surgery to manage complications of fistula, abscess, or relief of obstruction.

Diverticular disease

- Herniations or saclike outpouchings of mucosa through the muscle layers of the colon wall.
- Asymptomatic, diverticulitis with inflammation.
- Appears in weak points in the colon wall and reduces the diameter and increases pressure – can lead to rupture of the diverticula.
- Can lead to abscess formation and peritonitis.
- Increase in dietary fibre frequently relieves symptoms.
- Surgical resection may be required.

Peritonitis. Inflammation of the peritoneal cavity, covering of the:

- bowel and mesentery
- the omentum
- lining of the abdominal cavity
- perforation of any region leads to life-threatening peritonitis.

Causes:

- appendicitis
- Crohn's disease
- diverticulitis
- cholecystitis
- salpingitis.

A patient can be seriously ill with generalized peritonitis, as inflammatory fluid moves into the peritoneal cavity and causes hypovolaemia and may lead to toxaemia or septicaemia. This condition is most severe when contaminated with faeces, infected bile or pus and less severe in the absence of infection. The abdomen will be rigid and tender; bowel sounds will be absent. Treatment of peritonitis will depend on the cause.

Appendicitis is inflammation of the vermiform appendix, a projection from the apex of the caecum. A common surgical emergency, it affects 7–12% of children in the UK.

Causes:

- obstruction of the lumen with stool, foreign bodies, with consequent bacterial infection:
  - drainage of the appendix is reduced
  - increased pressure so appendix becomes hypoxic
  - bacterial microbial invasion
  - inflammation and oedema
  - gangrene.

Signs and symptoms

- A classic sign is a rebound tenderness, but this does not occur in all cases.
- There is abdominal pain in the right lower quadrant, but this may be vague at first and increasing over a period of 3–4 hours.
- Nausea and vomiting.
- Loss of appetite.
- Low-grade fever.
- Diarrhoea may occur in some children but is not always present.

Diagnosis can be assisted by abdominal X-ray or computed tomography, and an increase in white blood cell count. Appendectomy is the treatment for a simple or perforated appendicitis. Recovery is generally without complications, but can be more complicated if they occur.

Complications

- Perforation
- Peritonitis
- Abscess formation.

Liver failure

In liver failure there is a reduction in the functioning of the liver. The liver has great powers of regeneration and if injured can completely recover. When the process of regeneration is inadequate cells are being regenerated and damaged at the same time. Blood vessels and biliary ducts must be replaced as well as connective tissue, fibrous tissues are laid down to form the normal liver cells – known as cirrhosis. Liver failure only occurs when 75% of liver cells have died.

As cirrhosis develops blood supply becomes disrupted and collateral circulation develops from hepatic portal vein, back pressure is created in the portal system around oesophageal/gastric junction, which may burst. Fluid will also accumulate to cause ascites, discomfort and respiratory embarrassment.

Functions of the liver

- Converts glycogen, fat and protein into glucose.
- Stores protein.

- Breakdown of worn-out red blood cells and white blood cells and some bacteria.
- Renders dangerous substances harmless to the body – either breaks them down or transforms them into less harmful compounds.
- Produces bile salts used in small intestine for the emulsification and absorption of fats in the body.
- Stores copper, iron and vitamins A, D (involvement of the kidneys), E and K.
- Production of clotting factors – heparin, prothrombin, fibrinogen and albumin.
- Formation of urea – removal of ammonia.

Classifications of liver failure

- Fulminant liver failure: severe in onset, rapid in progress and also known as acute liver failure. From onset to jaundice to development of encephalopathy is 0–8 weeks.
- Sub-fulminant liver failure: from jaundice to encephalopathy in 8 weeks–6 months.
- Chronic liver failure: over 6 months in duration.

Causes:

- Poisoning due to overdose, e.g. paracetamol
- Drug induced, e.g. isoniazid, sodium valporate, anti-depressants, NSAIDs
- Viral hepatis
- Miscellaneous, e.g. Wilson's disease, Well's disease, Reye's syndrome.

Liver disease can also occur in the following infections:

- herpes simplex
- varicella zoster
- measles
- rubella
- coxsackie B
- adenoviruses.

Clinical features

- *Varices*: as pressure increases in the portal veins small veins open in the oesophagus and rectum to equalize pressure. The increased pressure shunts blood, and gets the veins wider and if they become too large may rupture:
  - 70% of patients with liver cirrhosis will develop varices
  - cause of life-threatening haematemesis when they rupture
  - painless, but extremely frightening for patient and relatives.

- *Encepalopathy*: amino acids are burned for energy and they leave behind toxic nitrogenous waste (ammonia), which is generally converted to urea by the liver; while other organs cope the brain deteriorates (Grades 1–5)

- *Jaundice*: urine testing is an early diagnosis, bilirubin appears in the urine.

- *Respiratory failure*: generally relates to coma grades 2–3 with hyperventilation and respiratory arrest. Ascites makes lung expansion difficult.

- *Bleeding*: clotting factors not being made, bruising may be visible.

- *Renal failure*: patients with fulminant hepatic failure go into renal failure, reduced BP episodes and hepatorenal syndrome, also excretion

of ammonia, an acid that damages the renal tubules.

- *Metabolic disturbances*: ammonia is acidotic to the body and a metabolic acidosis develops, abnormal metabolism of glucose due to reduced vitamin in take of thiamine (B_1), riboflavin (B_2) and pyridoxine (B_6).

- *Impaired drug metabolism*: drugs can act as double doses as cannot be converted by the liver quickly, reduced enzymes that render some drugs harmless.

- *Ascites*: seen in chronic liver failure.

- *Portal hypertension*: due to obstruction and liver cirrhosis.

Hepatitis

The different types of hepatitis are:

- obstructive
- drug induced
- infectious: an acute viral hepatitis is a common and sometimes serious infection of the liver – there are five subgroups:
  - A – enteric, faecal–oral transmission incubation is about 28 days, usually sudden onset
  - B – blood and sexual high risk groups incubation is 70 days insidious onset
  - C – 'delta agent' bloodborne transfusion
  - D – parenteral transmission plus? sexual + ? other
  - E – enterically transmitted, non-A and non-B.

Many other viruses affect the liver and cause hepatitis:

- yellow fever virus
- Epstein–Barr virus (EBV)
- Cytomegalovirus (CMV).

Investigations

- Liver function tests (see Section II)
- Pulmonary artery pressure measurement
- ICP monitoring
- Blood glucose level
- Liver biopsy
- Arterial blood gases
- Coagulation studies
- EEG.

Pancreatitis

Aetiological factors

- Alcohol, biliary disease, trauma, metabolic abnormalities, infection, drugs, etc.
- Initiating process
- Spontaneous, obstruction, bile, reflux, duodenal reflux (oedema, vascular damage, rupture of pancreatic ducts)
- Activation of enzymes
- Autodigestion
- Necrosis.

Diagnosis

Diagnosis is difficult due to differential diagnoses:

- pain
- tenderness over the abdomen
- reduced bowel sounds
- abdominal distension
- nausea/vomiting
- pyrexia
- hypotension
- blue brown discoloration of limbs (Grey Turner's sign), a late sign of pancreatitis.

Complications

- Starvation/malnutrition
- Absorptive and postabsorptive states
- Absorptive state – process of eating/ digestion
- Post-absorptive state – fasting no more than 12 hours:
- glycogenolysis in the liver
- glycogenolysis in skeletal muscles
- lipolysis in adipose tissues and the liver
- catabolism of cellular protein.

Immunological

HIV/acquired immune deficiency syndrome (AIDS)

HIV is spread by:

- blood transfusion
- IV drug use
- sexual contact
- artificial insemination
- in utero from mother – baby
- organ transplantation.

AIDS is fourth commonest cause of death world-wide.

Epidemiology

- 34.5 million people were infected with HIV in 2000.
- 24.5 million people in sub-Saharan Africa.
- Approximately 16 000 new infections occur daily.

- 33% of 15-year-olds in some countries will die of HIV.
- Deaths have fallen in wealthy countries.
- There are 2500 new diagnoses of AIDS a year in the UK.
- The majority of infections are transmitted via semen, cervical secretions and blood.

HIV in the UK

- Over 50% of infections are still due to sex between men.
- In 2000 32% of infections were due to heterosexual intercourse.
- Over half of those infected are women.

The virus

- First reported in 1981.
- Retrovirus – at least two types:
  - HIV-1 is less pathogenic, patients stay healthy and live longer than those with HIV-2
  - HIV-2 is a HIV-1 mutation and differs genetically from HIV-1; it is a more virulent strain.

Only survives in living host cells dying quickly once outside the body, it cannot survive on inanimate surfaces.

Pathogenesis

- A versatile virus, it does not immediately initiate an immune response
  - it surrounds itself by a protein shell and not recognized by the host's immune system
  - attaches itself to the receptor of certain T-cells
  - implants itself, replicates antibody cells
  - eventually reduces the effectiveness of the whole immune system.

- Main receptor is CD4 (T-helper cells), expressed on most T lymphocytes
- Virus attaches via its surface proteins (gp120) on the surface of the T-cell
- CD4 plays a major role in establishing an immune response
- Destruction of CD4 cells occurs.

Clinical features

- Incubation 2–4 weeks following infection.
- Initially there are no clinical signs, there might be some non-specific illness 6–8 weeks after exposure:
  - fever
  - arthralgia
  - myalgia, lethargy
  - lymphadenopathy
  - sore throat
  - mucosal ulcers
  - faint pink rash.

Seroconversion

- Median time of 10 years from infection to development of AIDS, some progress earlier, other up to 15 years
- Leads to immuno-suppression
- AIDS patients are susceptible to persistent opportunistic infections
- May have tumours such as Kaposi's sarcoma and/or Hodgkin's lymphomas.

HAART – highly affective antiretroviral therapy

- Combinations of drugs that act against reverse transcriptase and protease enzymes
- Effective in controlling HIV replications

- May show marked improvement in 4–8 weeks
- Full improvement takes about 6 months
- Involves multiple drugs, that have to be taken at the same time every day
- Psychological effects can be great to the patient, but compliance is generally good.

Effects of HIV

- Neurological disease
- Eye disease
- Mucocutaneous manifestations
- Haematological complications
- Gastrointestinal effects
- Renal complications
- Respiratory complications
- Endocrine complications.

Autoimmune disease

- The response of the immune system against self, protected by self tolerance
- Affects about 5–7% of the population
- May be:
  - organ specific
  - systemic.

Organ specific

- Immune response is directed to a target antigen unique to a single organ or gland.
- Manifestations limited to that organ.
- Organ may be subjected to direct cellular damage or may be stimulated or blocked by antibodies.

- Lympocytes or antibodies bind to cell membrane antigen causing lysis and/or an IR.
- The cellular structure of the organ is replaced by connective tissue and the organ function declines.

Organ specific diseases include:

- Addison's disease – adrenal glands
- Haemolytic anaemia – RBC membrane protein
- Graves' disease – over stimulation of the thyroid gland by thyroid-stimulating hormone (TSH)
- Hasimoto's thyroiditis – thyroid proteins uptake of iodine reduced production of thyroid hormones
- IDDM – pancreatic beta cells
- Myasthenia gravis – acetylcholinesterase receptors
- Pernicious anaemia – gastric parietal cells.

Systemic autoimmune diseases

- The response is directed towards a large number of target antigens and involves a number of organs and tissues
- A defect in immune regulation, which results in hyperactive T and B cells
- Tissue damage is widespread both from cell-mediated immune responses and from direct cellular damage caused by auto-antibodies
- Systemic autoimmune diseases include:
  - ankylosing spondylitis affects the vertebrae
  - multiple sclerosis affects the white matter in the CNS

- rheumatoid arthritis affects connective tissue IgG
- systemic lupus erythematosus (SLE) affects DNA, nuclear protein, RBC and platelet membranes. The response is directed towards a large number of target antigens and involves a number of organs and tissues.

Treatment

- Aimed at reducing the autoimmune response but leaving the rest of the immune system intact.
- Current therapies are palliative.
- Reduce symptoms to give a reasonable quality of life.
- Immunosuppressive drugs to slow down proliferation of lymphocytes.
- Increased risk of infection and cancer.
- Removal of thymus for myasthenia gravis.
- Plasmapheresis may help some patients.

Hypersensitivity

Cytotoxic hypersensitivity

This type of hypersensitivity involves IgM or IgG antibodies directed against antigens on the surface of the body's own cells. Antibodies bring about the destruction of the cells in the same way as foreign bacteria are destroyed.

Mechanisms of cytotoxic hypersensitivity:

- Once the antibody has bound to the surface of a cell there are three ways the cell can be damaged:
  - phagocytosis – antibodies bind to the surface of the cell, engage with fc receptors on phagocytic cells, facilitated by complement.
  - direct lysis of the cell coated with antibody
  - extracellular killing – due to the activation of phagocytosis neutrophils and macrophages release mediators or cytokines that brings about lysis and death of the target cell.

Types of cytotoxic hypersensitivity:

- Haemolytic disease of the newborn when the mother is Rh − and baby is Rh +
- Reactions to drugs, such as haemolytic anaemia following penicillin (uncommon)
- Reactions to tissue antigens, such as thyroid and endocrine tissues; antibodies directed against cells and molecules of a gland leading to damage or destruction
- diabetes – antibodies to the insulin-producing islet cells
- basement membranes – antibodies against the kidney (nephritis) affecting filtration capacity of the kidney
- myasthenia gravis – antibodies deposited in the neuromuscular junction.

Immune complex hypersensitivity

- When antigen combines with antibody in the body, immune complexes are formed.
- These immune complexes can be eliminated through phagocytosis and macrophages.
- The reaction can become exaggerated and lead to a tissue-damaging inflammatory response.

- When localized in a particular tissue the response is called an Arthus reaction.
- When spread throughout the body it is called serum sickness.
- The formation of immune complexes is a natural and protective process.
- It is only when the body is exposed to an excess of an antigen over a long period of time e.g.:
  - microbial organism
  - foreign antigen
  - autoimmunity to the body's own tissues.

Mechanisms of immune complex hypersensitivity:

- When a large amount of immune complexes are formed the phagocytes become overloaded leading to:
  - prolonged circulation of the complexes
  - deposited at vulnerable sites, e.g. the glomerulus of the kidney.
- Immune complexes trigger a variety of inflammatory processes:
  - degranulation of mast cells
  - interaction with platelets to form a clot or thrombus.
- Arthus reaction occurs in a variety of occupational lung diseases, the antigens are different but the mechanisms are the same:
  - farmer's lung
  - pigeon fancier's disease
  - maple bark stripper's lung
  - cheese washer's disease
  - furrier's lung.
- Allergic bronchopulmonary aspergillosis – a mixture of hypersensitivity and allergic reactions:
  - IgE-dependent allergic (type I)
  - an immune complex (type III).

- Serum sickness:
  - reaction like serum sickness can occur with some antibiotics
  - immune complex glomerulonephritis following infection with certain strains of streptococci, malaria, chronic hepatitis B infections
  - can also occur in SLE, which may be triggered by an infection of some sort.

Delayed-type hypersensitivity

- This type of hypersensitivity is not mediated by antibodies.
- It is mediated by T-cells alone, and these initiate tissue damage.
- The reactions are slow, may take up to 10 years to develop.
- There are three types:
  - contact hypersensitivity
  - tuberculin reactions
  - granulomatous reactions.
- In contact dermatitis and eczema, the most common agents are:
  - nickel
  - chromate (in cement)
  - hair dyes (p-phenylene diamine)
  - poison ivy and oak.
- The tuberculin-type:
  - tuberculosis sufferers and immunized patients have T cells that recognize tuberculin
  - if tuberculin is injected into the skin, T cells migrate to the site of injection.
- Granulomatous hypersensitivity:
  - Tuberculosis:
    - immunological granulomas are thought to be a physiological response to wall off the site of persistent infection

- can occur throughout the body wherever mycobacteria exist, and not just in the lungs.
  - Leprosy:
    - granulomatous skin lesions observed in leprosy
    - dependent on CD4 and CD8 cells which make different cytokines, e.g. interleukin (IL)-2, IL-4 and IL-10
    - the major cause of nerve destruction in this disease is the process of inflammation and cell infiltration.

Hypersensitivities can be:

- life threatening and can be fatal (asthma, anaphylaxis)

- degenerative, leading to severe debilitation, poor quality of life and may lead to death following a number of years coping with a particular disease/illness (autoimmune disease).

- an inconvenience with uncomfortable feelings of itching and upper respiratory swelling (eczema, hayfever)

- can be due to occupational disease which can lead to chronic diseases/illness of the lungs (farmer's lung).

- can mean that an injection or treatment is required that prevents the occurrence of the consequences (anti-D).

The broad focus of allergy and hypersensitivity denotes a variety of understanding and knowledge regarding its presentation, progress, mortality/morbidity and ultimately the interventions and treatments required.

The nurse is at the forefront of caring for patients with these conditions and as they vary from being fatal to just an inconvenience a broad range of skills are needed.

Burns

Burns can occur from intense heat or from radiation or electrical injuries. Severe burns lead to devastating physical and psychological effects, and a massive fluid loss from the circulatory system. Therapy ranges from initial resuscitation to eventual surgery and rehabilitation. Burns patients are most effectively treated by specially trained staff in an isolated environment controlled in temperature and humidity (Freebairn and Oh 1997).

Burns affect:

- Cardiovascular through loss of circulating fluid volume by a combination of hypovolaemic and cellular shock.

- Respiratory dysfunction due to:
  - airway injury
  - lung injury
  - cellular injury.

- Inflammatory process – the release of mediators.

- Metabolic – nitrogen loss.

- Burned tissue is easily colonized by bacteria – the immune system response is stimulated.

- Renal failure may occur due to renal hypoperfusion and associated with high mortality.

- Gatrointestinal ulcers can occur.

- Psychological – pain, severe illness, surgery, disfigurement, loss of independence and long-term care.

Here is the calculation of percentage of body surface area in children (Felon and Nene (2007)

Head front and back ½ of head by age in years

- 0 = 9½
- 1 = 8½
- 5 = 6½

- $10 = 5\frac{1}{2}$
- $15 = 4\frac{1}{2}$

Front and back 13%

Upper arm 2%

Lower arm $1\frac{1}{2}$

Buttocks $\frac{1}{2}$ $2\frac{1}{2}$ each side left and right

Genital area 1%

Upper leg $\frac{1}{2}$ of one thigh by age in years

- $0 = 2\frac{3}{4}$
- $1 = 3\frac{1}{4}$
- $5 = 4$
- $10 = 4\frac{1}{4}$
- $15 = 4\frac{1}{4}$

Lower leg $\frac{1}{2}$ of one lower leg

- $0 = 2\frac{1}{2}$
- $1 = 2\frac{1}{2}$
- $5 = 2\frac{3}{4}$
- $10 = 3$
- $15 = 3\frac{1}{4}$

The classification of burns

Generally refers to the depth of the burn:

1. Superficial dermal wound (1st degree burn) only involves the epithelial layer, very painful, resolves within 2 weeks with no scarring.
2. Deep dermal wound (2nd degree burn) involves epithelium and a varying degree of dermis, some scarring, healing is slow.
3. Full-thickness burns (3rd degree burns) leads to scarring and contractures, wound closure by grafting.

The greater the body surface burned the greater the fluid loss. Fluid losses are caused by an increase in capillary permeability that persists for 24 hours after burn injury, because of this fluid resuscitation is needed by intravenous infusion to restore the circulatory blood volume.

There are various recognized treatment options, here are just two:

1. The Muir and Barclay plan
   - The first 24-hour period is divided into 3-4 hour intervals followed by 6 hour intervals.
   - Albumin is the replacement choice in this regime and is given at a strength of 4.5%.
   - The amount to be administered in each time interval is determined by the formula 0.5/kg/% of total body surface area (TSBA) of burns.
2. The Parklands plan
   - This uses Hartmann's solution as the fluid of choice.
   - The first 24-hour period is divided as follows:
     • half of the calculated amount is given in the first 8 hours and the remainder over the following 16 hours
     • the formula used to calculate the volume for the 24 hour period is 4 ml/kg/% TBSA of burns.

The different properties of the two fluids between the Muir and Barclay plan consists of albumin, which is a colloid and because of this stays in the body longer due to the increase in colloid oncotic pressure. The Parklands plan gives crystalloid, a clear fluid with sodium chloride and other electrolytes. The colloid solution is administered more slowly and less is required.

The main physiological problems are:

- fluid output: which can be lost as fast as it is infused
- pain: analgesia would be required depending on whether burns are first, second or third degree.
- risk of infection: antibiotics would be needed
- input and output measure
- there is a massive water loss and flux of large amounts of fluids and electrolytes in the body tissues which manifests as oedema and circulatory hypovolaemia.

Monitoring should include:

- temperature, pulse, respiration and blood pressure
- oxygen saturation
- urine output
- CVP
- blood tests – arterial blood gases
- weight if possible.

Therapeutic intervention to sustain life is required urgently, the main three elements are:

- meticulous wound management
- adequate fluid and nutrition
- early surgical excision and grafting.

Electrocution

Patients suffering from electrocution and associated burns occasionally require hospital intervention (Critchley and Oh 1997).

Considerations:

- For a current flow the body must complete a circuit.
- Generally from sources to ground through the body.
- The physiological effects depend on the:
  - size of the current
  - duration of the current
  - the tissue traversed by the current.
- Most cases of electrocution occur in the workplace (60%) or at home (30%)

Types of injury:

- The injury is generally burns to the skin and internal tissues and organs.
- Depolarization of muscle cells:
  - sufficient currents can lead to cardiac asystole
  - VF and other arrhythmias may occur
  - MI has been reported.

- Tetanic contractions which can lead to long bone fractures.
- Vascular injuries – thrombosis or occluded blood vessels causing ischaemia and necrosis.
- Neurological injuries – central or peripheral, spinal cord injuries, unconsciousness.
- Renal failure – muscle necrosis.
- Other injuries:
  - may lead to falls or thrown
  - clothing to catch fire
  - rupture of the eardrum.

Management

- First aid and resuscitation
- Investigations – ECG, echocardiography, CT, EEG, X-ray of spine and long bones, haemoglobin, serum electrolytes, creatine kinase and urine myoglobin.
- Management – burns, ischaemic and necrotic tissue and injured organs, faciotomies and amputations.

Poisoning/Overdose

Poisoning or overdose is frequently intentional, accidental or iatrogenic or may result from criminal intent. Specific antidotes are available for only a very few number of poisons or drugs. Many patients will recover with supportive care.

Priority poisons

- Paracetamol
- Carbon monoxide
- Methanol
- Ethylene glycol
- Cyanide and paraquat are dangerous poisons.

General principles

Diagnosis:

- The time to diagnosis is imperative limiting the period from ingestion to supportive treatment is important.
- Always considered in the unconscious patient.
- Consult with relatives, friends, general practitioners and pharmacists who may provide valuable information.
- Administration of thiamine and glucose should be considered.

    Assessment and resuscitation

- airway and ventilation
- haemodynamic status
- conscious level and neurological signs
- body temperature
- body surface – head or body injury, venepuncture marks.
- investigations:
    - urinalysis
    - chest X-ray
    - electrolytes and creatinine
    - osmolality – may indicate ethanol, methanol or ethylene glycol poisoning
    - ABC analysis
- Drug levels, e.g. paracetamol and paraquat.

Drug manipulation

Decrease absorption by the administration of:

- emetics – ipecacuanha
- gastric lavage
- absorbent – activated charcoal (carbomix, medicoal)

- Cathartics – magnesium citrate/hydroxide, magnesium sulphate (milk of magnesia), sorbitol (sorbilax).

    Increase excretion

- Forced diuresis – diuretics
- Alkalosis – hyperventilation and/or sodium bicarbonate
- Increasing the acid of urine may increase the elimination of phencyclidine and amphetamines
- Extracorporeal techniques, e.g. haemodialysis.
- Administer specific overdose antidotes
- paracetamol – acetylcysteine, methionine (parvolex)
- anticholinesterase – atropine
- narcotic – naloxone (Narcan)
- benzodiazepine – flumazenil (Anexate)
- heparin – protamine sulphate
- digoxin – anti-digoxin antibodies (Digibind), atropine, phenytoin (Epanutin).
- warfarin – vitamin K_1.

Continued supportive therapy

- Care of the unconscious patient
- Vital functions are monitored and recorded
- Organ function is supported where possible
- The patient is rewarmed using humidified gases, space blankets and warmed infusion fluids
- Antibiotics are started if aspiration has occurred.
- Fluid and electrolytes and nutritional support are maintained.

Trauma

Neurological trauma

The skull is tough and takes quite a lot of abuse but the brain is well protected by bone and cushioned by cerebrospinal fluid (CSF). Many cases of skull fracture depend on age as the young and the old are vulnerable as their bones and blood vessels are fragile. An accident may result in:

- Laceration of the scalp – occurs when the brain is forced against the sharp ridges of the skull, the meninges and blood vessels are torn – bleed and increase the intracranial pressure (ICP).

- Fracture of the skull:
  - linear/simple fracture – two fragments which remain in apposition
  - comminuted – multiple linear fractures, but the fragments are not displaced
  - compound – communication with outside scalp wound, increased possibility of infection of bone and cranial contents
  - depressed – fragments are driven inwards, compressing or piercing the meninges or brain as well as the direct injury.

Slight or severe brain injury may or may not be associated with a fracture of the skull. However brain injury/trauma may lead to:

- Intracranial haemorrhage:
  - Subdural haematoma – damaged blood vessels on the surface of the brain, blood accumulates over several hours/days, therefore development of symptoms may be delayed. Occurs on average in 10–15% of head injuries generally due to contusion and lacerations.
  - Extradural haematoma – damaged blood vessels inside the skull and occurs in 2% of head injuries. 80% are due to fracture of the skull.
  - Intracerebral haematoma – damaged vessels inside the brain itself. Occurs in 2–3% of head injuries generally in the frontal and temporal areas.
  - Epidural haemotoma.

- Compression of the brain – resulting from a depressed fracture, oedema, haemorrhage, if untreated will progress into a deepening unconsciousness and a rising ICP.

- Supratentorial herniation – a critical condition associated with brain trauma whereby a portion of the cerebrum herniates through the tentorial hiatus (a space in the base of the brain stem). The rigid skull stops outward expansion therefore the brain has nowhere to go but down. This leads to compression of the brain stem – brain stem death may ensue (see earlier).

- Concussion – a brief period of unconsciousness due to jarring of the brain and its forceful contact with the rigid skull. As a result normal brain activity temporarily is interrupted and the patient will present a picture of shock. There is usually spontaneously reversal with no residual damage. The patient may be dazed, confused, restless and amnesic, complaining of a headache; vomiting may occur in the recovery period.

- Contusion – this is bruising of the brain, which causes haemorrhages in the region that is damaged, e.g. inflammation process. The patient may recover but may regress and it may take several weeks to recover. There may be residual scarring and impaired function.

- Contre-coup injury – this occurs when a stationary object hits the rigid skull and is stopped instantly. The softer brain rebounds back and forth within the skull.

Signs and symptoms

This depends on the nature and severity of tissue damage. May appear immediately or several hours later, as a sign of:

- cerebral oedema,
- intracranial bleeding
- ensuing brain compression
- elevation of ICP.

Symptoms may include:

- unconsciousness – either immediately or following a lucid interval
- headache and dizziness
- disturbed vision
- changes in pupillary reactions
- changes in vital signs
- disorientation and confusion
- motor and sensory deficits
- convulsions
- speech impairment
- neck stiffness
- hyperthermia
- CSF leakage
- 30% of patients have injuries in other parts of the body.

Autoregulation of the brain

The brain has its own method of maintaining homeostasis and this is by ensuring normal dynamics:

- brain tissue 80%
- CSF 10%
- cerebral blood flow (CBF) 10%.

When the brain is threatened by a rise in intracranial pressure the brain compensates, some of these mechanisms relate to the three areas mentioned above:

- CSF displacement cranial and lumber
- CSF production $\uparrow$ CSF re-absorption
- cerebral perfusion pressure (CPP)
- cerebral vascular resistance (CVR) leads to an increase in $\uparrow$ BP to maintain CPP above 60–70 mmHg
- CBF venous blood shunted away (can lead to further insult)

Cerebral blood flow (CBR) – CBF = CPP/CVR

- Parasympathetic stimulation $\downarrow$ heart rate
- Changes in action potentials
  - electrical – action potentials become sluggish or are blocked
  - chemical – neurotransmitters fail to be released at the neuromuscular junction e.g. acetylcholine.
- Changes in hormonal control fail to initiate a response:
  - failure to activate plasma membrane permeability
  - reduction in synthesis of proteins or regulatory enzymes – producing building blocks to produce haemoglobin or immunoglobulins of the immune system.
  - failure of enzymes activation or deactivation – digestive enzymes
  - reduction in secretory action – reduction in stress response, e.g. epinephrine (adrenaline) and norepinephrine (noradrenaline)
  - stimulation of mitosis – reduction in growth and repair.

Aims of care

- Frequent careful observations and neurological assessment
- Prevent complications
- Caring for the unconscious patient
- Rehabilitation
- Caring for the family
- Understanding of the neurological outcomes that can occur:
  - epilepsy
  - transient loss of consciousness
  - loss of limb movement, weakness, gait
  - loss of sensation, temperature, touch, pain
  - changes in sight (partial or complete blindness), hearing (deafness, tinnitus, vertigo), facial (Bell's palsy), lips/jaw movement
  - incontinence (faecal, urine)
  - loss of appreciation of size, shape, texture and weight (astereognosis) loss of cognitive thought, memory, speech, understanding, recognition, interpretation (prosopagnosia), learning ability
  - aggressive or antisocial behaviour
  - personality changes
  - hallucinations
  - in addition, the loss of ability to care for self which depends on age:
  - disturbances of speech:
    - dysarthria
    - dysphonia/aphonia
  - disorders of language – dysphasia
  - impairment of vision/ocular movement
    - hemianopia
    - quadrantanopia
    - diplopia
    - conjugate deviation of the eyes
  - persistent vegetative state (PVS)
  - locked-in syndrome
  - brain stem death.

Neurological patients require a lot of time and effort to enable them to return to a normal life. This involves initial treatment and interventions, then generally a lengthy period of rehabilitation. When neurological outcomes are the end result they can be serious as to affect a person's ability to continue a normal life (Table 4.5) but younger children have the ability to re-learn. When caring for a neurological child or adolescent it is important from the outset to deliver high quality care in an attempt to reduce the devastating effects of these outcomes.

Spinal trauma

The spinal cord consists of 31 pairs of nerves:

- cervical – C1–8
- thoracic – T1–12
- lumbar – L1–5
- sacral – S1–5
- coccygeal – C0

The higher the spinal cord injury the worse the patient outcome in relation to their ability to move (Table 4.4), and this depends also on whether the injury is complete of incomplete. There are about 20 spinal cord injuries each week in the UK, is most common age is 16–35 years, but children are often involved. The causes are:

- motor vehicle accidents 46%
- falls 21%
- penetrating trauma 15%
- sports injuries 14%
- diving accidents less than 2%.

Table 4.5 Neurological outcomes

Neurological outcome	Description
Confusion	Loss of concentration Memory impairment Misinterpretation Delusions Reduced intellectual functioning Anxiety and restlessness Compulsive behaviour Reduced alertness Forgetfulness Disorientation Hallucinations.
Dysamnesia	Loss of past memories Inability to form new memories Observed in subarachnoid haemorrhage or brain injury, lobectomy and Alzheimer's
Agnosia	Defect of recognition of objects both what it is and what it is for – the object may be recognized through other senses e.g. visual, auditory or touch, language.
Dysphasia	Impairment of comprehension or production of language Results from dysfunction of the left cerebral hemisphere Generally involving the middle cerebral artery or a tributary.
Alterations in muscle tone	Hyponia – decreased muscle tone passive movement occurs with little or no resistance, there is reduced excitability of the neurones, tire easily or are week. Hypertonia – increased muscle tone passive movement occurs with resistance, there is spasticity with an increased stretch reflex due to damage of the motor areas in the CNS, rigidity muscles are firm and tense.
Alterations in movement	Hyperkinesia – excessive movements, repetitive movements, compulsions, mannerisms Hypokinesia – decreased movements, loss of voluntary movements despite preserved consciousness, include: Paresis – partial paralysis, incomplete loss of muscle power Paralysis – loss of motor function Akinesia – decrease in voluntary movements, reduced time to do anything

Table 4.5 Neurological outcomes—cont'd	
Neurological outcome	**Description**
	Bradykinesia – slowness of voluntary movements, reduced time it takes to do a movement, all movements are slow, laboured and deliberate and cannot perform more than one movement at a time.
Seizures	Partial – locally, temporal lobe, involves the temporal lobe, the patient remains conscious or complex loss of consciousness
	Generalized – symmetrical multifocal

Spinal cord transection

Refers to severance of the spinal cord at the different levels of the spinal cord (Table 4.6) and can be complete, partial or slow. It is important to assess the level and completeness of spinal cord injury as this allows a prognosis to be made. If the lesion is complete from the outset, that is, there is no sign of spinal cord function below the level of

Table 4.6 Functioning and potential outcomes by level of spinal cord injury		
Level of injury	**Muscle functioning**	**Outcome**
Cervical C4 and above	Loss of all muscle functioning including muscles of respiration.	Usually death
	Injuries are usually total because of respiratory failure.	
Cervical C5	The phrenic nerve innervating the diaphragm is usually spared	Quadriplegia with poor pulmonary capacity
	Loss of intercostal muscle functioning often causes respiratory problems.	High level of dependency for activities of living.
Cervical C6–C8	Muscle movement of the neck	Quadriplegia but adequate muscles of the arms and hands are spared
	Some chest and arm movement remains	
	Therefore some muscles of respiration continue to function	Independence in feeding, some dressing and propelling of wheelchair.

(Continued)

Table 4.6 Functioning and potential outcomes by level of spinal cord injury—cont'd

Level of injury	Muscle functioning	Outcome
Thoracic spine T1–T3	Neck, shoulder, arms and hand muscle functioning intact Loss of muscle functioning from above nipple line and all of trunk and lower extremities.	Considered a quadriplegic if lesion above T3 Much more independence, intact arm function. Needs support in upright position because of loss of trunk muscles.
Thoracic T4 (nipple line), T10 (umbilicus)	More of the chest and trunk muscle functioning remains All neck and shoulder, arm and hand functioning intact.	Paraplegic – involves only the lower part of the body Can perform all activities, transfer easily Achieves mobility with a wheelchair.
Thoracic 11–Lumbar 2	Same as above Muscle function extends to upper thigh.	Bladder control located here and sexual erections Loss of voluntary bowel and bladder control but can have reflex emptying.
Lumbar 3 Sacral 1	Muscle functioning at all of upper body, chest and most of leg muscles.	Paraplegic with many muscles of mobility intact Loss of voluntary bladder and bowel control, but can have reflex emptying.
Sacral 2–4	Same as above but more leg functioning.	The centre for micturition is situated at this level Destroys the reflex arc to the bladder and bowel Results in flaccidity and complete loss of bladder and bowel control Loss of ability to have a reflex erection.

injury, recovery is far less likely than in an incomplete lesion. There are three types:

1. Sudden complete transection, which results all of the following below the level of injury:
   - total paralysis of all skeletal muscles below the level of injury
   - loss of all spinal reflexes below the level of injury
   - loss of pain, temperature, proprioception and the sensation of pressure and touch
   - absence of somatic and visceral sensations
   - unstable, lowered blood pressure due to loss of vasomotor tone
   - loss of perspiration, bowel and bladder dysfunction
   - abnormal, painful and continuous erection (priapism).
2. Partial transection – the patterns of incomplete injury can be viewed in Table 4.7.
3. Slow transection – there is no spinal shock (results from tumours, multiple sclerosis)

Spinal shock

This is an abrupt cessation of impulses firing from the higher centres which results in flaccid paralysis below the level of injury. Damage may lead to:

- paralysis
- paraesthesia
- weakness
- numbness
- pain.

The main effects of spinal cord injury (Table 4.6):

- loss of voluntary movement below lesion
- loss of sensation below lesion
- potential effects on respiratory system
- loss of normal control of sympathetic nervous system, affecting most of the body, including:
  - cardiovascular system
  - loss of ability to regulate temperature below lesion
- loss of normal bowel function
- loss of normal bladder function.

Respiratory trauma

- The most common is closed chest injury from a RTA, with associated extrathoracic injuries, all of which may be life threatening.
- Swift assessment and resuscitation are carried out simultaneously.
- Initial management is directed toward detection and correction of life threatening effects from the sustained injuries.

Direct chest injuries

- Knife wounds
- Injury due to a fall
- Road traffic accidents
- Violent incidents (beatings, boxing)
- Inhalation burns
- Blast injury.

  Effects:

- Ruptured aorta determined by:
  - widened mediastinum
  - left haemothorax
  - depressed left main bronchus
  - fractured 1st rib.
- Ruptured diaphragm
  - due to abdominal compression (risen since seat belts made compulsory)

Table 4.7 Incomplete/partial spinal cord injury

Type of injury	Cause of injury	Recovery
Anterior cord syndrome	The anterior part of the spinal cord is injured by flexion – rotation force causing dislocation or compression fracture of the vertebral body. Anterior spinal artery compression – spinal tracts are damaged by direct trauma and ischaemia	Results in loss of power Reduced pain and temperature sensation below the lesion
Central cord syndrome	Observed in older patients with cervical spondylosis A hyper-extension injury often from minor trauma compresses spinal cord Cervical tract serving arms suffer brunt of injury	Flaccid lower motor neurone weakness of the arms Relatively strong but spastic upper motor neurone leg function Sacral sensation and bladder and bowel function are partially spared
Posterior cord syndrome	Seen in hyper extension injuries with fractures of the posterior elements of the vertebrae Contusion of the posterior columns	Good power, pain and temperature sensation Profound ataxia due to loss of proprioception makes walking very difficult
Brown–Sequard syndrome	Results from stab injuries Common in lateral mass fractures of the vertebrae A hemi-section of the spinal cord occurs	Reduced or absent power Relatively normal pain and temperature sensation on the side of the injury The uninjured side has good power Reduced or absent sensation to pin prick and temperature

- risk of gut strangulation
- left sided rupture is more common, right difficult to diagnose due to the liver.

Disruption of major airways is frequently due to:

- respiratory distress
- subcutaneous emphysema
- haemoptysis.
- In the presence of ruptured bronchus a pneumothorax is common.
- Massive haemothorax
- Pulmonary contusion
  - bruising of the lungs
  - avoid over hydration.
- Myocardial contusion
  - common in blunt chest trauma
  - may result in arrhythmias – non-specific T wave changes to pathological Q waves
  - cardiac failure may be evident – generally should be managed as a myocardial infarction
- Oesophageal perforation due to penetrating injury, occurs rarely with closed chest trauma; the patient develops:
  - resrosternal pain
  - difficulty in swallowing
  - haematemesis
  - cervical emphysema.
- Systemic air embolism
  - more common in penetrating injuries – life threatening
  - uncommon, but is thought to generally be under-diagnosed
  - caused by a bronchopulmonary vein fistula.
- Cardiac tamponade
  - suspected in a patient with thoracic trauma with a low blood pressure and raised venous pressure
  - differential diagnoses are:

- tension pneumonothorax
  - severe heart failure
  - prolonged and inadequate treatment of shock
  - aspiration of the pericardial sac under ECG control.

Flail chest is disruption of the normal structure of the chest due to:

- fracture of three or more adjoining ribs in one or more places
- rib fractures with costochondral separation
- sternal fractures.

paradoxical movement occurs:

- on inspiration the intact chest expands, the injured flail segment is depressed
- on expiration the flail segment bulges outward, thus interfering with exhalation.

mediastinal shift occurs:

- during inspiration the increased intrapleural pressures on the unaffected side displace the mediastinum toward it
- during expiration the negative pressure on the unaffected side is less than on the affected side, and the mediastinum shifts toward the affected side (mediastinal flutter).

Changes in inspiration lead to reduced cardiac output.

Indirect injuries

- Pulmonary embolism
- Pulmonary oedema
- Carbon monoxide poisoning
- Hanging
- Obstruction

- Aspiration
- Drowning
- Anaphylaxis and asthma.

Unrelated injuries

Any conditions whereby the demand for oxygen outweighs supply can lead to unrelated trauma to the respiratory system due to:

- stress
- major trauma
- hypovolaemia
- diabetic ketoacidosis
- myocardial infarction
- pancreatitis
- liver / renal failure
- hyperpyrexia, hyperthermia, hypothermia.

Interventions

- Control any bleeding.
- Insertion of an IV cannula.
- Basic circulatory resuscitation is initiated.
- Administration of oxygen.
- Exclude or treat pneumothorax or haemothorax – insertion of 12 or 14 FG intravenous cannula inserted percutaneously in dire emergencies.
- Assessment of extrathoracic trauma, head, neck and abdominal injuries and significant concealed blood loss must be excluded.
- Gastric decompression – risk of regurgitation (vomiting or aspiration); extremely common in severe cases of chest trauma.

- Provide pain relief to relieve respiratory distress in patients with fractures of the ribs and/or sternum.
- Reconsider endotracheal intubation, ventilation if:
  - dangerous hypoxaemia and/or hypercarbia
  - significant head injury
  - gross flail segment and contusion.
- Respiratory distress.

4.2 Other conditions observed in children

Cancer in children

Tumours affecting children under 15 years of age are classified as 'childhood cancer' (Cancer Research UK 2010b).

- Childhood cancer is relatively rare: only 0.5% of all cancers.
- In the UK, 1 in every 500 children under 15 years will develop some form of cancer.
- Each year the UK sees approximately 1500 new diagnoses of childhood cancer.
- Leukaemias (blood cell cancers) and cancers of the brain (brain tumours) and central nervous system account for more than half the new cases each year.
- About 75% of childhood cancers are leukaemias, so it is the most common childhood cancer.
- Cancers of the brain and central nervous system are the most frequent

cause of death of all childhood cancers.

- Cancer is the leading cause of disease mortality in children under 15 years.

- About 300 children die from cancer each year in the UK.

- There are approximately 26°000 childhood cancer survivors in UK today.

Causes of childhood cancers

The causes of childhood cancers remain unknown. Specific correlates of childhood cancer include (Cancer Research UK 2010a):

- Rare genetic disorders such as Li–Fraumeni syndrome and Fanconi anaemia.

- Abnormal responses to infections during infancy (linked to an increased risk of some leukaemias).

- Link to viral infections such as EBV, hepatitis B and human virus 8. EBV is associated with an increased risk of Burkitt's lymphoma, Hodgkin lymphoma and nasopharyngeal carcinoma; hepatitis B is associated with an increased risk of liver carcinoma; and HHV8 is associated with an increased risk of Kaposi's sarcoma.

- Down's syndrome (linked to an increased risk of leukaemias).

- An inherited faulty gene (resulting in two types of retinoblastomas).

- Radiotherapy and/or chemotherapy (linked to an increased risk of developing a second primary cancer).

Potential risk factors (Cancer Research UK 2010b)

There are a number of possible risk factors that are suspected to contribute and these are:

- Parental, fetal or childhood exposures to environmental toxins such as pesticides, solvents, household chemicals.

- Parental occupational exposures to radiation or chemicals. Antenatal obstetric irradiation from X-ray examination during pregnancy is associated with an increased risk of the fetus developing any childhood cancer.

- Parental and fetal exposure to infectious agents.

- Genetic susceptibility.

- Parents' diet, smoking and alcohol use during pregnancy. Maternal smoking during pregnancy is associated with a slightly increased risk of all neoplasms.

- History of allergies is associated with a reduced risk of acute lymphoblastic leukaemia (ALL).

- Increased maternal or paternal age at childbirth is associated with an increased risk of ALL.

- High birth weight is associated with an increased risk of ALL.

- Breastfeeding is associated with a slightly decreased risk of ALL.

Survival rates

Due to significant advances in treatment over the last few decades, childhood cancer is no longer a fatal disease. Most children with cancer survive beyond the treatment period and the majority can be cured.

Advances in treatments and medical technologies have increased the survival rate such that nearly 80% of all children diagnosed with cancer will survive for five or more years (Cancer Research UK 2010a).

Types of cancers

The types of cancers can be grouped into two areas (Cancer Research UK 2010b):

- Malignant haematology (ALL, lymphomas).
  - ALL is the most frequently occurring blood disease in children, accounting for 79% of all leukaemias in children. Incidence is high in boys and girls at the ages of three and two years respectively. ALL is cancer of the lymphoid cells (white blood cells) in the bone marrow and the lymphoid organs of the body which are part of the immune system.
  - Acute myelogenous leukaemia (AML) accounts for 15% of childhood leukaemias and incidence rates are highest in infants under 1 year. AML is cancer of the myeloid blood cells which are produced in the bone marrow and which help fight bacterial infections.
  - Lymphomas account for 10% of all childhood cancers and incidence is twice as high in boys as girls. Lymphomas are tumours of the lymph tissues, which are part of the immune system. Rare before the age of 2 and incidence increases with age.

The types include: Hodgkin's disease (41%), which affects lymph nodes near the body's surface such as in the neck, armpit and groin area; non-Hodgkin's lymphoma (NHL) (44%) affects lymph nodes found deep within the body.

- Oncology (solid tumours):
  - *Childhood brain and CNS tumours* account for 25% of all childhood cancers overall:
    - The most common subgroup is astrocytoma (43%), which is uncorrelated to age or sex and is most frequently classified as 'low grade' (76%) rather than 'high grade' (14%).
    - Intracranial and intraspinal embryonal are the second most common subgroup, representing 19% of all childhood brain and CNS tumours. Intracranial and intraspinal tumours are commonly diagnosed in younger children and frequently appear as medulloblastomas/primitive neuroectodermal tumours (PNETs).
  - *Sarcomas* are tumours involving the bones and soft tissues.
    - 7% of childhood cancers are soft tissue sarcomas, which are much more frequently diagnosed in boys aged 3–8 years.
    - Soft tissue sarcomas are rhabdomyosarcomas, which are the most common type of soft tissue sarcoma in children (53%), peaking in prevalence at 3 years of age and decreasing thereafter. Rhabdomyosarcoma develops in muscles and is found in the heart, neck, kidneys, bladder, arms and legs.

- Only a small minority of all childhood cancers are caused by renal tumours (6%; the vast majority of which being nephroblastomas); bone tumours (4%; the majority of which being osteosarcomas and Ewing tumours); malignant melanomas and carcinomas occurring outside the liver, kidney and gonads (3%); retinoblastomas (3%; rarely found in children older than 5 years of age); and hepatic tumours (affecting only one in every million children and primary as hepatoblastoma).
- The other solid tumours that are less common, e.g. Wilms' tumour, neuroblastoma (cancer of the sympathetic nervous system which most often is found in the adrenal glands above the kidney).

Signs and symptoms

These can vary according to the type of cancer. With leukaemias, the cells are abnormal cells that cannot help the body fight infections so for this reason children with ALL often have infections and fevers. Some of the common symptoms are:

- fever
- fatigue
- frequent infections
- paleness
- swollen or tender lymph nodes
- easy bleeding or bruising
- tiny red spots under the skin (known as petechiae)
- bone or joint pain.

Symptoms arising from CNS tumours

- Raised intracranial pressure
- Focal deficits (including seizures)
- Papilloedema.

The initial presentation of symptoms arising from CNS tumours present challenges to reaching a timely diagnosis because they are easily mistaken for common childhood conditions, such as migraine, gastrointestinal disorders and behavioural problems. The prevalence of the three most common symptoms in childhood CNS tumours according to tumour location are provided as follows (Wilne et al 2007):

- supratentorial tumours: unspecified raised ICP symptoms, seizures and papilloedema
- posterior fossa tumours: nausea/ vomiting, headache, abnormal gait/ coordination
- spinal cord tumours: back pain, abnormal gait/coordination, spinal deformity
- brain stem tumours: abnormal gait/coordination, unspecified cranial nerve palsies, unspecified pyramidal signs
- central tumours: headache, abnormal eye movements, nausea/vomiting.

Treatment for cancer

- Chemotherapy is the primary treatment used to cure many childhood cancers. It destroys cancer cells and shrinks tumours.
- Surgery for biopsy or excision of tumour.

- Radiation – most common mode of delivery is external beam therapy or teletherapy.
- Bone marrow transplantation.

Routes of administration for chemotherapy

- Mouth
- Subcutaneous injections
- Intramuscular injections
- Intravenously (most commonly used route – usually via a long term central venous access device (CVAD) or implantable port (porta-cath)
- Intrathecally (directly into the central nervous system).

Administration of chemotherapy

- Cytotoxic drugs can produce mutagenic, carcinogenic or teratogenic effects so safety precautions are essential.
- Oral cytotoxic drugs should not be handled due to the possible absorption through the skin membrane.
- Children should have a drink following an oral dose to remove any residue from mouth.
- Chemotherapy should be prepared by competent personnel using protective clothing in a laminar airflow room.
- Drugs should be packaged to avoid leakage or tampering.
- Chemotherapy should only be administered by nurses who are competent and have received adequate training.

- Please ensure that you adhere to your hospital policy on the safe practice for handling and administering cytotoxic drugs. Aseptic technique should be used at all times.
- Use protective aprons and gloves.
- Close observation of the administration site for extravasation is essential as this is a serious issue that can result in skin ulceration, blistering and necrosis.
- Nurses who administer cytotoxic drugs must be aware of the hospital policy on extravasation and an extravasation kit must be available.
- If accidental spillage occurs, access to area restricted, full protective clothing worn, absorbent paper used to clean up spillage, area washed down with soap and water, and all waste disposed of in an identified cytotoxic disposal bag for incineration.
- If contamination of the skin or eyes occurs, skin should be washed thoroughly with soap and water, and eyes irrigated with 0.9% sodium chloride and eye wash.
- The incident should be reported according to local hospital policy.
- Any local or systemic symptoms arising after the administration of chemotherapy should be reported to occupational health.
- If drugs are not intended for immediate administration, they should be stored according to local policy.
- Pregnant women should not have contact with these drugs and should avoid contact with the body fluids and excreta of children receiving chemotherapy.

- Unused drugs should be returned to the pharmacy.
- Parents who administer chemotherapy in the home should be educated on how to manage accidental spillage.

Potential side-effects

Chemotherapy is used to destroy rapidly dividing and mutating cancer cells by interfering with cell division, causing cell death. Therefore in addition to cancer cell destruction, many normal cells are destroyed, causing a wide range of side effects.

- Nausea and vomiting. The gastrointestinal side effects of cancer treatment vary depending on the strength and type of the prescribed treatment.
- Vomiting is a common side effect of intensive courses of treatment and may be alleviated with antiemetics, nasogastric nutritional supplementation or parenteral nutrition.
- Other side effects affecting the gastrointestinal system include oral thrush and mouth ulcers, which can be treated and staved off with good dental habits, antiseptic mouth wash, and the use of oral antifungal medication during neutropenic phases (Children's Cancer and Leukaemia Group 2010).
- Children receiving bone marrow suppression treatment involving chemotherapy face increased risk of infection due to immunosuppression.
- Where blocks of treatment are prescribed for solid tumours, children are highly likely to develop neutropenia 7–10 days after the onset of treatment.
- Neutropenia does not ordinarily develop in children receiving maintenance treatment for ALL.
- IV broad spectrum antibiotics are the first course of treatment in neutropenic patients.
- Anaemia and thrombocytopenia arising from bone marrow suppression treatment may require blood transfusion (Children's Cancer and Leukaemia Group, 2010).
- Loss of hair on all parts of the body. Alopecia is, in most cases, a reversible side effect of cytotoxic drugs and cranial irradiation. Wigs, headscarfs and hats may help alleviate the social and emotional difficulties experienced by children with alopecia (Children's Cancer and Leukaemia Group, 2010).
- Damage to ovaries and sperm cells. Impeded growth, brain hormone deficiencies and neuropsychological sequelae are common late effects of radiotherapy.
- Cumulative toxicities such as cardiotoxicity, and renal damage may develop as late effects of cytotoxic drug treatments.
- In cases where fertility may be compromised, sperm banking is offered and endocrine replacement therapy may be used to encourage puberty.
- Childhood cancer survivors face an increased risk of developing secondary tumours later in life (Children's Cancer and Leukaemia Group, 2010).
- Pain.
- Diarrhoea or constipation.
- Pancreatitis.
- Impaired liver function.
- Swelling and oedema.

Immunity during cytoxic treatment

Immunosuppressed children whose antibody status does not confirm chickenpox immunity and who are suspected of not having immunity to measles face serious risk of death if either of these diseases is contracted.

Live vaccine (MMR or BCG, for instance) must not be given during cytoxic treatment. Instead, children suspected of having had direct contact with either disease should receive passive immunization within 48 hours.

Psychosocial impact of cancer on child and family

- Cancer treatment represents a significant and protracted life experience in the lives of sick children and their families.
- Although there is a strong chance of cure, the illness course can be unpredictable with some children experiencing relapse after the intensive treatment, then recovery, then relapse again.
- Chemotherapy, radiotherapy and surgery impart considerable challenges on children's emotional health and psychosocial development, and create a host of physiological side effects resulting in pain and discomfort.
- Children with cancer face psychosocial and developmental challenges arising from disruptions to their everyday participation in their home, school and community environments.
- Where treatment is successful, its consequences on the body often far outlive the cancer itself: disrupted growth, cardiac problems, reproductive damage and diminished endocrine function are a handful of protracted effects experienced by childhood cancer survivors.
- Clinicians should aim to understand children's symptoms and difficulties from the child's perspective, but may be unable to fully do so where a child's ability to articulate their needs and experiences is compromised by distress, undeveloped self-awareness or difficulty with expressing themselves through traditional routes of conversation (Ruland et al 2009).
- The quality of life of children with cancer has been shown to be diminished by fears about the future, reduced ability to participate in routine activities and significant pain caused by the illness and treatment process (Eiser et al 2005).
- Parents of children with cancer are known to suffer from high levels of depression and anxiety immediately following diagnosis, with adverse effects on their physical and mental well-being occurring over longer periods of time (Eiser et al 2005).
- Research suggests that adolescents tend to experience more emotional distress, academic difficulty and social isolation than children in younger age groups (Ruland et al 2009).
- The uncertainty can be hard to handle for many children and they need good psychosocial support:
  - help with developing a routine
  - needing information to understand
  - needing explanations to prepare for procedures
  - preparation for possible side-effects

- allowed choices over everyday decisions
- allowed to be involved in decisions about their care and treatment
- help with adjusting to side effects
- help with maintaining normality (school work, friends, family nearby, favourite pillow, etc.).

Long-term management: shared care model

Cancer treatment usually takes place over a period of several years and involves combinations of care in the home, the clinic, and the hospital. In order to alleviate the practical difficulties for families of receiving care in a specialist centre the concept of shared-care was devised (Hooker and Milburn 2000).

- Shared care involves the provision of cancer care by both specialist paediatric oncology centres as well as local children's services.

- Good communication is essential for the success of the shared-care model.

Meningitis

Viral meningitis is generally aseptic and not usually serious. Bacterial meningitis is septic, has an increased mortality, and if untreated almost always fatal (see Table 4.8).

Symptoms

- Severe headache.
- Malaise.
- Fever.
- Vomiting.
- Photophobia.

- Convulsions.
- Irritability.
- Meningeal irritation:
  - neck and spinal stiffness
  - pain
  - resistance to extending the knee when the thigh is flexed (Kernig's sign).
- Apathy.
- Drowiness.
- Progressing to unconsciousness.
- In immunosuppressed patients these signs may be absent and mental confusion may be the predominant feature.

Differential diagnosis

- Meningeal irritation can occur without meningitis – may be a feature of other types of severe infection.
- Subarachnoid haemorrhage.
- Cerebral abscess.

Causal organisms

- Meningococcus – eight strains – dies quickly outside of the body, five strains are carriers rather than cases. A, B, C strains are the most common:
  - A strain almost eradicated
  - B strain responsible for most infections
  - C is increasing over recent years
  - incubation period of 3 days, the source is generally human nasopharynx–blood stream–meningitis and spread via infected respiratory secretions
  - sometimes epidemics.
  - treated with benzylpenicillin
  - swelling is most marked in the parietal, occipital and cerebellar regions.

Table 4.8 Differences and similarities between meningitis and encephalitis

	Meningitis – inflammation of the meninges	**Encephalitis – inflammation of the brain substance**
Differences	Bacterial – serious and can be fatal	Viral – serious and can be fatal
	Antibiotics – benzylpenicillin, ampicillin, chloramphenicol, gentamicin, cephalosporins	Antibiotics – acyclovir
	Organisms that cause the inflammation	Organisms that cause the inflammation in blood and CSF
	Epidemics can occur and can be serious in children	Epidemics very uncommon
	Bacterial meningitis is a notifiable infection	Not a notifiable disease
	CSF findings – protein and pressure increased, glucose is reduced or absent, turbid or clear (this varies between bacterial and viral meningitis	CSF findings – increased protein and pressure, fluid clear, glucose normal
Similarities	Clinical features – fever, malaise, anorexia, cerebral dysfunction, altered conscious level, abnormal behaviour, seizures, headaches, nausea/vomiting, tremor, positive Kernig's sign	Clinical features – headaches, neck stiffness, seizures, drowsy, confused leading to unconsciousness, fever, septicaemia, photophobia, positive Kernig's sign, purpuric rash
	Diagnosis – lumber puncture, blood cultures	Diagnosis – lumber puncture, blood cultures
	Differential diagnosis – cerebral abscess, subarachnoid haemorrhage	Differential diagnosis – cerebral abscess, subarachnoid haemorrhage
	Antibiotics if TB suspected	Antibiotics if TB suspected
	Treatment – steroids, sedatives, analgesia, isolation, artificial ventilation / care of the unconscious patient	Treatment – steroids, sedatives, analgesics, isolation, artificial ventilation/care of the unconscious patient

- *Haemophilus influenzae* – a parvobacterium, common in the normal respiratory tract, but tends to be more common in children/infants 1 month–4 years old. Treatment is with chloramphenicol.

- *Streptococuus pneumoniae* – (pneumococcus) a normal commensal of the upper respiratory tract. There are many types, not all of them infective, and it is generally observed in:
  - the middle aged and elderly
  - reduced general health
  - pneumococcal infection of the lungs, sinuses and middle ear as a secondary infection

  The infection is usually treated with benzylpenicillin. The infection generally restricted to the anterior lobes of the lung.

- *Myobacterium tuberculosis* – 100 cases/year in England and Wales. Treatment generally involves rifampicin, isoniazid, and ethambutol pyrazinamide.

Diagnosis

- History – infectious ear, sinuses or contact.
- CSF examination – appears cloudy, turbid, with an increased white blood cell count, protein and pressure. Glucose is reduced.
- Blood cultures.
- Nose and throat swabs.
- Chest X-ray.

Treatment

- Antibiotics as above.
- Steroids.

- Sedatives if patient is fitting or agitated.
- Isolation if meningococcal is suspected.
- Artificial ventilation may be required if unconsciousness results.

Complications/sequelae

- Encephalopathy.
- Cranial nerve palsy.
- Cerebral infarction or abscess.
- Obstructive hydrocephalus.
- Subdural effusion of sterile or infected nature.

Encephalitis

This is inflammation of the brain substance leading to oedema/necrosis or haemorrhage and an increase in ICP, and it differs from meningitis in a number of ways (Table 4.8).

Causes

- Herpes simplex
- Herpes zoster
- Measles/mumps – can be caused by vaccinations and known as post-vaccination encephalitis
- Viral infection, which is very serious and has a high mortality:
  - rubella
  - arbovirus
  - polio
  - enterovirus
  - EBV
  - cytomegalovirus.

- Bacterial
  - tuberculosis
  - syphilis.

The most common method of transmission is in the bloodstream; less common is via nerves and can lead to brain damage and cranial nerve damage. The spread of the infection is faecal or oral route but can be spread via direct contact with respiratory secretions.

Symptoms

- Sudden or gradual
- Fever
- Malaise
- Anorexia
- Cerebral dysfunction
- Altered level of consciousness
- Abnormal behaviour
- Seizures
- Headaches
- Tremor
- Positive Kernig's sign.

Diagnosis

- Lumbar puncture, which will have increased protein and pressure, fluid may be clear
- Stool specimen, which will contain the enterovirus
- Blood serum antibodies
- CT scan.

Treatment

- Isolate the patient
- Aciclovir
- Steroids may be beneficial.

Cerebrovascular accident

Interruption of the blood supply to the brain due to:

- any injury to nerve cells and/or pathways to the brain
- Increase of pressure within the cranium.

This results in loss of, or reduction in, the function of the part of the brain affected and the organs and tissues supplied by the effected nerves, due to:

- thrombosis – rare in children
- haemorrhage – bleeding within the brain due to cerebral aneurysm
- abrupt hypertensive episode, often precipitated by activity
- rupture of an atherosclerotic vessel
- embolism – leads to maximum immediate neurological deficit:
- clot detached from the heart following a MI or subacute bacterial endocarditis.

Risk factors and prevention

- Hypertension
- Diabetes
- Heart disease – rare.

Blood flow to the brain

The brain requires 20% of the body's total circulating volume.

The major arteries are:

- middle cerebral artery
- carotid artery

- vertibrobasilar artery
- anterior cerebral artery
- posterior cerebral artery.

Blood to the brain is supplied by the carotid arteries situated in the neck, which branch off from within the brain into multiple arteries, each of which supplies a specific area. The vertebral arteries supply the posterior part and the brain stem – even a brief disruption in blood supply can cause neurological deficit.

Symptoms will vary depending on the area that has been affected, ranging from dysphasia to hemiplegia.

Abnormalities caused:

- Middle cerebral artery area:
  - some loss of field of vision right hemiparesis
  - lack of awareness of affected side
  - facial numbness
  - weakness in arm more than leg.
- Carotid artery area:
  - weakness and hemiplegia on opposite side, numbness, sensory changes, visual disturbances
  - headache or altered level of consciousness.
- Vertebrobasilar artery area:
  - one side weakness, numbness around mouth and lips, altered vision both eyes, double vision, dysphasia.
  - ataxia
  - dysphagia
  - loss of memory.
- Anterior cerebral artery:
  - weakness and numbness especially lower limbs or loss of motor power and co-ordination
  - incontinence, confusion, personality change.

- Posterior cerebral arteries:
  - visual disturbances, sensory impairment
  - dyslexia
  - paralysis usually absent.

Types of stroke

Transient ischaemic attack:

- temporary paralysis lasting 10–15 minutes
- presenting with speech difficulty or numbness
- sudden onset recovery within 24 hours.

Reversible ischaemic neurological deficit:

- resolves within 72 hours
- partial non-progressing stroke
- neurological deficit does not develop further into a complete stroke.

Progressing stroke / stroke evolving:

- symptoms fluctuate for 24–76 hours
- complete stroke
- once occurred the stroke is considered complete, but children can relearn and so eventual deficit may not be so severe as observed in adults.

Symptoms

- Specific changes in brain function will depend upon the location and extent of the damage.
- Symptoms are typically on one side of the body, but may be isolated to specific functions and may include:
- Loss of movement/paralysis of limb.
- Decreased sensation, numbness, tingling, weakness.

- Decreased vision.
- Language difficulties/dysphasia.
- Swallowing difficulties.
- Inability to recognize affected side of the body.
- Loss of memory.
- Vertigo, loss of co-ordination.
- Personality changes, depression/apathy.
- Consciousness changes, sleepy, lethargic, comatose.
- Loss of bladder / bowel control.
- Dementia, impaired judgement, limited attention span.
- Facial paralysis, uncontrollable eye movements, lid drop.
- Seizures, unpredictable movements.

Myasthenia gravis

Myasthenia gravis is a disorder of neuromuscular transmission characterized by:

- Abnormal weakness and fatigue of some or all of the muscle groups
- Weakness worsening on sustained or repeated exertion, or towards the end of the day and relieved by rest.

This condition is a consequence of an autoimmune destruction of the nicotinic postsynaptic receptors for acetylcholine. Myasthenia gravis is rare, with a prevalence of 40 per million. The tendency for patients to carry certain histocompatibility (HLA) antigens and the increased incidence of autoimmune disorders in first degree relative suggests an immunological basis.

Aetiology

Antibodies appear in the receptor sites resulting in their destruction. These antibodies are referred to as acetylcholine receptor antibodies (Ach R antibodies) and are found in the patient's serum.

The role of the thymus:

- Thymic abnormalities occur in 80% of patients.
- The main function of the thymus is to effect the production of T-cell lymphocytes, which participate in immune responses.
- Thymus function is noted in a large number of disorders which may be associated with myasthenia gravis, e.g. systemic lupus erythematosus.

Clinical features

- 90% are adults – but can occur in children.
- The disorder may be selective, involving specific groups of muscles.
- Several clinical subdivisions are recognized:
  - Group I – ocular muscles only 20%
  - Group IIA – mild general weakness 30%
  - Group IIB – moderate generalized weakness – 30%
  - Group III – acute fulminating – 20%
  - Group IV – severe upon mild or moderate at onset – 20%.
- Approximately 40% of Group 1 will eventually become Group II. The rest remain purely ocular throughout the illness.
- Groups IIB, III and IV develop respiratory muscle involvement.

- Bulbar signs and symptoms:
  - ocular involvement produces ptosis and muscle paresis
  - weakness of the jaw muscles allows the mouth to hang open
  - weakness of facial muscles results in expressionless appearance
  - on smiling, buccinator weakness produces a characteristic smile (myasthenic snarl).
  - may result in:
    • dysarthric speech, dysphonic speech
    • dysphagia
    • nasal regurgitation of fluids
    • nasal quality to speech.
- Limb and trunk signs and symptoms:
  - weakness of neck muscles may result in rolling of the head
  - limb muscles tend to be involved proximally
  - movement against a constant resistance may demonstrate fatigue
  - limb reflexes are often hyperactive and fatigue on repeated testing
  - muscle wasting occurs in 15% of cases.

Treatment

- Anticholinesterase drugs – interfere with cholinesterase, the enzyme responsible for the breakdown of acetylcholine allowing enhanced receptor stimulation. As a result more acetylcholine is available to effect neuromuscular transmission.

- Cholinergic overdose (can be masked if atropine is being taken) will result in generalized weakness – cholinergic crisis:
  - muscle fasciculation
  - increased secretions – sweating
  - respiratory difficulty
  - papillary signs – miosis.

- Steroids – prednisolone for those patients who do not respond well to anticholinesterase therapy.
- Thymectomy.
- Plasmapheresis.

Guillain–Barré syndrome (GBS)

Sometimes referred to as acute idiopathic post-infectious polyneuropathy and the condition occurs following viral infection but also with other infections, for example mycoplasma, Gram-negative infection and following surgery or trauma. Fifty percent of patients describe an infectious illness in the 4 weeks prior to the onset of neuropathy. It is a cell mediated immunological reaction directed at peripheral nerves comprising of an acute demyelinating polyradiculopathy.

GBS includes a progressive, flexic motor weakness with progression manifesting over days and weeks. Patients often present with minor sensory disturbances and autonomic dysfunction is not unusual. On CSF examination, there is no evident cell count increase but protein levels typically rise gradually. Nerve conduction studies show slow conduction velocities with prolonged F waves. Another manifestation of GBS is muscle tenderness and back pain. However, other causes of muscle weakness and back pain must be excluded before a diagnosis of GBS is finally made. There is generally a history of an infectious illness then there is:

- loss of feeling
- ascending weakness and areflexia
- Sensory, autonomic and brainstem abnormalities may also be seen

- gradual ascent of paraesthesia from the feet, then upper legs, thighs, buttocks, and abdomen
- in severe cases respiratory and bulbar involvement occurs.

GBS is the most common cause of acute motor paralysis in children.

Overall mortality rate in childhood GBS is estimated to be less than 5%. A major contribution to mortality and morbidity in children presenting with GBS are respiratory muscle weakness and autonomic dysfunction, for example arrhythmias, hypotension. Full recovery within 3–12 months is experienced by 90–95% of paediatric patients with GBS. Between 5 and 10% of individuals have significant permanent disability. The outcome is more favourable in children than in adults and deaths are rare if diagnosed and treated early, even though the recovery period can be long – often weeks to months. Recurrence can occur sometimes many years after the initial bout.

The child is more susceptible to complications such as:

- pneumonia
- septicaemia
- pressure ulcers
- pulmonary embolism
- ileus
- constipation
- gastritis
- dysaesthesia – impairment of touch sensation.

Management

- In cooperative children older than 5 years, respiratory function measures, such as vital capacity or maximal inspiratory force, is useful. This measure is unfortunately difficult to monitor in young less than 5 years and any uncooperative child. Experienced paediatric respiratory therapists can be very valuable in these measures.
- Experienced pulmonary care is vital if neuromuscular weakness is affecting pulmonary function. Possible interventions include CPAP, BPAP, mechanical ventilation, or cough-assist devices.
- Blood gases are not helpful in assessing neuromuscular respiratory failure and only become abnormal when there is no longer any respiratory reserve, so that other means of assessing respiratory function, such as respiratory rate and dyspnoea on lying supine are far more valuable early indicators of respiratory dysfunction.
- Chest radiographs can be obtained to look for signs of infection.
- Cardiac monitoring is essential to detect any signs of cardiovascular instability and treat any arrhythmia.

Treatment

- Is mainly supportive with management of the paralysed patient.
- Occasionally ventilation and tracheotomy may be required.
- IV gammaglobulin.
- Plasmapheresis, it is important that this treatment is started within 14 days of onset of symptoms for it to be effective.
- Steroids are sometimes used, but this has not been shown to be useful.
- Regular chest physiotherapy.
- Monitoring of $paCO_2$ for early signs of respiratory failure.

- Continuous cardiovascular monitoring for early detection of autonomic dysfunction.
- Nutritional support especially if ileus present from autonomic dysfunction.
- Adequate analgesia for muscle pains, etc.
- Regular pressure area care.
- DVT prophylaxis due to reduced mobility.

GBS patients require a lot of time and effort to enable them to return to a normal life.

Cardiomyopathy

Cardiomyopathy is a disorder of the cardiac muscle that can be acute, subacute or chronic. It is often of an unknown aetiology but can occur at birth or in childhood. There are many different types of cardiomyopathy:

- Dilated cardiomyopathy – characterized by dilatation and impaired contraction of the left ventricle or both ventricles.
- Hypertrophic cardiomyopathy – characterized by left and/or right ventricular hypertrophy, which is usually asymmetric and involves the intraventricular septum.
- Arrhythmogenic right ventricular cardiomyopathy – a familial myocardial disease characterized pathologically by right ventricular (RV) myocardial atrophy and fibrofatty replacement, a progressive heart muscle disease that with time may lead to more diffuse RV involvement and left ventricular (LV) changes and may culminate in heart failure.

- Restrictive cardiomyopathy – the least common and defined as heart muscle disease that results in impaired ventricular filling, with normal or decreased diastolic volume of either or both ventricles (Richardson 1995). Treatment is usually palliative.

Nursing considerations in cardiomyopathy

Care of the patient with cardiomyopathy may present the nurse with many challenges; the presentation of cardiomyopathy within a family may range from the asymptomatic patient who requires no treatment to sudden cardiac death and heart failure. It is important to remember that nurses will encounter patients who are living with a cardiomyopathy at various stages of disease progression.

Heart failure

When the heart fails, its ability to contract efficiently is reduced and it can no longer respond to increased filling pressure by contracting more strongly. The heart is not strong enough to pump blood efficiently around the body and various organs receive insufficient blood supply. The kidney then activates the renin–angiotensin–aldosterone system and causes salt and water retention and oedema. Breathlessness may occur due to oedema of the lung tissue – pulmonary oedema.

Fluid collects in the body tissues and causes systemic congestion. The brain is protected and receives its oxygen and blood supply at the expense of other organs, which are starved, and this may lead to fatigue. This condition is generally not curable, but it can be kept under control with the use of drugs. There is a failure of the heart to eject blood efficiently from the ventricles, resulting in elevated intra cardiac pressures.

- The increase in pressure in the left side of the heart causes pulmonary congestion.
- Increased pressure on the right side causes systemic venous congestion and peripheral oedema.

Examination:

- Peripheral cyanosis
- Distended neck veins
- Oedema of the ankles
- Rales at the lung bases
- Gallop rhythm of heart
- Enlarged liver
- Dyspnoea
- ECG: Normal sinus rhythm, q waves and left axis deviation may be present
- Chest X-ray: enlarged heart, diffused density in the lung bases.

Renal disease

Because the kidney filters in blood, it is directly linked to every other organ system. Therefore, renal conditions that lead to renal failure can be life threatening. Two different causes:

Glomerulonephritis

Inflammation of the glomerulus caused by:

- immune responses
- toxins or drugs

- vascular disorders
- systemic diseases.

  Classification of glomerulonephritis:

- acute glomerulonephritis
- rapidly progressive glomerulonephritis (RPGN)
- chronic glomerulonephritis.

Nephrotic syndrome

Excretion of at least 3.5 g protein in urine per day:

- hypoproteinaemia, hyperlipidaemia and oedema
- caused by loss of plasma proteins across the injured glomerular filtration membrane
- reduced protein leads to oedema.

  Treatment involves:

- normal-protein, low-fat diet
- salt restriction
- diuretics
- steroids
- occasionally albumin replacement.

Renal failure

Classification of renal dysfunction

- Renal insufficiency refers to a decline in renal function to about 25% of normal or GFR of 25 to 30 ml/min.
- Renal failure refers to significant loss of renal function.
- End stage renal failure (ESRF) is when less than 10% of renal function remains.

Different types:

- Acute renal failure (ARF) – prerenal, renal, postrenal
- Chronic renal failure (CRF)
- ESRF.

ARF

- Causes (prerenal)
  - Failure of blood supply to the kidneys.
- Causes (renal)
  - Generally structural abnormalities to the kidneys:
    - ATN, depends on severity and duration
    - pre-renal causes which may last up to 6 weeks
    - glomerulonephritis
    - drug-induced nephrotoxicity.
- Causes (post-renal)
  - More likely to be CRF, interstitial nephritis
    - malignant hypertension
    - blood transfusion.

Clinical features

- asymptomatic
- oliguria
- increasing blood urea
- nausea, vomiting
- confusion
- loss of appetite.

Recovery is in three phases:

- oliguria 1–3 weeks
- diuresis volume depletion may occur
- recovery.

CRF

The kidney has many important regulatory functions, but renal symptomatic changes do not become apparent until the renal function declines to less than 25% normal.

Causes:

- glomerulonephritis
- diabetes mellitus
- chronic pyelonephritis
- polycystic kidneys
- hypertension.

Clinical features:

- gastrointestinal tract – anorexia, nausea and vomiting, hiccups
- skin – itching, uraemic frost
- blood – anaemia, tendency to bleed
- bones – inadequate vitamin D, bone pain, pathological fractures
- cardiovascular system – hypertension, coronary artery disease
- nervous system – uraemic neuropathy leading to apathy, confusion, irritation, tremours and seizures.

Management of renal failure

- Blood and urine analysis – check haemoglobin for anaemia, electrolytes, creatinine and urea, urine testing for protein
- Fluid and electrolyte balance – potassium – ECG changes, sodium, phosphate and calcium balance, fluid and diet intake is strictly controlled, fluid output
- Acidosis – metabolic acidosis begins to develop when GFR decreases by 30–40%, maintained by respiratory system removal of carbon dioxide.

Renal replacement therapy

- Haemodialysis – intermittent, traumatic to the circulation, reduced blood pressure.
- Haemofiltration – continuous, less traumatic to the circulation.
- Peritoneal dialysis – intermittent generally at home at night, managed by the patient.
- Transplantation – various success, there has been more success recently with live donors due to the advances in live organ retrieval, requiring the donor to only undergo keyhole surgery.

Renal failure accounts for a small group of patient deaths. Death can sometimes be easy to predict because dialysis has been discontinued. They can suffer from pain during the last days and this underscores the necessity for medical and nursing staff to be skilled providers of modern palliative care. If the symptoms of ESRF are poorly managed it leads to misery at the end of life. Knowledge of palliative care in these instances is essential.

Sickle cell disease

Sickle cell disease (SCD) is a chronic hereditary haematological disorder. SCD is characterized by sickle-shaped (crescent-shaped) fragile red blood cells with impaired ability to transport oxygen. The crescent-shaped RBCs hinders blood flow which results in vaso-occlusion, anaemia, infarction, and necrosis of body organs and joints.

Pathological processes of SCD

- Haemolysis precipitates vascular endothelial damage by causing anaemia and nitric oxide functional deficiency.
- Haemolysis may also contribute to the development of pulmonary hypertension and stroke.
- Vaso-occlusion, the other main pathological process of SCD, can result in acute pain, organ damage and chronic ischaemia.

Incidence

SCD is found in just over 1 in every 2000 neonates, making it the most frequently occurring genetic condition in England.

- People of African and African-Caribbean origin have substantially higher prevalence rates, though, as it is estimated that this group may see 1 in every 300 infants born with SCD (Streetly et al 2010).
- Cases of SCD are also more commonly diagnosed in families of African-Caribbean, Middle Eastern, Indian and eastern Mediterranean origin.
- There is wide variation in the prevalence of SCD according to geographic area: as most ethnic minority groups are found in London and other urban centres, high-density areas face significantly higher rates of SCD. South-east London, for example, showed a prevalence rate of 3 in 1000 screened infants; Cumbria and Lancashire, on the other hand, hold a prevalence rate of just 0.12 in every 1000 infants (Streetly et al 2010).

- A child with sickle cell trait (HbSA) is a carrier of the disorder and does not have the disease (HbSS).

Screening for SCD

In 2006, the National Health Service (NHS) had fully implemented a neonatal sickle cell disease (SCD) screening programme across hospitals in England. The newborn dried blood-spot screening programme currently offers sickle cell disease (SCD) screening to infants of all ethnicities at 5–8 days of age (Streetly et al 2010). While the frequency and expression of symptoms varies widely from one individual to the next, improvements in diagnostic and treatment technologies have greatly improved patients' prognoses (Telfer et al 2007).

Signs and symptoms

Rarely displayed before 6 months but are usually symptomatic by the age of 1 year. The majority of hospital admissions for SCD arise from:

- acute pain arising from vaso-occlusion or severe anaemia
- severe anaemic crisis arises from the production and destruction of RBCs and pooling of the blood in the spleen.

Acute complications (Dick et al 2006)

- Infants with undiagnosed SCD frequently present with acute splenic sequestration or sudden death from pneumococcal sepsis from splenic hypofunction.
- Infants 9–18 months of age may present with dactylitis.

- Stroke occurs in approximately 5–10% of children with SCD.
- Acute chest syndrome, biliary disease, renal disease, osteomyelitis, avascular necrosis, ophthamalogical conditions, priapism and leg ulcers are other complications arising from SCD.
- It is important to bear in mind that the frequency, duration and type of symptoms and complications are highly variable between individuals. This variability may be due in part to secondary effector genes which contribute to conditions and complications arising from vaso-occlusion.

Management of SCD

SCD manifests in various ways depending on the individual. Some children suffer from severe symptoms and frequent hospitalization, while others experience relatively few symptoms (Dick 2008).

Assessment

- Observe, and record vital signs. Report fever, increased respiratory and pulse rates and low blood pressure.
- Assess level of pain using pain assessment tool. Pain is an extremely important indicator of a sickling crisis and should be acted upon immediately.
- Blood analysis is required where fever climbs above 38.5°C in order to rule out chest infection, urinary tract infection, meningitis and cholecystitis.
- Observe extremities for mottling, cooling or cyanosis.

- Observe mental status for alterations.
- Observe and record urinary output.
- If chest infection suspected, include a chest X-ray.
- If stroke suspected, assess neurological symptoms (e.g. transient weakness, paraesthesiae), and include magnetic resonance scan.
- If acute chest syndrome suspected or haemorrhage include a high resolution CT scan.

> **!**
> Abdominal palpation should be avoided in case of splenic sequestration as may cause splenic rupture.

Management of an acute episode

- Intravenous hydration. Hydration is extremely important for the prevention of red blood cell sickling and for delaying the vaso-occlusive ischaemia cycle. It is normally recommended that children consume 1.5–2 times what is normally required to maintain adequate daily hydration.
- Administer oxygen. Oxygenation will help break the hypoxia-metabolic-acidosis-sickling cycle.
- Ensure bed rest and keep child warm
- Administer pain medications as prescribed. Acetaminophen or ibuprofen is used to treat mild to moderate pain; this can be supplemented with codeine where required. Severe pain may require morphine, hydromorphone or methadone. As patients with SCD

are at increased risk of developing normeperidine-induced seizures, meperidine should not be prescribed (Simon et al 1999).

- Administer antibiotics as prescribed.
- Administer blood transfusion if prescribed.
- Acute chest syndrome is any new change on chest X-ray that may be caused by infection or sickling of red cells. It is the most common cause of morbidity among children with SCD. Early intervention for the treatment of acute chest syndrome may involve pain relief, oxygenated ventilatory support, physiotherapy, antibiotics and blood transfusion. Pneumococcal infection is 600 times more prevalent in children with SCD when compared to the population norm, and its rapid onset in the immunocompromised child can result in death where immediate treatment is not received (Dick 2008).
- Acute stroke: exchange transfusion may be required following treatment to include magnetic resonance scan.

Long-term management

Patients with SCD in the UK are almost exclusively managed by the acute care sector. While this route of care is currently not seen as ideal, it is supported by sickle cell and thalassaemia centres, which deliver information, genetic counselling and health advice in certain high-prevalence communities (Dick et al 2006).

- Patient and carer education is extremely important for drug treatment adherence, pain management and knowledge of crucial signs and symptoms.

Education should focus on preventative strategies, the identification of early warning symptoms, and timely responses to pain. In particular, issues relating to hydration, medication compliance and serious symptom recognition should be discussed with patients and included as regular components of care (Simon et al 1999).

- Avoid cold and dehydration.

- Part of long term management an annual review is recommended

- Penicillin prophylaxis (or an equivalent alternative) should be taken on a twice daily basis throughout childhood and beginning at 3 months of age.

- As SCD causes a rapid rate of erythropoiesis, daily folic acid supplements are recommended (Simon et al 1999).

- Children with SCD are immunocompromised and should therefore receive routine immunization, in addition to annual influenza vaccines, pneumococcal vaccine and polysaccharide vaccine (the last of which beginning at 2 years of age and continuing every five years) (Dick 2008).

- Pneumococcal hepatitis and annual influenza immunizations should be offered. In cases where the child may be travelling to affected areas, malaria prophylaxis is strongly recommended.

- Continual hip or shoulder pain should be investigated for avascular necrosis through an MRI scan. If avascular necrosis causes considerable pain or develops to stage III or higher, a referral to an orthopaedic surgeon should be made (Dick 2008).

- Stroke is a serious complication of sickle cell anaemia (SCA), occurring most frequently in 2–5-year-old patients who carry homozygotic expressions of sickle cell disease (HbSS) (Roberts et al 2009).

- Stroke and progressive cerebrovascular disease are preventable complications of SCA through transcranial Doppler ultrasound (TCD) screening. UK guidelines for the management of SCD in children recommend yearly TCD screening, beginning at three years of age. Scans should be repeated within 2 months where high-risk or conditional cerebrovascular disease is identified (Dick 2008).

- Regular blood transfusions may be required for the treatment of children who remain at high risk of developing cerebrovascular disease. Blood transfusion therapy should occur throughout childhood as a secondary preventative measure against stroke.

- Children with SCD should receive liver function tests annually. Ultrasound of the liver and biliary tree should follow-up complaints of abdominal pain. Symptomatic biliary disease may be treated with elective cholecystectomy.

- Children should undergo yearly measurements/laboratory work-up of blood pressure, urea, creatine and electrolytes in order to monitor signs of kidney disease. Further renal investigation may be required where hypertension or elevated creatine/urea levels are found.

- Hydroxyurea should be offered to children with two or more episodes of acute chest syndrome in the last 2 years. Where only one episode occurred but which required ventilator support, hydroxyurea is also the recommended course of treatment. Myelosuppression is the most common reported side effect of hydroxyurea (Dick 2008).

- Visual symptoms should receive immediate attention by an ophthalmologist.

- Infected leg ulcers should be treated with debridement, antibiotic therapy and appropriate pain relief. Persistent cases may respond well to oral zinc sulphate treatment.

- Minor occasions of priapism should be treated with pain relief, warm baths, and emptying the bladder prior to sleep. Stuttering priapism should be treated with oral etilefrine (Dick 2008).

- Bedwetting which occurs over the age of 6 should be treated with basic measures or through specialist management where necessary in children 7 years and older (Dick 2008).

Children with SCD do not often undergo bone marrow transplantation because of difficulty in establishing a matched sibling donor, and because of the efficacy of hydroxyurea in reducing painful episodes and acute chest syndrome. Children eligible for bone marrow transplantation must be at least 16 years of age and must fulfil clinical requirements relating to severity, frequency and type of signs and symptoms requiring treatment.

Long-term prognosis

- Life expectancy (between 50–60 years), has improved considerably due to early recognition, improvements in diagnostic/treatment technologies

and better management of acute episodes.

- Where SCD is managed carefully with regular antibiotic compliance, proper hydration and annual medical tests, patients can expect reduced complications and symptoms.

- However, patients do experience complications in response to the treatment itself (e.g. transfusion treatments), and the pathophysiology of SCD, for many patients, causes significant disability and premature death (Simon et al 1999).

4.3 Mental ill health in children

The level of mental issues are on the increase in children with problems such as adolescent/child suicide, substance misuse, behaviour problems, teenage pregnancy, bullying, attention deficit hyperactivity disorder and social communication disorders. Some of these issues are a reflection of changing values within society whilst other issues have been around a long time but which were under-diagnosed or not recognized.

Attention deficit hyperactivity disorder (ADHD)

ADHD (also known as hyperkinetic disorder [HKD]) is a common neurological developmental disorder. It is estimated that between 3–9% of children and adolescents in the UK meet the Diagnostic and Statistical Manual of

Mental Disorders 4th Edition (DSM-IV) criteria for ADHD, with HKD thought to occur in 1–2% of children in the UK according to International Classification of Mental and Behavioural Disorders 10th Revision (ICD-10) criteria, that affects at least 3–5% of children in the UK (National Institute for Health and Clinical Excellence (NICE) 2008). However, as no diagnostic criteria have been agreed upon amongst clinicians in the UK, widely divergent prevalence rates abound: recent epidemiological studies estimate rates spanning between 0.5–26%. In the UK, children as young as 3 years of age have been diagnosed with ADHD, although it is more commonly identified in a child's early years of primary school.

Assessment of ADHD

Considerable variation exists in the clinical assessment and treatment of ADHD in children in the UK. The inconsistency in diagnosis and treatment of children with ADHD represent significant barriers to effective management. ADHD is characterized by a cluster of symptoms:

- reduced attention span
- hyperactivity
- impulsivity.

While it is common to observe all three types of behaviours within a child, some children will show stronger symptoms of hyperactivity/impulsivity or poor concentration. Identifying ADHD-related behaviours in preschool-aged children poses difficulty because impulsivity, short concentration and hyperactivity are observed in neurotypical *as well as* ADHD children in this age group (Harpin 2005).

Assessing ADHD in children

This hinges on behavioural observation, specially designed rating scales and parental reports and history taking.

- The ADHD Rating Scale (ADHD-RS) and the Conners Parent and Teacher Rating Scales are commonly used because of their correspondence with DSM-IV criteria.

- The Strengths and Difficulties Questionnaire (SDQ) is another common assessment tool in the UK.

- When assessing girls, it is important to bear in mind that symptoms normally observed in children with ADHD – such as hyperactivity and difficult behaviour – may be less prevalent in school-aged girls, despite having intellectual difficulties and learning problems in the classroom (Steer 2005).

Diagnosis of ADHD

Clinicians in the UK currently use the ICD-10 and the DSM-IV as two primary means of diagnostic assessment. The ICD-10 is more suitable for use in people whose symptoms and level of impairment are more severe, while the DSM-IV is broad-spectrum in its assessment and is designed to identify ADHD subtypes. To reach a clinical diagnosis of ADHD, the following criteria must be met (NICE 2008):

- A fulfilment of the diagnostic criteria outlined in the DSM-IV or ICD-10.

- A case history or observation in various settings which identifies moderate impairment in the child's social, intellectual or psychological functioning.

- Impairment of the above description which persists across two or more settings (e.g.in the school, home or community setting).

Combined-type ADHD

Where elements of reduced attention span, increased activity level and increased impulsivity are all present in a child's behaviour, he or she may be diagnosed with combined-type ADHD.

Comorbid disorders

ADHD does not exist in isolation from other related disorders, and children may have comorbid conditions such as learning/social/communication difficulties, anxiety, poor motor control and mood disorders. Approximately 65% of children with ADHD live with comorbid disorders affecting them on neurological developmental levels. The most common associated disorders in ADHD children are listed below:

- dyslexia
- developmental coordination disorder (DCD)
- conduct disorder
- oppositional defiant disorder (ODD)
- autism spectrum disorder
- Tourette's syndrome.

Impact of ADHD on the child and adolescent

- Many children with ADHD experience depression, frustration and poor confidence.
- Tend to experience poor concentration and/or hyperactivity/impulsivity which causes some degree of impairment in various settings and circumstances (such as in school, at home and during a range of different activities).

- Children in primary school years experience delayed social skills and poor academic achievement which sets them apart from their peer group (Harpin 2005). This can result in poor self-confidence and creates difficulties in the home and classroom.

- May also experience sleep difficulties which negatively impact upon their behaviour during the day.

- As ADHD children develop into their preteen and adolescent years, hyperactivity and other behaviours that once showed in the child's temperament may be replaced with poor concentration, impulsivity and a distorted sense of self.

- Discontinuation of academic studies, poor school performance, unplanned pregnancy and juvenile delinquency feature more frequently in the lives of ADHD pre-teens and adolescents, and many of these issues *contribute to* and/or *result from* poor social relationships within an individual's peer group and academic circle (Harpin 2005).

Impact on the family

- Parents and families of children with ADHD experience increased stress, guilt surrounding the decision to medicate their child, and higher rates of divorce, paternal alcoholism and maternal depression.

- As children with ADHD require more behavioural supervision, emotional support and school-related guidance from their parents, relationships within the home can become strained.

- Previous research has shown that siblings of school-aged children with ADHD experience significant anxiety over disruption caused by the ADHD child to the home environment, and often share the responsibility of caring for and protecting their ADHD sibling.

- Diagnosing and treating ADHD in children is important because of its positive impact on mitigating parental stress and promoting healthy parent–child relationships.

Management and treatment of child with ADHD

Children with ADHD require multidisciplinary care that gives equal consideration to their education needs, home environment, psychological wellbeing and medical treatment. It is generally recommended that children and adolescents diagnosed with ADHD receive drug treatment as part of a first-line, multimodal course of care which includes social, psychological and behavioural interventions.

Medication

Prior to beginning a drug treatment plan for children diagnosed with ADHD, baseline medical data should be gathered which includes (NICE 2008):

- full physical examination including heart rate, blood pressure, growth chart plotting, cardiovascular exam and ECG (where history of cardiovascular problems are present)

- substance misuse risk assessment

- mental health and social skills assessment.

Medication usually methylphenidate hydrochloride, a psychostimulant manufactured under the trademark name Ritalin. Licensed for use in children 6 years and older. It is available in once-daily or immediate release (2–3 times daily) doses. If a child does not respond to the medication after one month, treatment should be stopped.

- Common side effects include disrupted sleep, headache, depressed appetite, abdominal discomfort, dizziness, tachycardia, stunted growth, heart palpitations and increased blood pressure (NICE 2006).

- The numerous side-effects of short-acting stimulants may contribute to poor compliance.

- If a child with ADHD cannot tolerate or does not respond to methylphenidate hydrochloride, a combined behavioural, medical and psychological intervention which uses atomoxetine is the recommended second-line course of treatment (NICE 2008).

- The use of methylphenidate hydrochloride is ordinarily discontinued once a child reaches late adolescence. However, the discontinuation of drug treatment should only be considered upon completion of an individualized assessment overseen by the child's paediatrician, psychiatrist or primary care physician.

A prescription requiring multiple dosing throughout the day may cause embarrassment for children in the school, poor compliance or missed doses. One solution to this problem is the use of sustained-release formulations of methylphenidate hydrochloride (e.g. Concerta XL or Equasym XL), which work with comparable efficacy to their multiple-dose counterparts but only require once-daily dosing (Steer 2005).

As some studies have shown growth to be thwarted by stimulants such as methylphenidate hydrochloride, the child receiving stimulants should be monitored for signs of delayed growth (Harpin 2005).

In cases where comorbidities or moderate to severe symptoms are present, dexamfetamine or atomoxetine are recommended (NICE 2006).

A pharmacological alternative to short-acting or sustained release stimulants, tricyclic antidepressents (TCAs), selective serotonin reuptake inhibitors (SSRIs) and other medications are prescribed when psychostimulants are not well tolerated (Steer 2005).

Concerns about drug misuse and poor compliance suggest that the pharmacological treatment of ADHD be supported by patient education and close monitoring (Steer 2005). Clinical need remains the primary determinant of drug therapy, and the ADHD child should be reassessed at least annually to ensure that their course of treatment meets their present needs.

Behavioural and psychological interventions

Behavioural interventions

- Once a diagnosis has been made, it is important that parents, educators and health care professionals work with the ADHD young person from a holistic perspective.

- Health care professionals should support parents and children through behaviour modification techniques for managing symptoms in conjunction with drug therapy.

- Behavioural management approaches that, for instance, seek to simplify the child's required tasks or guide behaviour through positive and negative reinforcement techniques are effective in mitigating conduct problems and boosting self-confidence and school performance.

- Behaviour therapy should be provided both at home and in school.

- Increase parents and child's knowledge of ADHD through educational resource materials.

- Provide dietary and fitness advice.

- Refer parents to parenting skills programmes.

Psychological interventions

These recommend psychological treatment for children with moderate to severe ADHD:

- When appropriate approaches are used in combination with prescription medication, parents report higher satisfaction with their child's treatment plan, and medication is often only required in reduced doses (Steer 2005).

- Treating all facets of ADHD in children requires extensive liaising with professionals from health, social and education services.

- Nurses who are specially trained in treating ADHD or in the field of neurodevelopmental disorders are uniquely positioned to refer families to specialist services, recommend child and adolescent mental health services and provide referrals to community-based parenting programmes.

> ⚠ The UK has seen a 22% rise in methylphenidate hydrochloride prescriptions in the last decade alone, and the NICE recognizes a risk of methylphenidate hydrochloride misuse within individuals and communities (Blew and Kenny 2006). Nurses working with families, schools and communities should therefore be vigilant to the potential for misuse or abuse, and should seek to educate children and their families about the dangers of prescription drug misuse.

Behaviour and emotional difficulties

The latter decades of the twentieth century have seen significant increases in the prevalence of childhood psychosocial disorders in the industrialized West. Historical trends drawn from suicide rates, retrospective studies, self-harm prevalence, clinical records, mental disorder diagnoses, and health/social service use point to an increase in public awareness of mental health as well as an increase in the absolute prevalence rates of mental health problems and disorders (Collishaw et al 2010).

Increase in depression and anxiety

Collishaw and others (2010) compared scores from two nationally representative studies which measure the prevalence of depression and anxiety in adolescents in England.

- The prevalence of youth- and parent-rated emotional problems significantly increased in adolescents in England between the time of the first (1986) and second (2006) points of data collection, with the overall prevalence of depression and anxiety in young people doubling in the last two decades (Collishaw et al 2010).

- This change was quite substantially more pronounced in girls than in boys, with previous studies in the UK lending support to the finding that adolescent girls are more prone to suffering from depression and anxiety than boys in their peer group.

- Compared to the 1970s and 1980s, today's rates of childhood mental health problems remain high and thus require targeted research and services aimed at reducing them.

Factors predisposing children to behavioural and emotional problems

Learning disabilities

- British children and adolescents with intellectual disability are significantly more likely to have any psychiatric disorder, and 14% of all British children with a psychiatric disorder are intellectually disabled (Emerson and Hatton, 2007).

- Children with specific speech and language difficulties (SSLD) are at increased risk of developing psychosocial and mental health comorbidities such as conduct disorder, social problems and poor self-confidence (Lindsay and others 2007).

Chronic illness or physical disability

- Behavioural difficulties and mental health problems are present as comorbidities in 20–30% of children with chronic illness or physical disability. Such comorbidities include poor attention, depression, anxiety, affective disorder and psychosocial problems (Darke et al 2006).

- Duchenne muscular dystrophy (DMD), the most common neuromuscular disease in children and is most frequently found in boys, is associated with psychosocial and behavioural problems as well as cognitive problems resulting in learning and communication difficulties (Darke et al 2006).

- Children with neuromuscular disease with comorbid autism spectrum disorder, Becker muscular dystrophy or severe/moderate learning disability were significantly more likely to have carer-reported problems affecting their behavioural, communicative and psychosocial functioning (Darke et al 2006).

Socially disadvantaged

- Social disadvantage was correlated with increased rates of all conduct disorders, all emotional disorders and ADHD (Emerson and Hatton 2007).

- Boys, pre-adolescents, children with special educational needs, low socioeconomic status, poor maternal educational attainment and family size of three or more children were correlated with the presence of a persistent conduct disorder (Office for National Statistics 2008).

- It appears that aggression, defiance and behavioural difficulties in children are quite frequently associated with parental marital problems, depression, academic difficulty, social isolation/bullying, bereavement and broader problems within the family (Parentline Plus 2009).

- Aggressive behaviour in younger children was found to be linked to feelings of low self-worth, while in older children aggression appears to be tied to low self-worth as well as self-harming behaviour and drug/alcohol misuse (Parentline Plus 2009).

- Aggressive behaviours are more frequently acted out in the family/home environment, with young adolescents aged 13–15 years showing aggressive behaviours more frequently than other age groups (Parentline Plus 2009).

- There is a positive relationship between feelings of safety and risk-taking behaviour for example substance misuse, anxiety and negative feelings about relationships.

Behaviour problems

Parents of young children often seek advice on how to cope with a range of behavioural difficulties, ranging from eating, sleeping, and toileting problems to managing aggressive behaviour and include:

- conduct and oppositional disorders (disruptive behaviour disorders)

- ADHD
- sleeping, eating, toileting problems (e.g. tantrums, failure to thrive, enuresis, encopresis)
- emotional problems (e.g. anxiety, depression, panic attacks, phobias, obsessive compulsive behaviour)
- anorexia nervosa
- self-harm
- substance misuse (e.g. alcohol, solvents, drugs).

Assessment of behavioural problems

Social, emotional and behavioural difficulties in children vary in strength and frequency of expression according to context. For instance, teachers' and parents' reports of a child's behaviour and development may differ with regard to the nature, frequency and duration of problem behaviours. Therefore it is essential that the child/young person are assessed carefully by an appropriately qualified professional.

- Assessing the child and family is the first step.
- Establish rapport and show empathy.
- Tone should be warm and friendly.
- Approach should be respectful, interested and accepting.
- Adopting a 'one-down' position – asking the child to tell you something of which he/she knows more than you do or acknowledging the parents as experts on their children (Barker 2004)
- Use open questions and direct requests for the expression of feelings.
- Ask how often the problem is occurring.

- Assess how extreme is the problem.
- Identify how long there has been a problem.
- Does the child show other problems.
- Assess are the child's behaviour and emotions appropriate for their developmental level.
- Assess does the child have any sensory disabilities.
- Elicit the child's view on the problem.
- Identify if there is something that triggers the problem, e.g. an event or person.
- Determine how the problem usually resolves or what the consequences are each time.
- Determine what family life is like and observe interactions between family members.
- Determine what actions parents use to manage the child's behavior.
- Assess the quality of the parent–child relationship.
- Identify if any traumatic events or major life events have occurred recently, e.g. divorce, bereavement, separations, unemployment.

Formulating the management and treatment plan

Before assigning a diagnostic label to the child's problem, it is more important to systematically formulate the management and treatment plan by considering the following (Barker 2004):

1. Predisposing factors: what pre-existing factors contributed to the development of the problem?

2. Precipitating factors: why did the problem appear at that particular time?
3. Perpetuating factors: what is maintaining the problem?
4. Protective factors: what are the child's and family's strengths?

Management strategies that parents can use

Feeling stressed, overwhelmed and demoralized are common experiences of the parents of children with behaviour problems. Parents must look after their own mental health before addressing the well-being of their children. Parentline compiled a list of recommendations for parents seeking help in dealing with their children's aggressive behaviour. The following strategies are recommended (Parentline Plus 2009):

- Parents should be advised to seek out professional, family or community-based support and make time to address their own emotional needs and responses.

- Identify signs of escalating aggression by discussing the child's behavioural and emotional difficulties with the child's teacher or other adults in regular contact with the child.

- Consider how the child's social group, school experiences and family relationships affects his or her ability to cope with stress.

- Involve the child in all aspects of exploring and dealing with their aggression through supportive, pro-active conversation which takes place outside of an aggressive episode.

- Use language which emphasizes constructive behavioural resolution rather than language which conveys non-acceptance of the child as an individual.

- Replace criticizing, problem-focused statements with language which offers encouragement and ways of moving forward.

Therapeutic approaches

Many minor and some major behavioural problems clear up with some assistance at a family level. Some behavioural difficulties can be managed and eventually eliminated with the appropriate family centred therapy. Since children and young people's behavioural and emotional problems often have multiple causes, it may be necessary to use more that one form of treatment:

- family therapy
- counselling
- behaviour therapy
- individual psychotherapy
- problem-solving skills training (PSST)
- group therapy
- hynotherapy
- pharmacotherapy
- educational measures
- speech and language therapy
- day treatment
- inpatient and residential treatment.

Counselling

It is estimated that over 400 approaches to counselling have been developed and are used in practice, causing considerable confusion amongst health care professionals over which approach to adopt when addressing patients' needs. Rather than learn specific types of counselling, it is useful to begin by understanding the primary categorizations into which counselling techniques fall:

- Person-centred/Rogerian – One of the most frequently used approaches in the UK. Supports the patient in reaching desired outcomes on their own terms. Exemplified for use in children by play therapy.

- Psychodynamic – another very commonly used approach in the UK. Draws on the work and theories of Freud to relate present circumstances to past experiences and unconscious processes.

- Behavioural – examines current behaviours and encourages targeted goal-setting. Draws on learning theory.

- Cognitive – focuses the patient on their thought patterns, behaviours and ways of looking at problems in order to bring about resolution through cognitive and behavioural change.

Key skills in counselling

Fulfilling the emotional aspects of patient care can be a challenging task for busy nurses, but any extra attention paid to this issue can have a far-reaching impact on a patient's wellness and recovery. Addressing patients' emotional needs is a skill which can be developed by reflecting on one's communication strategies as an approach to delivering patient-centred care. Specific techniques for developing counselling and communication skills as a nurse include:

- Engaging with the patient through active listening, such as

by: demonstrating your understanding with your body language; repeating important words or phrases that the patient used; clarifying information by rephrasing and recapping what was said.

- Gathering information sensitively: encourage information sharing by asking open-ended questions which cannot be answered with a simple yes or no; avoiding leading questions which may plant answers in a patient's mind; avoiding questions beginning with 'why' so as to avoid coming across in a confrontational manner.

- Treating patients with empathy by seeking to understand their condition through their words and experiences rather than through your own assumptions of what their situation must be like.

Counselling children on health and illness

- Counselling and educating children on health and illness requires the provision of information and support in a developmentally appropriate manner, and for this reason such interventions differ substantially from those aimed at adult patients.

- A 'patient-centred' approach which encourages agency and values the unique experiences of the individual is supported by a number of studies on children's health counselling.

- The process of counselling children on health-related issues should be collaborative in nature (i.e. involve parents, child and practitioner) and identify coping strategies and ways of managing the child's medical condition and treatment process.

- Counselling and health education interventions for children which have gained significant attention in recent studies include interventions which address obesity/nutrition, chronic illness, smoking prevention and childhood cancer (Theunissen et al 2004).

Counselling children with chronic illness

Children with chronic illness are an overlooked group in counselling and communication literature, despite the fact that they have unique and urgent psychosocial needs. Suggested techniques for supporting chronically ill children through counselling and health education include (Chesson et al 2004):

- Using play therapies, drawing and pretend play to help children and pre-adolescents act out their emotions and experiences in a way that is more natural for their developmental level.

- Communicating problems over a number of short sessions in order to build a comfortable relationship over time.

- Eliciting the child's thoughts, fears and concerns over an unrelated activity, such as while playing with toys or a game.

- Being clear about the extent to which certain information may be kept confidential or may be shared with the child's parents or wider health care team.

- Assisting the child in coming to terms with a decision that has been made about their medical treatment that may cause anxiety or upset in the child.

- Where appropriate, encourage chronically ill and hospitalized children to interact with other children on the ward in order to build confidence and social skills.

- Be aware of common emotional responses that children of different developmental stages have toward their illness and its treatment. For example, older children may experience feelings of shame and unfairness toward being ill, and often want to appear 'normal' to their peers. Younger children may have difficulty articulating their feelings, and may experience significant fear and anxiety toward treatment processes and medical environments.

Motivational interviewing (MI)

MI is a counselling technique used by health care professionals to help patients bring about a desired behaviour change. MI has shown some success in facilitating behavioural change in the paediatric health care setting (Suarez and Mullins 2008).

MI has been used in a range of health care settings for the treatment of substance abuse, medication and treatment compliance, eating disorders, lifestyle change and smoking cessation (Knight et al 2006).

- Motivational interviewing has an end goal in mind such as long-term lifestyle change or medical treatment adherence and uses a number of communicative and counselling approaches to help patients achieve positive change.

- Is a counselling technique that helps individuals identify behaviours and attitudes which support or prevent them from achieving a desired outcome.

- Clinicians using MI should adopt an empathetic, non-judgemental and reflective approach to their interactions with patients, aiming to encourage intrinsic behavioural change.
- May have an educational component, but it does not view the process of information giving as a pivotal motivating agent.
- Healthcare professionals require skills training in MI for effective implementation.

MI technique

- Balancing the provision of guidance, support and direction with the need to create space to listen to the patient's concerns in a non-judgemental and empathetic way.
- Identifying and exploring the reasons behind a patient's ambivalence toward behaviour change.
- Recognizing that motivation to change is an intrinsic process that cannot be imposed on the patient

through coercive argument, verbal agreement or extensive information-giving.

- Reflecting back aspects of the patient's language which are self-motivating, solution-focused and indicative of an intrinsic desire to change.
- Understand that behaviour change is an iterative process during which a patient may stall, move between or regress within the following six stages: precontemplation, contemplation/change consideration, preparation and commitment, action/change engagement, sustained change engagement, and lastly, habitual change engagement leading to the resolution or complete termination of an unwanted behaviour.
- Establishing a relationship of trust and mutual collaboration by summarizing and reflecting the patient's language and by providing empathetic feedback and support.
- Encouraging the patient to speak about factors in their daily life that may prevent or facilitate the desired change. This will also have the effect of addressing any contextual factors which impact upon a patient's progress or willingness to change.

Section 5

Psychosocial and ethical care

5.1 Professional and practice issues

Philosophy

Nursing philosophies are in a constant state of development, debate and reformation. Nursing philosophy, therefore, is not prescriptive and does not seek to provide steadfast rules to be adhered to; rather, it serves as a platform for professional development and reflection, and as a method of finding meaning in the nursing profession (Sellman 2010). Good patient care is:

- A central feature of nursing philosophies across all disciplines and areas of practice (Haggerty and Grace 2008).
- Achieved by meeting patients' needs on an individualized basis, which becomes easier with experience and the building of clinical wisdom.
- One's personal nursing philosophy, which includes good patient care, will therefore grow stronger as practical experience and 'clinical wisdom' is gained.

'Clinical wisdom' can be applied to everyday nursing practice by drawing from past experiences to make sound judgements and decisions on current situations. It further implies a moral commitment to one's actions; that one has a personal conviction to the ideals and philosophies that shape one's nursing practice. Past experiences and compounded practical knowledge that constitute clinical wisdom also support nurses' abilities to determine which courses of action are advantageous to individual patients (Haggerty and Grace 2008).

When caring for patients, it is important to balance the use of procedural guidelines and standards of care with the provision of individualized care and a reliance on personal moral values (Haggerty and Grace 2008). Key points about philosophy and nursing are:

- It is important to always uphold professional guidelines and codes of conduct, especially when they regard patient safety and care (McCurry et al 2009).
- Nursing is a highly 'doing-based' profession, requiring strong interpersonal and communicative skills as well as an ability to make decisions and adapt to changing situations (Lykkeslet and Gjengedal 2006).
- Nurses' knowledge can be described as flexible, adaptive and action-based.
- The integrative nature of nursing knowledge demands that applied skills be blended with experiential learning in order to respond to unique or unusual patient cases.
- With regard to patient care, nurses should remember the importance of treating patients as people and of showing a personal commitment to supporting patient health, wellbeing and safety.
- Nurses can improve upon their practice by reflecting on past experiences
- Barriers to good care include: staff shortages, time restrictions, opposing personal values and limited autonomy in the workplace.
- Experienced nurses have noted that these barriers can be overcome

through task prioritization, team work, reflective thinking, value cohesion and motivation to inspire positive change (Miller 2006).

Ensure a high standard of professional care by:

- Caring for others and supporting their health and wellbeing.
- Maintaining and preserving human dignity.
- Treating patients with compassion and showing a positive regard for the needs and wellbeing of others.
- Applying skills and knowledge in a manner that prioritizes patient health and wellness.
- Empathetic approach to understanding patients' needs and experiences.
- Demonstrating a commitment to care through integrity in one's behaviours and words (Miller 2006).
- Facilitating 'humanization, meaning, choice, quality of life, and healing in living and dying' for all individuals receiving care (Willis et al 2008).
- Advancing nursing practice by drawing from, and identifying linkages between lines of theory, inquiry and evidence across the discipline (Willis et al 2008).

Professional code of ethics

The International Council of Nurses' (ICN) *Code of Ethics for Nurses* (International Council of Nurses 2005) framework states that nurses have an ethical obligation 'to promote health, to prevent illness, to restore health and to alleviate suffering' (p. 1). This obligation must be carried out with due regard for human rights and personal dignity, regardless of creed, colour, gender or any other defining personal or social characteristic. These same ethical principles are outlined for nurses and midwives in *The Code: Standards of conduct, performance and ethics for nurses and midwives* (Nursing and Midwifery Council 2008).

Nurses' relationships with their colleagues, patients and patients' families should be guided by the following four principles of ethical conduct:

1. Nurses and people:
   - Respect the values, beliefs and human rights of all individuals.
   - Uphold the principle of informed consent by explaining procedures in full detail in developmentally appropriate language.
   - Always protect patients' and families' confidentiality insofar as doing so is within legal bounds.
   - Confidential information may only be shared with others in special legal circumstances.
   - Patients must be treated as unique individuals.
   - Patient–practitioner boundaries must be maintained at all times.
2. Nurses and practice:
   - Ongoing professional skills development should be undertaken throughout the course of one's career.
   - Looking after one's personal health is a prerequisite to caring for others.
   - Tasks requiring a high level of clinical skill should only be undertaken when one has the necessary professional competence to do so.

- Deliver care at its highest possible standard.
- Practise thorough record keeping, provide evidence-based care and maintain an up-to-date skill set.

> **Nurses' competencies** are outlined by the Nursing and Midwifery Council UK in the regulatory guidelines *Essential skills clusters* (Nursing and Midwifery Council 2007) and An Bord Altranais (Republic of Ireland). All nursing procedures should adhere to the outcomes and proficiencies contained within the *Standards of proficiency for pre-registration nursing education* (Nursing and Midwifery Council 2004).

3. Nurses and the profession:
   - A safe and equitable work environment is both the prerogative and responsibility of nurses.
   - Nurses have an obligation to participate in professional development activities, such as research, management, education and the development of clinical standards.
   - Practise honest communication and behave with integrity.
   - Respect your professional position, your colleagues and those under your care by providing unprejudiced, unbiased care.

Principles/processes

The provision of medical treatment to children should follow the four principles approach to care – respect for autonomy, beneficence, non-maleficence and justice (Baines 2008). The principles are closely linked to key concepts such as accountability, advocacy, consent and safeguarding children.

Respect for autonomy

Nurses caring for very young children should act in ways that respect their *developing autonomy*; this can be accomplished by encouraging young children's participation in decision-making activities, and is supported by parents who encourage their child to participate in discussion about their care. Please be aware that some children are not autonomous because they are wholly dependent on their parents to care for them and make decisions on their behalf. This is especially true for infants and children with severe developmental delay.

Beneficence – best interest of the child

In a healthcare setting, beneficence is achieved by providing care that has been designed with the child's best interests in mind. The principle relies on an assessment of the child that identifies treatments which are believed to benefit the child's health and wellbeing.

- In cases where children cannot advocate for what they feel is in their own best interest, a holistic assessment of how best to go about supporting the child's mental, physical and emotional wellbeing should be carried out with all stakeholders.
- Parents of severely developmentally delayed or disabled children should feature prominently in assessments to

determine what is in these children's best interests (Birchley 2010).

- At the same time, children irrespective of their age or developmental abilities, may still be able to express their opinions toward medical treatment and therefore their views must always be sought and heard.

- While treatments are only carried out with the child's best interests in mind, it is very important to acknowledge the child's feelings and explain to the child in developmentally appropriate terms why the treatment and actions are needed.

- Determining what is in the best interests of a child should not be based on clinical outcome alone (Birchley 2010). While some treatment options will have clinically superior outcomes, their social or emotional consequences may not be worth their clinical advantages.

Respecting the child's dignity

Dignity is emerging as a central aspect of biomedical ethics and the philosophy of medicine (Lundqvist and Nilstun 2007). Valuing our own and others' dignity demands recognition of unconditional human worth that is intrinsic to an individual's unique identity, experiences, preferences and needs. External factors, such as injury, loss or negative opinions of others, can cause emotional changes in an individual which result in a weakened self-image and diminished level of self-respect. Children and young people who are seriously ill or injured and who have to rely on others for their care are more vulnerable to devaluing their worth as individuals.

- Children's dignity can be promoted by ensuring privacy.

- Ensuring child's body is not exposed beyond what is necessary.

- Ensuring that a child's assent to procedures is always obtained.

- You can respect and support children's sense of dignity and self-worth by encouraging participation and informed consent.

- Involve children in discussions about their care.

- Communicate information in an interactive and developmentally appropriate way.

- Encourage children to share their questions, concerns and opinions during discussions about possible treatment pathways.

- Sometimes patients in long-term care fear being perceived as a nuisance to their caretakers, this may repress the desire to express their feelings and needs (Lundqvist and Nilstun 2007). Therefore special care must be directed toward eliciting the input and feedback of children in long-term or highly dependent care.

Ethical and legal issues

A child's ability to consent to medical treatment depends on the child's understanding and developmental stage:

- Very young children who lack the intellectual capacity to comprehend treatment options and their consequences are deemed incompetent and are thus unable to give consent for their own treatment (Parekh 2006).

- In the UK, there is no definitive legal age at which incompetent children at once become competent. For children approaching middle childhood, competence to consent is usually determined by the child's doctor, who also considers contextual factors, such as the severity and nature of the treatment options (Parekh 2006).

- In the UK, children under 16 years of age cannot give consent to their own medical treatment unless they have been deemed Gillick competent. Children in middle/late childhood and early adolescence are ordinarily considered Gillick competent, otherwise known as Fraser competent.

- In the Gillick case, the judges held that 'parental rights were recognised by the law only as long as they were needed for the protection of the child and such rights yielded to the child's right to make his own decisions when he reached a sufficient understanding and intelligence to be capable of making up his own mind', (Gillick v West Norfolk and Wisbech Area Health Authority (1985) 3 All ER 402 1985).

- Gillick-competent children can comprehend information about medical treatments, weigh the advantages and disadvantages of each, and arrive at an informed decision about their care.

- For treatment decisions that are unlikely to have such grave consequences, therefore, a young person under 16 can consent to treatment provided he or she is

competent to understand the nature, purpose and possible consequences of the treatment proposed.

Refusal of treatment

Ethical dilemmas arise when children do not consent to medical treatment which, if not delivered, would prevent the best interests of the child from being achieved. There are various reasons why a child may refuse consent to medical treatment. Fear of unknown or unwanted outcomes, moral or cultural conflicts, relationships with medical staff, previous negative experiences, unsatisfactory and lack of information may contribute to a child's refusal (Vasey 2009).

- Children must be given adequate opportunity to deliberate on proposed treatment before further action.

- All attempts should be made to outline the social, ethical and medical consequences of treatment and its refusal.

- Children must receive full information about a treatment or procedure in developmentally appropriate terms before nurses can reasonably seek to advocate (Parekh 2006)

Legal position

Although 16–18-year-olds have the right to consent to medical treatment in the absence of parental consent, subsequent cases have retreated from this position, particularly where they have involved treatment refusal by the young person. Gillick competence is contextually dependent; for example, a child's ability to give informed consent to a major surgical procedure may be unreliable even at the Gillick-competent stage if their decision-making process appears to be largely motivated by an emotional response (Parekh 2006). Regardless of a child's developmental stage, a court maintains the right to give consent to a child's medical treatment in cases where the following two conditions are present:

- Both the parents and child refuse treatment
- The treatment in question is very strongly in the child's best interests, as determined by the child's doctor and ruled by the courts.

Gillick-competent adolescents can consent to their own medical treatment in the absence of parental consent; however, in cases where Gillick-competent minors *refuse* consent, their refusal can be overridden by parental consent until the child reaches 18 years of age (Vasey 2009).

Thus if a child *refuses* consent to their own medical treatment and it is in their best interest, parental consent in favour of the treatment overrides the child's refusal (Parekh 2006).

The ethical justification for allowing courts and/or parents to commit a child to medical treatment despite his or her refusal to give consent stems from the belief that in many cases, a child's refusal is a consequence of their developmental immaturity, especially in cases where lifesaving treatment is refused.

Similarly when parents may be asked to make decisions on behalf of a very young or severely developmentally disabled child, parental authority is never justified when parents make decisions that are clearly in conflict with the best interests of the child. In these instances, the treatment outcome will be decided by the courts under the advice of the physician (Baines 2008).

Advocacy

Advocacy is an integral part of a nurse's role. In children's nursing it is essential as children are vulnerable and unwell. Children are vulnerable to having their rights infringed, as the environment is adult controlled. Nurses have a professional responsibility to act as the child's advocate in conjunction with the parents. Advocacy can be demonstrated in different ways:

- Enabling the child to express their wishes
- Promoting child's right to self-determination
- Protecting the child's safety and wellbeing
- Representing child's wishes to other adults
- Speaking on behalf of infant/child
- Supporting child's needs and wishes
- Acting as a mediator.

Parents may also need nurses to act as their advocates. Some parents may find it difficult to speak on behalf of their child due to: shy personality; respect for professionals; lack of knowledge; feeling intimidated; uncertainty about rights; and lack of familiarity with hospital regulations. Nurses tend to build good relationships with parents because they provide continuous care. So nurses' presence and familiarity with the family can help them feel more inclined to voice their concerns. Nurses can play a valuable role by:

- Representing the expressed wishes of the parent
- Speaking on behalf of the parent
- Providing parents with opportunities to express their concerns
- Helping parent to present their concerns to the doctor.

Confidentiality

Children are entitled to the same level of confidentiality as adults. Therefore if a child tells you something in confidence, then you must not share this information with others. The only exception is in the case of child protection issues. The decision to breach confidentiality should never be taken lightly. The child who has expressed the desire to keep information confidential should be informed of your decision to inform parents and the reason for doing so.

Strategies of care

Partnership model

The partnership model developed by Anne Casey in 1988 was fundamental to the introduction of the concepts of parent participation and partnership nursing as core principles for nursing children in hospital or the community. Parent participation may be seen as the care-giving activities performed by a parent/guardian for a child in the hospital setting. These concepts have evolved to a more inclusive term of family-centred care (FCC), which recognizes the importance of including both the child and families' needs in planning and delivering high quality care. This should be underpinned by communication and negotiation of roles.

Key characteristics of FCC

- The family must be viewed as the constant in the child's life:
  - Admission to hospital disrupts family life and routines

  - Parents / primary carer want to provide emotional support
  - Children of all ages desire their parents' emotional support
  - Parents know their child best, know their child's preferences and can provide assistance in communicating with their child
  - Children from 3 upwards are usually capable of expressing their preferences and their views should be sought on all matters that affect them
  - Assessment process should include both child's and family's needs.

- Parents'/primary carer's preferences for participation may vary considerably so daily negotiation is essential:
  - Planning of care should include both child's and family's preferences on how they would like to be involved in care delivery
  - Care plans should document families' role and preferences
  - Listening and sharing information is essential for building collaboration and good relationships
  - Families' situation may alter daily therefore assessment and negotiation should be on-going
  - Some families may be reluctant to perform technical nursing care and their preferences should be accommodated
  - Families need assurances that nurses will provide the care for their child when they are unable to be there
  - Nurses need to be aware of the importance of being there alongside families as a caring human presence
  - Discharge planning should begin early so as to ensure that

community support services are tailored to meet family's and child's needs

- Ensure parents and/or child are instructed in the management of care required for discharge so discharge is not delayed unnecessarily
- Ensure that parents and/or child are capable of performing the procedure safely, and know what to do in case of an adverse event occurring.

■ Families from different cultures have unique social, cultural and linguistic needs and different understandings of FCC:
  - Families have diverse needs and different forms of coping
  - Some families especially dual earners may find it difficult to be present with their child at all times
  - Hospital stays can be very expensive, e.g. car parking, food, and travel
  - Families will require emotional, physical and some financial support
  - There needs to be space for siblings on the ward so that they can visit or accompany a parent if desired.

■ Hospital system and policies need to be flexible and responsive to families needs:
  - Services and resources should be designed and delivered around the child and family
  - Families need resources and facilities for washing, eating, sleeping and relaxing
  - The impact of resident parents on nurses' workload needs to be acknowledged by hospital management

- Staffing levels need to be optimum so that nurses have time to meet families' needs
- Care should be evaluated frequently so that care plans are kept up-to-date and relevant to child and families' needs.

Caring for siblings' needs

During the child's illness the siblings can feel neglected or abandoned. They can also feel guilty because they are well and not ill in hospital. Parents may experience difficulty meeting siblings' needs. There are general principles for helping take care of siblings that apply:

■ Speak to the parents and encourage them to involve the siblings.

■ Elicit siblings concerns and provide explanations to dispel any myths or misconceptions (e.g. that they caused the illness).

■ Include siblings in discussions early on and keep them informed using simple explanations.

■ Whenever possible emphasize the positive side of treatments.

■ Allow siblings into hospital to share experiences.

■ Encourage parents to take turns staying at home or in hospital.

Education/school activities

Most hospital or wards that care for children have the service of a school within the hospital staffed by school teachers. For children who are bed bound, the teacher will visit each child and ensure that homework is provided.

- Ensure that schooling continues is beneficial for children as it promotes normality and daily routine.
- Chronic illness can cause serious disruption to schooling so maintaining progress in school work is essential.
- Children education should not be disadvantaged by hospitalization.
- Hospital teachers can liaise with school teachers to plan that education will continue and the child is provided with appropriate schoolwork.

Play in hospital

Play is an integral aspect of childhood, child development and a basic need of all children. The first 5 years of a child's life is a period of rapid development in physical, mental and social skills such as walking, talking, understanding and imitating. One of the most important ways in which a child learns to develop these skills is through play. It is an activity that assists in the normal development, as children learn physical, mental and social skills through play. It is a universal activity in all cultures so child's freedom to play must be preserved in hospital.

- All children irrespective of gender, culture or racial origin, background or individual ability, should have equal access to play experiences while in hospital (Department of Health and Children 2004, Department of Health 2004).
- Hospitals are alien environments for many children because they encounter unfamiliar people, treatments, medical equipment and language. Play helps reduce the adverse effects of hospitalization by acting as a diversion and refocusing

attention away from stressors and unfamiliar environment.
- Play specialists play a key role in facilitating children's opportunities for play and preparing children for procedures through therapeutic play.

Means of play

- Toys, e.g. games, soft toys, jigsaws, computer games, mp3 players, games consoles
- Creative materials
- Music and dance
- Dressing-up clothes
- Puppets
- Clown therapy
- Pet therapy.

Functions of play

- Fun activity for children
- Mental, physical and social stimulation
- Integral to child development and acquisition of skills
- Provides opportunity for self-expression (Wikstrom 2005)
- Encourages creativity and imagination
- Provides outlet for emotion
- Allows children to practise roles and situations
- Helps provide or restore normality
- Helps nurses to build a relationship with the child
- Helps the child to assimilate new information
- Helps the child to adjust to and gain control over a potentially frightening environment

- Play material such as dolls and props useful for explaining procedures
- Using play to explain procedures, lessens the stress caused by fear of the unknown, enhances child's coping abilities and promotes cooperation (Brewer et al 2006)
- Assists coping with painful procedures
- Helps provide distraction
- Pet therapy programmes are useful aids for enhancing well-being and in promoting normalcy (Kaminski et al 2002).

Integrated care pathways (ICPs)

Over the last two decades, ICPs have become increasing popular for healthcare systems in Europe and worldwide. Integrated care pathways are documented policies and guidelines for *delivering* integrated care. ICPs have been adopted for variety of health conditions and patient populations. Although integrated care contributes to improved clinical outcomes and patient satisfaction, more empirical evidence is needed to demonstrate clinical efficacy (Allen et al 2009, Doocey and Reddy 2010).

Functions of ICPs

- Organizational tools that direct the flow of care in cases where patients require multidisciplinary intervention.
- Often consist of care matrices and protocol documents.
- Are process-based and temporal, often taking the form of a set of clinical benchmarks charted on a timescale.
- Define possible treatment pathways for patients with conditions requiring multiple clinicians' expertise.

- Promote adherence to clinical guidelines (Middleton et al 2001).
- Documentation reduces variation in care by defining the roles and responsibilities to be assumed by each member of the care team.
- Clinicians working with ICP models can expect a high degree of protocol-driven guidance (Allen et al 2009).

Advantages to ICPs

- Models of care that support multidisciplinary teamwork and collaboration.
- Most valuable when applied to conditions and patient populations which follow predictable trajectories of care.
- Offer valuable guidelines for clinicians whose mixed disciplinary backgrounds present challenges to caring for patients with multiple healthcare needs.
- Practitioners can more freely share patient information in an atmosphere of collaborative work care plans and benefit patients as they consider needs from a holistic perspective.
- Beneficial for guiding complex, multidisciplinary decision-making processes, and for improving communication between patients and clinicians (Allen et al 2009).
- Most appropriate for: high-risk conditions and areas of care which are poorly implemented or in need of reform (Middleton et al 2001).
- Because they require systemic change and policy development, ICPs are most effective when implemented on an organizational level (e.g. within specific wards or integrated into hospital-wide policies).

- Successful ICPs have a strong medical focus and are managed by elected facilitators who liaise with clinicians in the care team (Middleton et al. 2001).

Challenges to using ICPs

- Paucity of research is thought to contribute to the slow rate at which ICPs have been made available for implementation. For healthcare practitioners, this creates a situation whereby the implementation of integrated care is encouraged, but a framework for doing so is immaturely developed or unavailable (Doocey and Reddy 2010).

- Major goal of integrated care is to bridge the gap between primary and secondary care, yet this has taken a minor role in what is currently observed in practice (Panella et al 2009).

- ICPs are not useful to *all* cases requiring multidisciplinary care; complex or infrequently occurring conditions, for example, can actually be impeded by prescribing to the protocol-driven guidelines of ICPs (Allen et al 2009).

- If participating agencies and institutions are new to integrative care, they may lack the policies and guidelines required for many of the activities that integrated care inspires (Doocey and Reddy 2010).

- Children's nurses working in multidisciplinary, integrated care teams may encounter ethical and organizational dilemmas involving (Doocey and Reddy 2010):
  - Competing philosophies/ approaches to care
  - Emphasis on integrated primary and secondary care collaboration

  which blurs previously established roles and decision-making pathways
  - Poorly developed transitional pathways for children progressing to adult services and for hospital patients migrating to home- or community-based care.

Widening the focus of ICPs

- Practitioners and researchers want to widen the focus of integrative care so that it includes a stronger emphasis on the use of evidence-based, multidisciplinary treatment guidelines (Panella et al 2009).

- Aim of the integrative approach is to respond to developed countries ageing demographics by developing stronger transitional links between acute and chronic care.

- Integrative care is therefore in the process of expanding beyond its original goals of cost-containment and collaboration to include provisions for organizational reform (Panella et al 2009).

5.2 Psychosocial Issues

Attachment and loss

The concept of attachment is one way of describing the closeness-seeking and care-eliciting behaviours of children to their main carer. John Bowlby (Bowlby et al 1956, Bowlby 1952, 1980) was an eminent psychiatrist who developed a theory to explain the process of attachment and separation.

Bowlby defined attachment as need for the infant/child to stay in close proximity to the primary care-giver usually the mother and to be comforted by her presence, sound and touch. Attachment theory is based on the following, that:

1. Attachment behaviour and the internalization of how the care-giver will respond is most acutely developed between 6 months and 5 years of age
2. Children who are able to predict the availability of their care-giver will suffer less fear and alarm in frightening situations than children who cannot predict the behaviour of their care-giver
3. The child's experience of seeking care and receiving protection is pivotal to continued healthy development.
4. Linked to attachment is the development of basic trust – the child experiences the world as nurturing, reliable and trustworthy.
5. Another term used to denote attachment is bonding. The bond between a child and parent is usually established within the first year of life.

Attachment figure

Defined as any person with whom the child has an emotional bond and these are most often the child's parents or main caregivers.

- The child will seek out or search for their attachment figures when they are feeling fearful, frightened or anxious (Cassidy and Shaver 2008).

- The child will seek out physical and emotional closeness to their attachment figures when strangers, strange places or strange situations face them.

- Being admitted to hospital means the child is confronted by all three so it is important that you identify those adults to whom the child is psychologically attached in order to provide emotional security during their illness.

Features of attachment behaviour

- Crying
- Calling
- Stranger anxiety
- Separation anxiety.

Secure attachment

If the child experiences their carer as responsive, nurturing, supportive and available, they are cooperative, easily comforted and eager to explore new situations. Most children are securely attached to their primary carer usually the mother, and if left alone may become clingy when mother returns.

Insecure attachment

If the child experiences their carer as unresponsive, detached, distant, and unavailable they become insecure and display behaviours that are termed as:

- Avoidant – show little distress when the parent is absent. When the parent returns they tend to avoid interacting. The mother/parents are often insensitive to their child's signals – they avoid close contact, and are often angry and irritable.

- Ambivalent – show frequent distress whether the mother is present or absent. When the parent returns, they show ambivalence by intermittently seeking closeness and then angrily rejecting the parent. The mother/parents are often insensitive to their child's signals, but are not as rejecting as avoidant mothers.

- Disorganized – child demonstrates a mixture of avoidance, anger and behavioural issues. The mother/parents are often insensitive to their child's signals, avoid contact, do not display affection and alternate between being present or rejecting.

Consequences of insecure attachment

- Harmful consequences for a child's emotional welfare and development
- Can develop delay in thinking, talking and social development
- Have difficulty interacting with their peers
- Have behavioural and social difficulties.

Promoting the process of attachment

The strength and quality of the emotional bond affects the emotional behaviour of the child and is fundamental to the child's psychological wellbeing.

- Parents need time to develop an attachment to their baby so nurses can help facilitate and support this relationship.
- Nurses can help mothers become more aware of their babies behaviour and learn how to respond.
- New mothers are usually anxious and the provision of advice and

guidance to their babies' responses will reduce anxiety.

- Parents who show mutual reciprocal interaction and affection with their babies are showing attachment.

Reducing separation anxiety

- Children under the age of 5 years are particularly vulnerable.
- Children begin to show separation anxiety from 8 months.
- The impact of separation is increased if there has been a poor quality relationship with the parent.
- Parents of young children should be able to sleep alongside their child.
- Parents of older children should be provided with accommodation so that they can stay with their child in hospital.
- Babies and young children who experience long stays in hospital will form attachments so they need to be provided with a primary nurse carer.
- Unaccompanied children need particular care to ensure that they are not left alone for long periods.

Effects on a child admitted to hospital

Most children experience hospitalization as a stressful event. Numerous studies have reported that children have concerns about experiencing pain, mutilation, immobility, separation from significant others, loss of control, and disruption to normal activities. The experience of illness itself causes disruption to children's sense of well-being and consequently hospitalization may represent a threat to children's independence, usual self-caring abilities and self-control (Coyne 2006).

Reaction to hospitalization

Children can have many fears about hospital and procedures. However this does not mean that all children will appraise the same events as stressful. Hospitalization affects children differently depending on age. For example children under 7 years may experience behavioural manifestations such as separation anxiety, sleep disturbances, changes in eating and feeling apathetic, withdrawn or aggressive. Preschool-aged children may experience difficulty understanding information about hospitalization and separating imaginary events from reality. Strategies to reduce the adverse effects of hospitalization are:

- Children need to be prepared for procedures and preadmission programmes should be offered to all.
- Children seek order and security in an environment that is alien to them. Therefore promote a safe environment in the hospital by encouraging children to bring in familiar items from home.
- Family-centred care should be encouraged, supported and facilitated.
- Minimize the disruption to children's normal routines, and separation from family and friends, by maximizing the children's contact with outside friends, family and school and minimizing the adverse aspects of the hospital environment.

- Children view intrusive procedures, blood tests, and pain as particularly threatening and very stressful. This indicates the importance of sufficient preparation, age-appropriate explanations and use of relaxation techniques prior to invasive procedures.
- Involve children in discussions around the delivery of their care.
- Encourage involvement in daily care decisions as this will help foster good self-esteem in children.
- Support children's play activities and attendance in school and homework.

Ensure ward environment is child-friendly by:

- Have signage at appropriate level and in simple terms.
- Ensure décor is child-friendly by using murals on walls, patterned curtains, and bright colours.
- Keep ward temperature at optimum level and ensure adequate ventilation.
- Ensure child has a consistent primary nurse if possible as care from multiple healthcare professionals is anxiety provoking.
- Document children's food preferences and ensure choice in food provided.
- Ensure that children have free time in the day for relaxation and quiet time.
- Ensure that play facilities and resources are freely available and suitable for all age groups.
- Only have the minimum number of lights on at night-time to encourage restful sleep.
- Turn down the ring tone on ward phones at night-time to reduce noise levels.

- Keep noise to a minimum at night by reducing talk and whispering.
- Perform as many nursing observations as possible together to minimize disturbing the child unnecessarily.

Children's right to be heard

The past decade has seen a growing recognition of the importance of children's rights and the need to listen to and consult with children both at a national (Department of Health and Children 2000a,b,) and international level (United Nations 1989, Department of Health 2003, Royal College of Paediatrics and Child Health 2000). The United Nation Convention on the Rights of the Child (1989), which was ratified by the UK in 1991, and Ireland in 1992, clearly stated the right of every child to self-determination, dignity, respect, non-interference, and the right to make informed decisions. Both the National Service Framework (NSF) for England (Department of Health 2004) and National Children's Strategy (2000) for Ireland directs healthcare services to give children greater choice and participation in decisions about their health and care.

The Children's National Service Framework states that:

Children and young people should receive care that is integrated and co-ordinated around their particular needs, and the needs of their family. They, and their parents, should be treated with respect, and should be given support and information to enable them to understand and cope with illness or injury, and the treatment needed. They should be encouraged to be active partners in decisions about their health and care, and, where possible, be able to exercise choice (Department of Health 2003, p 9).

- This policy emphasizes that all children, regardless of ability, race, or ethnic background, have the right to express their views on what happens to them and to have those views taken seriously by the adults delivering services.
- Therefore health professionals have a responsibility to listen to children's views and involve them in discussions that directly affect them.

Communicating with children

Cognitive developmental level rather than age or health condition, is most strongly linked to the way in which children conceptualize health and illness. Good communication with children and their families can have a number of positive effects.

- Children's need for information has been confirmed in many studies.
- Information prepares them for what to expect and helps with their participation in decision making.
- Information helps parents to understand and cope with their child's illness.
- Parents appreciate health professionals who allow them to express their concerns and expectations about their child's hospitalization and treatment.
- Health professionals who take time and explain information clearly demonstrate respect for the family.

- Children generally prefer to be included in information sharing, but there may be times when they do not want to participate particularly when they are feeling unwell.

- Young children aged about 6 years and younger often prefer to be present but for the discussion to be held between their parent and health professionals. This is because they have difficulty understanding some words or because they are afraid of hearing bad news. They prefer their parents to be present so they can:
  - explain the information in simpler terms
  - help child understand what is planned for them
  - help allay the child fears and concerns
  - be an advocate for the child by asking questions on his/her behalf
  - act as a mediator in situations where the child is afraid to question care.

Making healthcare consultations 'child friendly'

Many consultations are held with the child and family beside the bedside which can be very frightening and intimidating for many children. Try to imagine what it is like for a child and take measures to make the situation easier.

- Ask the consultant to reduce the number of staff that accompany him/her into the child's room.

- Ask the leading doctor to sit on a chair beside the bed so he/she are on same level as the child.

- Use child's first name and include him/her in the discussion (according to child's preference at that time).

- Children aged 4 years and older will usually like to participate in the consultation.

- Sometimes a child may remain quiet and say very little, so allow the child time to speak and be patient and use gentle coaxing to help child participate.

- Remind health professionals to be careful with their comments as a child is listening and not to use potentially alarming statements.

Using non-verbal signals to communicate

Children are acute observers of adults and easily notice when an adult is impatient or not being genuinely friendly. Therefore it is important to be aware of your non-verbal and verbal skills when communicating with a child. There are specific skills which can help:

- Ensure you are on the same level as the child.

- Adopt an open posture by leaning towards the child and arms unfolded.

- Make eye contact.

- Use child's name.

- Ask parents for help with communicating as they will know what special words child uses, and they will be able to help with explaining the information.

- Find out what the child knows and understands and use this as a base for your explanations. It will help you identify misconceptions, which you can rectify.

- Try to use simple words and short sentences.
- Use visual aids and toys to help explain procedures/care.
- Use open ended questions such as 'can you tell me more about. . .' 'is there anything you are worried about?
- Wait for a reply while maintaining open posture and calm gaze.
- Use nonverbal behaviour such as nodding to show that you are listening.
- Use facilitative responses (such as mm, uh-huh) to encourage child to continue speaking.
- Repeat what the child has said to show that you are listening and to ensure that you have heard the child correctly.
- Observe the child for signs of anxiety, e.g. fidgeting, loss of gaze, worried look, sighing. If evident try to find out what is worrying him/her. You could use phrases such as: 'you look a bit worried. . .have you any questions which I could help answer' or 'Some children worry about the operation, are you feeling like that?'

Building rapport with the child

It is important to build a trusting relationship with children and their families. Children who are included feel happier and better informed patients tend to have less anxieties and fears. You can build rapport by chatting informally and being friendly with a child. Prior to a procedure, you can:

- Allow child time to adjust to the need for the procedure and do not proceed unless you have the child's agreement.
- Ask the child who he/she would like to accompany them if the procedure is held in another room.
- Ensure child privacy is protected by preventing exposure of body parts and by having the curtains drawn and a sign on the door.
- Provide explanations beforehand and throughout the procedure so that the child is aware of what is happening to them.
- Use distraction to help child cope with the procedure.
- Praise the child's efforts so that they feel valued and important.
- Provide reassurance and allay any fears the child expresses.

Children's participation in decision making

Children have a right to voice their opinions and to have those opinions taken into consideration in the delivery of their care. Children who are involved feel valued, comfortable and less anxious. Children are often seen as lacking the competence to take part in decisions, but there are many levels a child can be involved. Some decisions may require reasoning beyond the capabilities of some young children, but the same could be said for adults.

- Children want to participate in decisions about their care such as: medications, treatments, timing of procedures.
- Children have identified an age range from 9–18 years as to when they should be actively involved in decision making.

- When decisions are major such as a surgical decision, children want to be included but to share the decision-making with parents and health professional.

- Most young children prefer to be included but not necessarily to have responsibility for the decision.

- It is generally accepted now that children from as young as 2 years old can be involved in some form of decision making.

- Children's participation will vary according to type of decision and capability and preferences.

- Children want to be treated with respect and to be given opportunities to have a say without necessarily having full control over decision-making.

- Children of all ages can express their views given the right environment and support from adults.

Involving a child in decision making, ensure that:

- Treatment options are understood by everyone.

- Child encouraged to voice preferences.

- Parents' opinion elicited and heard.

- Everyone's preferred options are heard and acknowledged and discussed.

- Final decision made and agreed by all parties.

- Check later that all are happy with the decision made.

- If not happy with decision, reconvene the meeting and discuss options again.

- It is essential that all are happy with the decision, with the child being the most important person.

Types of decisions

Sometimes health professionals see decisions equating to treatments and operations, when there are many other daily care decisions which a child can be involved in. These include: time to get up, what activities they can play, what they would like to eat, what clothes they want to wear, etc. For many children the fact that they have to endure the treatments in order to get better can leave them feeling a significant loss of control and independence. Providing choices gives back some measure of control and indicates respect to the child.

Key points

- Allow child a choice wherever possible.

- Allow sufficient time for the child to decide on option.

- Child's preference should be sought and taken into account.

- Listen to child's concerns and respond appropriately.

- Never force care or procedures on an unwilling child.

Social services provision

Social care services operate in hospitals, community centres, residential care homes and other service or community-based settings. The services support people with financial difficulties, housing problems, disabilities, mental or emotional health problems, children or families under stress, foster families, homeless people and people who require assistance with daily activities in the home.

Most social services operate within local councils and in conjunction with NHS organizations or providers. Depending on the type of service required, services can be accessed directly or through a referral and assessment process which must be initiated by a GP or designated professional. An online search for social care services in the UK can be contacted at:

http://www.direct.gov.uk/en/Dl1/ Directories/Localcouncils/index.htm

Parents seeking advice and information on childcare, disability services, parenting, education, housing, financial support and early years services should be directed to their local authority. Parents, families and young people are also entitled to receive from their local authorities the following services:

■ Assistance with finding affordable childcare during a child's preschool years

■ Assistance with funding early years childcare for children with disabilities or special education needs

■ Specialist support to families from disadvantaged backgrounds that may require housing assistance, emergency employment schemes or emergency childcare provisions.

Child support services and charities

Voluntary organizations such as Action for Sick Children, UK (www.actionforsickchildren.org/) and Children in Hospital Ireland (www.

childreninhospital.ie) have made significant efforts to promote better standards of hospital care for children and their families and to safeguard children's rights. Visit these websites and you will notice how the key principles, although sometimes worded differently are recommending the same approach for children. There are many charities and organizations in the UK that provide a broad range of supports for children and families such as:

■ information and advice

■ training

■ counselling and bereavement support

■ assistance with accommodation

■ assistance with securing resources in the community

■ provision of home care services

■ emotional support and support groups

■ workshops and educational resources

■ financial assistance

■ online resources

■ rehabilitative services

■ parenting programmes.

Child protection

The UK's Department of Health defines child maltreatment as the infliction of harm on a child and/or a failure to prevent such harm from occurring (Asmussen 2010). From 2008 to 2010, child abuse in all four regions of the UK (England, Scotland, Wales and Northern Ireland) rose steadily in terms of the total numbers of new registrations

(Vincent 2008). Neglect was the most common registration category (of physical abuse, emotional abuse, sexual abuse or neglect) in all four UK areas during this time period (Vincent 2008). Abuse (physical, emotional and sexual) and neglect constitute child maltreatment and should be taken very seriously when suspected or substantiated in the clinical setting (Tingberg et al 2008).

Classification of child maltreatment

- Physical abuse: Inflicting physical force on a child through violent behaviours. Inducing illness or fabricating physical symptoms. May involve shaking, hitting, burning, throwing or other violent acts.

- Emotional abuse: An outcome of all other types of abuse, yet can also occur in isolation. Defined as ongoing treatment aimed at controlling, devaluing, isolating, shaming, intimidating or bullying the child in a way that causes psychological harm.

- Sexual abuse: Coercing, inviting or forcing sexual behaviours and activities with a child, including indecent exposure, forced intimate contact, sexually inappropriate acts, sexual grooming or viewing pornography, prostitution, and rape.

- Neglect: Failing to care for a child in a way that supports their physical, emotional, social and psychological needs. Inadequate or inappropriate food, shelter, supervision, medical attention and emotional support all constitute neglect.

Characteristics of those who abuse children

Child abuse has no single cause and it is likely that numerous personal, social and cultural factors play a role in its manifestation in adults' relationships with children (Asmussen 2010). Research consistently shows that psychological and socioeconomic characteristics influence the likelihood of certain individuals committing abusive acts toward children.

- Majority of child abuse is committed by family members or other individuals who are known to the child.

- Certain types of sexual abuse such as indecent exposure and attempted abduction are primarily committed by strangers.

- Mental health problems, learning difficulties, prior experience of abuse during childhood, substance abuse, poverty, cultural attitudes to punishment, and inadequate social support services have all been shown to play a role in the lives of adults who abuse children (Asmussen 2010).

- Parents who harm their children may suffer from mental health or substance abuse problems, be highly critical of their child, avoid routine health checks or treatments for their child, provide inappropriate or inadequate supervision, suffer from or contribute to domestic violence, or fail to ensure that their child regularly attends school (London Safeguarding Children Board 2010).

- Children suffering from abusive relationships may behave in developmentally inappropriate ways and/or regard their parents with fear and intimidation.

- Because children have difficulty comprehending inappropriate behaviour and often rely on an abusive adult for guidance and care, many children do not regard their abuser's behaviour as harmful, inappropriate or abusive (Asmussen 2010). This makes it difficult to determining whether a child is being abused and underscores the importance of regular child protection training for health and social services professionals.

'Hard to engage' children are defined as children who are highly vulnerable to continued harm, abuse or neglect because of any of the following conditions or circumstances: learning disabilities, cognitive difficulties, targeted rejection or abuse within sibling groups, previous time in social care, and risk-taking lifestyles adopted in adolescence (Thoburn 2009).

'Hard to change' parents are defined as parents of abused or neglected children who may have a role in their child's harm but who resist engaging with social services because of any of the following conditions or circumstances: mental health problems, prior abuse during childhood, being a lone parent of a child with behavioural or emotional difficulties, addiction, abusive romantic relationships, previous time in social care, and a mistrust of social services due to cultural reasons or previous negative experiences (Thoburn 2009).

Education and training for healthcare staff

Health and social service professionals providing care are well positioned to speak directly with abused or neglected children about their experiences and issue a child protection referral (Thoburn 2009).

- Nurses rely on their hospital's child protection protocol when seeking guidance on how to deal with a suspected case of maltreatment (Tingberg et al 2008).

- Health professionals should be kept up-to-date with their organization's child protection policy

- It is essential that practitioners who regularly work with children receive regular education and training in child protection such that its detection and referral are realistic possibilities.

- Knowledge of how to go about reporting suspected harm and knowing what to expect from the investigation process was beneficial to nurses who have dealt with child protection concerns in the workplace (Tingberg et al 2008).

Safeguarding procedure

Health practitioners working in England, Scotland or Wales should adhere to the child protection procedures and policies of the local authority presiding over their place of work (National Society for the Prevention of Cruelty to Children 2010).

- One of the most effective ways of supporting abused or neglected children during an initial disclosure is to ask child-focused, non-leading questions in a sensitive and developmentally appropriate manner (Thoburn 2009).

- Children's nurses, social workers and other practitioners who believe that a child in their care is suffering significant harm, should consult their agency's child protection protocol, discuss their concerns with their manager or agency's child protection advisor and make an immediate referral to their local authority's child protection services.

- The Local Safeguarding Children Board (LSCB) procedures (http://www.legislation.gov.uk/uksi/2006/90/contents/made) should also be consulted during this process.

- Children must not be discharged from hospital until a multi-agency plan to safeguard their wellbeing has been drawn up and the child's home has been found to be safe by child protection services.

Action following a referral

The child protection process is a formal procedure undertaken to evaluate suspected abuse and develop a set of actions for rehabilitation and prevention of future harm. A professional involved in the care of a child suspected of abuse or neglect should request that child protection services be initiated by social services.

- Following a child protection referral (National Society for the Prevention of Cruelty to Children 2010): the child protection team of the child's local authority will decide within one working day whether to:
  - Drop the referral altogether or refer the case to other services or conduct initial assessment within one week of the referral. Following initial assessment, a child may begin receiving social, medical or psychological services according to their needs.
  - Or apply for an emergency court order if the child is suspected of being in immediate danger.

- Police may also take immediate action at any stage and without a court order, remove the child from their home and place them in emergency care for no more than 72 hours.
- Child may also be placed on the child protection register as a precautionary measure while remaining in the family home.
- Following the core assessment, some children may be taken into care while their case undergoes legal care proceedings.

Case conference

Undertaken when there is known or suspected abuse in order to discuss any concerns about the child's welfare. Involves a confidential meeting between parents, child protection officers and all other social, educational, health and community-based professionals involved in the child's care.

Case management and review

A process of overseeing progress on a child's protection plan while tracking any legal proceedings which arise from the initial investigation. A social worker with a background in child protection ordinarily manages this process.

Interventions for stopping parents from abusing their children

- Home-based support, group-based parenting support and out of home care are currently used as interventions for stopping parents from abusing their children (Asmussen 2010).

- Specialist interventions may be required in cases where parents are suspected of harming their child but are resistant to engaging with the child protection process.

- Health professionals should be alert to signs of resistance, avoidance or disengagement, and should report these issues when making their referral to child protection services (Thoburn 2009).

- Home-based support can improve parent–child relationships and disciplinary patterns by offering individualized recommendations after a period of observation in the home.

- Group-based parenting support can produce similar outcomes, but it takes the form of parent education programmes whose efficacy is somewhat limited to parents who physically abuse their children.

- Out of home care, also known as foster-care placement, is ordinarily reserved for exceptional circumstances and in cases where all other viable options have been explored. Out of home care produces poor long-term outcomes for children yet remains a common intervention in the UK.

Health promotion in children and families

Health promotion is a method of enabling patients to achieve optimal health through patient autonomy, supported decision-making and education (Casey 2007). The integration of children's services in the areas of health, education, law, community services and social welfare is a strong priority of child welfare policies in the UK (Robinson and Cottrell 2005). Initiatives to bolster multidisciplinary children's work include the *NHS Plan* (2000), the Department of Health's *National Service Framework for Children* (2004) and legislation for multi-agency collaboration proposed by the Children Act (2004).

Health promotion

- Views health and illness as multidimensional constructs which both reflect and contribute to an individual's family life, community involvement and work/school environments.

- Health has broadened its original definition (the absence of illness) to include mental, physical, social and psychological wellbeing.

- Health of children is defined as the extent to which they can meet their full potential, satisfy their needs and develop into healthy young adults (Harris 2010).

- Children's social contexts – their homes, schools, families and communities – can be used in combination with clinical information to form a holistic indicator of their health and wellbeing.

- Focus should be on strategies that will promote the health of all children within the context of the family, school and community.

- Children's nurses should expect to be involved in collaborative work that encourages multidisciplinary care and problem-solving.

- All professionals working in the community need to work

collaboratively to promote the child's health and welfare.

■ Reduction in hospital admissions and hospital stays means that families may require more support from community services such as: general practitioner, community paediatrician, health visitor, public health nurse, and social worker.

Principles of health promotion

The theory behind an integrative approach to understanding human health states that the social, psychological, behavioural and biological domains of human life influence disease pathways; therefore, the promotion of health is a multidisciplinary endeavour (Harris 2010).

Each of the four domains are:

■ *Biological*: Human growth and development; clinical indicators; the role of biological processes in the development of illness and disease; the role of genetics in health and illness.

■ *Psychological*: Emotional and intellectual aspects of human experience; includes self-confidence, personality, cognitive aptitude, developmental level and mental health.

■ *Social*: Peer groups, families, community networks, schools, religious organizations and residential areas.

■ *Behavioural*: Contextually relevant (school behaviours, home behaviours, etc.) and related to developmental level. Includes issues regarding choices across the lifespan, educational attainment and risky versus health-positive behaviours.

Current conditions requiring health promotion

Many improvements in health outcomes are due to public health measures such as sanitation and water supplies. In the past many children died from illnesses caused by appalling sanitary conditions. Conditions such as ringworm, head lice, scabies and chronic ear discharges were common. Such conditions still exist today but are less prevalent. The conditions of concern today are chronic illnesses, accidents, obesity and mental health wellbeing.

Chronic illnesses such as:

■ asthma

■ diabetes

■ cystic fibrosis

■ cardiac disease

■ sickle cell disease.

Accidents such as:

■ road accidents

■ home accidents

■ injuries

■ poisoning.

Child health clinics have seen an increase in:

■ overweight and obesity

■ mental health issues, e.g. self harm, depression, anxiety disorders.

Approaches to health promotion

Health promotion can be described as nursing interventions that aim to educate and empower patients to prevent illness, increase overall health and manage existing conditions. Health-promoting activities can belong to one of three approaches: the traditional approach, the alternative approach (health deficits model) and the innovative approach (health assets model) (Whiting and Miller 2009).

Traditional approach to health promotion encompasses five sub-approaches which are widely used in current nursing practice (Whiting and Miller 2009). These are:

- *Medical approach*: Focuses on the prevention of illness rather than the achievement of health. Preventative procedures are emphasized according to individual risk.

- *Behavioural change approach*: Like the medical approach, the behavioural change approach focuses on the eradication and prevention of illness; however, a stronger emphasis is placed on behavioural change as opposed to preventative procedures.

- *Educational approach*: Enables patients to arrive at their own decisions about their care through patient education, participatory discussions and shared decision-making.

- *Client-centred approach*: Gives patients the opportunity to steer the focus of their treatment toward issues of personal concern. This is a responsive model which views patients and practitioners as equal players in the care process.

- *Societal change approach*: Seeks large-scale social change through health campaigns and educational programmes within schools, youth organizations and other social institutions.

The alternative approach (health deficits model)

This approach takes the form of government-driven programmes that respond to population health problems rather than anticipating or preventing such problems from developing in the first place. Interventions based on the alternative approach are designed as a response to 'health failures' which were criticized for their unidimensional treatment of population health (Whiting and Miller 2009). The emergence of large-scale government campaigns and representative surveys have contributed to health promotion by providing new means of reaching and identifying at-risk populations (Whitehead 2009).

The innovative approach (health assets model)

Aims to decrease a reliance on medical interventions by encouraging patient education, autonomy and personal responsibility. This approach maps and rewards health-positive behaviours in order to bolster self-esteem and encourage the continued practice of desired behaviours (Whiting and Miller 2009).

Combining approaches

Often, two or more of these approaches may be required when trying to promote healthy behaviour. For example, with childhood obesity, interventions focusing on education alone are not sufficient in sustaining new health behaviours, so it is important to combine educational interventions with discussions about ways of producing positive behavioural change in the child's life (Giles-Corti and Salmon 2007).

- A substantial body of research suggests that most parents have a sound understanding of what constitutes 'healthy, nutritious or beneficial' food (Jones et al 2008).

- Children's poor dietary habits therefore appear to be more complex than a reflection of parental knowledge of healthy eating.

- Children's eating patterns are a reflection of their social background and family food environment; parental preferences, cultural influences, media exposure and beliefs and attitudes toward food dictate what and how often a child eats (Jones et al 2008).

- Because children's eating patterns and activity levels are closely tied to those of their parents, consultations should consider the views and needs of parents and children alike by including them as equal participants.

- Obese and overweight children benefit from an ecological approach to treatment which considers the child's home routine and family environment when encouraging long-term lifestyle change (Limbers et al 2008).

5.3 Palliative care of a child

Caring for a dying child

The NHS delivers palliative care to children when curative treatment is no longer a viable care pathway (Cochrane et al 2007). Its primary aim is to improve quality of life by alleviating pain and suffering. The palliative care philosophy is a comprehensive approach to care which treats the emotional, physical, social and spiritual dimensions of a child and family needs.

Based on data from 2001–2005, it is estimated that half of all deaths of children aged 0–19 years were from causes which were likely to have required palliative care. Excluding neonatal deaths, approximately 18 000 children in the 0–19 age group are likely to require palliative care services in the UK annually (Cochrane et al 2007). In 2005, approximately 75% of 0–19-year-old non-neonatal deaths from conditions likely to require palliative care occurred in hospital (Cochrane et al 2007).

Conditions requiring palliative care (Cochrane et al 2007):

- congenital malformations, deformations and chromosomal abnormalities

- diseases of the nervous system

- neoplasms

- conditions arising during the perinatal period.

Palliative care provision

Palliative care provides relief to children from the following categories/conditions (Goldman 2007):

1. Where curative treatment is likely to fail; this especially applies to patients with malignant cancers or who have a high probability of secondary organ failure.

2. Cystic fibrosis or HIV/AIDS, which cause premature death and require protracted courses of intensive treatment.

3. Progressive conditions, such as metabolic diseases and mucopolysaccharidoses, for which curative treatment is never an option.
4. Cerebral palsy, severe neurological disability, illnesses or trauma resulting in severe disability, or otherwise non-progressive conditions which have a high potential for life-limiting complications.

The Association of Children's Palliative Care (ACT 2003) determines palliative care to be appropriate for children with any of the following conditions:

- Life-limiting conditions that have unclear prognoses or which do not respond to curative treatment

- Conditions requiring protracted courses of invasive treatment but which may still lead to premature death

- Progressive diseases for which palliative care is the only treatment option

- Conditions that are not progressive but which cause neurological disability and may result in serious health complications.

Symptoms that may arise:

- Fatigue and pain are the most commonly experienced symptoms of terminally ill children irrespective of disease and both tend to increase in frequency and severity near the end of life.

- Fatigue is often a side-effect of opioids while pain arises from the advancing disease process.

- Fatigue in the dying child is not ameliorated by rest, and can also arise organically from anaemia, pain, cytokines or psychological aspects of the child's condition.

- Nausea, vomiting, pain and constipation are commonly experienced symptoms during the palliative phase, but they typically respond well to drug treatment.

- Loss of appetite, weight loss, fatigue, decreased mobility and poor speech are also commonly experienced symptoms at this stage, yet are less amenable to drug treatment (McCulloch et al 2008).

- Children with CNS tumours tend to suffer from headache and other neurological symptoms as they near the end of life (McCulloch et al 2008).

- Children with solid tumours experience significant end of life pain caused by neuropathy and bone pain. Combined treatments of opioids and adjuvant medications are often required in these cases (McCulloch et al 2008).

- Caring for children dying of life-limiting brain tumours is complicated by a cluster of associated symptoms. In addition to having the highest mortality rate of all malignant neoplasms in children, brain tumours cause cognitive impairment, speech and language difficulties, problems with swallowing and paralysis (Zelcer et al 2010).

Providing individualized care

- Little research exists on the psychological and emotional responses that are commonly experienced by terminally ill children (McCulloch et al 2008). So it is essential that care is individualized to the child's needs and their preferences respected.

■ Children with life-limiting conditions have care needs specific to their particular condition, family background and non-medical (social, emotional, spiritual) needs.

■ Recent medical advances in diagnostic technologies and drug treatments have led to a growing population of children requiring intensive palliative care services.

■ Interventions gaining popularity in the treatment of this patient population include nasopharyngeal airways, tracheostomies, assisted ventilatory support, home-based care plans, and enteral feeding for severely neurodisabled children (Hain and Wallace 2008).

■ Nurses must provide care that is tailored to the child's symptoms and particular treatments to meet the unique needs of each child and family.

Pain control

Palliative care for children involves active symptom management to relieve any pain or unnecessary suffering. Parents whose child dies comfortably fare better during the grieving process, and patients benefit from an improved quality of life arising from better sleep, improved nutrition, faster healing and improved ability to cope with therapy (Friebert 2009). Pain management has multifaceted functions and is crucial to ensuring patient comfort and well-being.

■ Relief of pain is a basic human right, and human dignity and respect requires that treatable pain is relieved.

■ Thorough and accurate pain assessment is essential for child's quality of life. Severity, frequency and nature of pain should be assessed prior

to mapping a pain relief care plan (see pain assessment tools in Section 2).

■ Use pharmacological and non-pharmacological interventions for pain relief as outlined in Section 3.

■ Some practitioners and families may be reluctant to administer pain medications because they are fearful of opioids leading to dependency or hastened death. In such instances, they should receive reassurance and support about the importance of ensuring optimal pain relief.

■ Drug disposition and metabolic effect are influenced by a child's physical development, making drug prescribing a particularly challenging aspect of pain management.

■ Pain and symptoms should undergo regular review in order to identify any new development or changes to a child's condition.

Routes of administration available

Route of administration requires careful consideration when providing pain relief and other therapeutic interventions to terminally ill children. Nearly all children would choose to endure pain rather than experience relief through injection, yet many children have difficulty swallowing medication, and many drugs used in palliative care are not suitable for oral administration. However, the drugs used in palliative medicine have been developed in recent years to allow for administrative routes which are more comfortable for children. These routes include (Hain and Wallace 2008):

■ Transdermal delivery system: i.e. fentanyl. The smallest available dose delivers the equivalent of 90 mg/day of p.o. morphine; transdermal fentanyl is unsuitable as a starting dose or for dose titration.

- Matrix patches use the transdermal delivery system to reduce drug delivery into daily dosages, allowing for starting doses and titration. Fentanyl and buprenorphine can be effectively administered via this route.
- Buccal medications tend to be easily tolerated by children. This route is particularly amenable to opioids and benzodiazepines.

Common medication used in the palliative care of children include (Hain and Wallace 2008):

- morphine
- diamorphine
- fentanyl
- buprenorphine
- tramadol
- codeine
- gabapentin.

(Please refer to *BNF for Children* or local policy and guidelines for indications, dosage, contraindications and interactions.)

Caring for the psychological needs of the child, parents and family

Psychological care

With significant advances in medical and nursing care, the death of a child is not so common as in the past. When a child is diagnosed as requiring palliative care,

it can be a time of great sadness, distress, shock, and anger for families. It can be a rollercoaster for many parents as they try to come to terms with the fact that their child has a life-limiting condition. Dying children and their families have complex care needs that move beyond the medical realm to include social, emotional and spiritual aspects of care (Longden and Mayer 2007).

- Discontinuation of active care is made smoother by coordinating the commencement of palliative care services.
- Decisions concerning home care interventions, ambulance transportation, end of life care plans and bereavement support should be discussed with families and shared within care teams (Longden and Mayer 2007).
- One of the most important aspects of end-of-life care is empowering parents and children by allowing them to make decisions concerning place and time of death, family involvement, therapeutic interventions and bereavement support (Longden and Mayer 2007).
- It is vitally important that healthcare professionals listen and respond to children and families preferences.
- Parents must be given sufficient opportunity to discuss with clinicians their concerns, questions and fears regarding their child's death. Neglecting this aspect of palliative care can have disastrous emotional consequences for bereaved families (Midson and Carter 2010).
- Parents should be invited to discuss their wishes about place of death and after death arrangements in a non-crisis environment (Midson and

Carter 2010). Providing an opportunity to discuss these issues empowers parents to make decisions and gain a sense of autonomy and control over the dying process.

■ Anticipatory grief may be endured by parents of children approaching the end of life, while others may feel intense grief over having 'given up' on pursuing curative treatment for their child (Raphael 2006).

■ Psychologists, counsellors, chaplains and social workers are excellent sources of advice for clinicians (Midson and Carter 2010).

■ Religious and spiritual support should be ongoing and may occur in the form of baptisms, counselling and bereavement support.

Communication with the dying child and family

■ It cannot be emphasized enough that each child and family responds differently, their emotions and responses can fluctuate daily and they require empathetic sensitive care.

■ Honest and regular communication with the child and family about the disease process and course of treatment is very important (Goldman 2007).

■ Ongoing communication and honest dialogue about what to expect from the dying process must be included in the care given to all families during the palliative phase.

■ Communication should be compassionate and supportive at all times, but information about a child's prognosis should not be imparted with unrealistic optimism (Raphael 2006).

■ Anticipate that children and parents will ask challenging questions about their prognosis and eventual death. Do not try to avoid being involved in discussions about these topics; instead, accept that they will be difficult conversations, and try to learn from the shared experiences of more seasoned members of the care team (Midson and Carter 2010).

■ Involving the child in discussions about their wishes and concerns about the dying process is important to ensuring that children's desires are included in care plans.

■ Child's developmental level is unique, and this should be considered throughout all planning and implementation of care.

■ It is important to help children live meaningfully and according to what they feel is important for their own lives.

■ Maintaining a sense of routine and purpose in daily activities is another important aspect of supporting the dying child.

Palliative care services

Despite inadequate palliative service provision in hospitals, the majority of terminally ill children still die in hospital. There are several drawbacks to hospital as a place of death such as: limited privacy, poor palliative care skills among staff, limited family accommodation and a curative, as opposed to palliative, philosophy of care (Davies 2005). Although a paucity of research exists on paediatric palliative care services and on the suitability of palliative care services for children and families (Taylor et al 2010), we do know that home-based end-of-life care is preferred by many families (McCulloch et al. 2008). Likewise, most healthcare professionals believe that, where possible, terminally ill children should die in the home (Davies 2005).

Home-based palliative care

- There has been a move away from hospital/hospice care to the provision of care in the community because it is generally believed that children are best cared for at home and within families wherever possible.

- Home-based palliative care reduces the need for travel, is more comfortable for families and gives parents and children a sense of privacy and control (Longden and Mayer 2007).

- Hospices offer similar advantages through private rooms and family accommodation.

- Whichever setting in which palliative care is delivered, it is a personal decision that ultimately lies with parents and children.

Provision of respite

- Due to the burden of caring, respite or short breaks from caring are an essential component of providing care to a child with a life-limiting condition and their family (DOH 2008).

- Respite care may include: informal help from friends and family, home help, night sitter, attendance at a day care centre, admission to a specialist palliative care inpatient unit, admission to a community hospital or admission to a hospice (ACT 2003).

- Respite care provides parents and families with a break from the physical and emotional toll of caring for the child.

- Because of the progressive nature and neurological impairments of children with malignant brain tumours, parents of this group may be more likely to seek hospice support during the palliative phase (Breen 2010).

- When planning palliative and respite care, the preferences of the child and parents should be reflected in all decision-making.

Involvement of community and primary care services

- In the UK, palliative care within the home is managed by a paediatric outreach nurse, a representative from a hospice outreach team or a member of a children's community nursing team. This individual is responsible for coordinating the patient's hospital care team, primary care team and tertiary care.

- Service provision appears to be much better for children within oncology.

- Professional services and support must be coordinated and responsive to the needs of individual children and families (Craig et al 2008).

- Palliative care is not limited to only those services provided by specialist practitioners in the hospital or community.
- Teachers, community groups and the family doctor can liaise with the palliative care team and provide excellent support to sick children and their families (Goldman 2007).

When a child dies

- Following death in hospital, a bereavement coordinator will be introduced to the family and will liaise with the family, the healthcare team and any relevant community-based services, such as support groups or religious organizations (Longden and Mayer 2007).
- After the child's death, the care team should maintain professional contact with the family for a number of weeks and show support by attending the child's funeral (Goldman 2007).
- Following a child's death at home, clinicians should maintain professional contact with the family and offer to arrange bereavement counseling with the hospital's services or community support groups.
- Research has shown that parents benefit emotionally and psychologically from remaining with their child's body after death, and from being given control over their child's body (Davies 2005).
- It is important to support parents' wishes to be with their child at the time of death, either in privacy or in the company of family.

- Healthcare practitioners should inform parents of their right to decide what happens to their child's body after a planned death has taken place.
- Parents should be supported with whatever course of action they decide upon, even in cases where they wish to remain with the body for some time before proceeding to mortuary or funeral home services.
- Removal of a child's body should be paced according to the parents' wishes alone, and should not be rushed because of pressure from a mortuary or funeral home (Davies 2005).

Spiritual care

Spiritual care gives the child and family an opportunity to examine the impact of the illness on their belief systems. They need to be given the opportunity to ask questions:

- Why me/us?
- Why now?
- What have them or I done to deserve this?

As a children's nurse, by staying with this sort of spiritual pain and not being afraid of the questions asked by the patient or their family is a helpful and sensitive response. Offering the support of a relevant religious figure may not be appropriate for all, but listening and being present will be appreciated.

Cultural diversity

Making nursing practice relevant to people of many cultures is a constant challenge to nurses. Cultures differ with regard to:

- meaning of an illness
- attitude to pain, symptoms and to medication

- ways of coping with illness
- attitude to place of care, physical and emotional care
- role of the family
- rituals around death, the funeral and bereavement.

Last offices

This is the care given to a deceased child, which is focused on fulfilling religious and cultural beliefs as well as health and safety and legal requirements. It should be remembered that this is demonstration of respectful, sensitive care given to the child.

- It is important that the bedside nurse knows in advance the cultural values and religious beliefs of the patient and family, as there are considerable variations between people from different faiths, ethnic backgrounds and national origins in their approach to death and dying (see Table 5.1).
- Individual preferences should be determined and patients should be encouraged to talk about how they may wish to be treated upon dying. In the case of the unconscious child, the bedside nurse should consult the family members.

Table 5.1 Last rites and religious influences

Religion	Last rites
Baha'i	Treat body with great respect after death as believe in afterlife
	Routine last rites are appropriate
	Cremation is not permitted
	Burial should take place within an hour's journey from place of death
Buddhism	Believe in rebirth after death, therefore state of mind at moment of death is important in determining the state of rebirth
	Some form of chanting may be used to influence the state of mind at death so that it may be peaceful
	May not wish to have sedatives or pain killing drugs administered at this time
	Peace and quiet for meditation and visits from other Buddhists is appreciated
	If Buddhists are not in attendance, then a Buddhist minister should be informed of the death as soon as possible. Routine last rites are appropriate
	Cremation is preferred
Christian Science	There are no rituals to be performed

Table 5.1 Last rites and religious influences—cont'd

Religion	Last rites
Christianity Anglicans Roman Catholics Free Churches	Routine last rites are appropriate for all Christians
Hinduism	Want to die at home. This has religious significance and death in hospital can cause great distress
	May wish to call in a Hindu priest to read from the Hindu holy books and to perform holy rites. These may include tying a thread around the wrist or neck, sprinkling the person with water from the Ganges, or placing a sacred tulsi leaf in their mouth
	Their belief in cremation and body being returned to nature may involve a dying person asking to be placed on the floor during their last moments
Islam	May wish to sit or lie with their face towards Mecca. Moving the bed to make this possible is appreciated.
	Family may recite prayers around the bed. If no family are available, any practising Muslim can assist.
	May wish the Imam (religious leader) to visit
	After death, the body *should not be touched* by non-Muslims. Health workers should wear disposable gloves to touch body
	The body should be prepared according to the wishes of the family
	If family are not available, the following procedure should be followed:
	Turn the head towards the right shoulder before rigor mortis begins. This is so that the body can be buried with their face towards Mecca.
	Do not wash the body, or cut hair or nails
	Wrap the body in a plain white sheet
	Muslims are always buried, never cremated
	The body will be ritually washed by the family and Muslim undertakers before burial
	Funerals take place as soon as practicable, as delay can cause distress. If a delay is unavoidable, explain the reasons carefully to the relatives

(Continued)

Table 5.1 Last rites and religious influences—cont'd

Religion	Last rites
	If the death has to be reported to the Coroner, they should be informed that the patient is a Muslim and be asked if the procedures can take place as soon as possible
	If the family wish to view the body, staff should ask the mortician to ensure that the room is free of any religious 'symbols'
	Postmortems are forbidden unless ordered by the Coroner, in which case the reasons for it must be clearly explained to the family
	Family may request that organs removed should be returned to the body after examination
Jehovah's Witness	No special rituals for the dying but they will usually appreciate a visit from one of the Elders of their Faith
	Routine last rites are not appropriate
Judaism	In some cases the son or nearest relative, if present, may wish to close the eyes and mouth
	The body should be handled as little as possible by non-Jews
	Depending on the sex of the patient, a fellow male or female washes and prepares the body for burial. Usually three members of the community are present. Traditional Jews will arrange for this to be done by the Jewish Burial Society
	If, however, members of the family are not present, most non Orthodox Jews would accept the usual washing and last rites performed by hospital staff
	The body should be covered with a clean white sheet
	The family may wish for the body to be placed with the feet pointing towards the doorway and to light a candle
	Some Orthodox Jewish groups may wish to appoint someone to stay with the body 'watcher' from the time of death to the burial, which usually takes place within 24 hours
	If family wish to view the body, staff should ask the mortician to ensure that the room is free of any religious 'symbols'
	If the death has to be reported to the Coroner, they should be informed that the patient is Jewish and be asked if the procedures can take place as soon as possible
	Orthodox Jews are always buried but non Orthodox Jews allow cremation

Table 5.1 Last rites and religious influences—cont'd

Religion	Last rites
	The funeral has to take place as soon as possible
Mormons	There are no rituals for the dying, but spiritual contact is important
	The church has 'home teachers' who offer support and care by visiting church members in hospital
	Routine last rites are appropriate
	The sacred garment, if worn, must be replaced on the body following the last rites.
	Church burial is preferred, although cremation is not forbidden
Rastafarianism	Visiting the sick is important and often made in groups. Family members may wish to pray at the bedside
	Apart from this, there are no rites or rituals, before or after death
	Routine last rites are appropriate
	Burial is preferred
Sikhism	May receive comfort from reciting hymns from the Guru Granth Sahab, the Sikh holy book. Family or any practising Sikh may help with this
	Generally, Sikhs are happy for non-Sikhs to attend to the body. However, many families will wish to wash and lay out the body themselves
	If members of the family are not available, in addition to the normal Last Rites hair or beard should be left intact and not trimmed
	If the family wish to view the body, staff should ask the mortician to ensure that the room is free of all religious 'symbols'
	Apart from stillbirths and neonates, who may be buried, Sikhs are always cremated. This should take place as soon as possible
	There are no objections to postmortem examinations

- Catheters and other appliances should be removed (except in a Coroner's case where local guidance should be sought).
- Relatives should be asked whether jewellery should be left on or taken off.
- Wash the patient unless requested not to do so for religious/cultural reasons. It may not be acceptable for the nurse to undertake this task or sometimes, a relative or spouse may want to help.

- Body is dressed in a shroud or other garment (refer to local policy).
- Local policy should be followed with the identification of the body and their property identified and stored.
- Patient is then wrapped in a sheet and the sheet secured.
- Notification of death card is taped outside the sheet (refer to local policy).
- Request a porter to remove the body.
- Screen off appropriate areas from view of other patients and visitors when the body is being removed.
- Update nursing records, transfer property and patient records to appropriate administrative staff.
- Give bereaved family member's information booklet regarding contacting hospital about viewing the body, collection of death certificate, etc.

Sudden death of an infant, child or adolescent

Sudden death refers to a child who has died unexpectedly from accidents or illness. Sudden death includes suicide, murder, accident, illness, 'cot death' or sudden infant death, and also covers all age ranges. Sudden death(s) robs the relatives of any preparatory grief. The relatives may require more support and counselling than those who have known for some time their relative was dying. Emergency department deaths are more likely to be unexpected by the family.

Needs of survivors bereaved by sudden and unexpected death

Death and loss are an unavoidable part of life. People may show no manifestations of grief at the time of death but experience normal grief prior to death occurring (Purvis and Edwards 2005). With sudden death, it is imperative that nurses are aware of a family's distress, acknowledge this and have an understanding of needs of those who are suddenly bereaved. Families' experiences may have a powerful effect on their process of grieving and professionals' responses to them play a valuable part in the crisis.

- Viewing the body – equipment should not be in view and there should be privacy and a member of staff staying with them in the room being supportive and compassionate.
- Signing of papers is necessary but not an initial priority.
- Member of staff should accompany the family, offer support, give information and provide a separate room for them to wait.
- Survivors need accurate information about death and to talk about their experiences:
  - Breaking bad news of the death of a family's relative is one of the most difficult and sensitive things a nurse has to learn to do.
  - Poor communication skills can leave families confused and angry at the way news was broken.
  - Families need to be reassured that all appropriate actions were taken to save their loved one, and that being able to witness the resuscitation was helpful for them to cope with their grief.

- Offering sedation is the least helpful because it inhibits the bereaved person's expressions of grief.
- Consistencies with the usage of words:
  - Explanations should be clear of medical jargon, gentle and sincere.
  - The word 'dead' should be used, instead of terms such as 'passed away'.
  - The word 'dead' or 'died' can help the bereaved person from not denying the death and leads to less confusion.

Brain stem death

The brain stem is collectively the mid-brain, pons and medulla oblongata. It is between the cerebrum and the spinal cord, the medulla oblongata being a direct upward continuation of the spinal cord. Brain stem death occurs whereby structural brain damage is so extensive that there is no potential for recovery and the brain can no longer maintain its own internal homeostasis and there is a complete loss of brain stem function.

- It is the permanent loss of the function of the brain stem, which results in a combined, irreversible loss of the capacity for consciousness and breathing.
- It is a diagnosis of death accepted by both the medical and legal profession.
- Most frequent causes of brain stem death are intracranial haemorrhage, cerebral hypoxaemia and trauma.

Brain stem criteria

- The patient is brain stem dead and mechanically ventilated.

- Age is irrelevant to whether patients are selected to be potential organ donors, but what is essential is that the patient's clinical condition coupled with their blood results are within satisfactory parameters on the day of donation. This will be assessed by the relevant medical team.
- That the medical and nursing staff have no known objections from the family, or coroner.

Brain stem death tests

For brain stem death tests to take place, the patient will be deeply unconscious and require ventilatory support. The tests take place under certain preconditions:

- Normal blood gases, urea and creatinine, potassium (K^+) and sodium (Na^+), temperature.
- No sedation, analgesia or muscle relaxants for 24–48 hours (or longer).
- Patient has a specific condition that causes brain stem death.
- Diagnosis of brain stem death is by two independent and suitably qualified doctors.
- Two sets of tests are performed.
- Prior to commencement of brain stem tests, the patient must meet with certain preconditions. These preconditions are designed to ensure that the patient's unconscious state is caused by an irreversible structural brain damage and that their current status has not been influenced by other factors, e.g. use of muscle relaxants or an existing metabolic disorder.
- Tests have been designed to look at the most basic brain stem functions and assess their responses.

Tests consist of the following:

Eyes	Pupils do not react to light
	Eyelids do not move when the corneas are stimulated
	There is no movement of the eyes when 20 ml ice-cold water is injected in the ear canals
Cranial nerves	There is no motor response within the cranial nerve distribution to stimulation of any somatic area
Oral	There is no gag or cough responses to tracheal suction
Respiratory	There is no stimulation of breathing after a period of removal from the ventilator (preoxygenate with 100% oxygen to prevent hypoxia. If CO_2 has risen above 6.65 kPa, which exceeds the threshold for respiration, it can be assumed that no respiratory effort has taken place during the period of discontinuation of ventilation

Two doctors, a consultant in charge of the patient's case and a second doctor of senior registrar status conduct these tests separately or together to make the diagnosis of brain stem death. Once brain stem death has been confirmed, the possibility for organ harvest for transplantation should be considered. If a patient is going to become an organ donor, it is necessary to continue ventilation until organ retrieval takes place.

Potential organ donation

Children in the UK often die or suffer prolonged dependency because of a lack of organs for transplantation. Therefore, if a young or middle-aged patient with a fatal condition has healthy kidneys, liver, heart or corneas, it might be relevant to discuss organ donation with the medical team. Suitable organ donors include:

- victims of severe head injury
- severe subarachnoid or intracerebral haemorrhage.

Patients who are unsuitable for organ donation are:

- when brain death criteria fulfilment is uncertain
- where there has been a significant hypotension or hypoxic episode during a fatal injury
- where there is a history of previous disease affecting the potential donor (e.g. hypertension, diabetes, hepatitis B, alcohol abuse)
- where the patient has received drugs or other treatments, which might have affected the organs to be transplanted
- in the case of the kidneys, where there is persistent oliguria.

Clinical management of the potential organ donor

Following brain stem death diagnosis, significant pathophysiological changes will occur, which may lead to complications, and this may in turn lead to potential damage to the donor's organs. Once a family have made the decision to donate their child's organs, it is the duty of the medical and nursing team to ensure the donor's organs have the best possible outcome.

Common complications of children who have been diagnosed as brainstem dead include:

- hypotension
- hypothermia
- hypernatraemia
- hyperglycaemia
- acidosis
- diabetes insipidus
- disseminated intravascular coagulation
- pulmonary oedema.

Routine monitoring of a brain stem dead patient should include:

- ECG
- arterial blood pressure
- oxygen saturation
- temperature
- central venous pressure
- fluid balance
- arterial blood gases
- pathology, e.g. biochemistry, haematology.

Care of the donor and family

The physiological manifestations of brain stem death are complex. The effects include profound hypotension, cardiac arrhythmias, hypothermia, pulmonary oedema, diabetes insipidus and clotting abnormalities. Maintenance of a patient's status quo during this time can prove to be often difficult and multifaceted. Furthermore, organ donations are sometimes lost because of the rapid deterioration in the donor clinical condition.

Potential donors need intensive nursing and complex medical care once brain stem death has confirmed. Their combined care will ensure that the organs are maintained at a high quality pre donation and thus ensure that the families wish for donation is fulfilled. It is important to note that the longer the gap between diagnosing brain stem criteria, the more problems may arise in the child's clinical condition and medical management.

Often family members of potential donors choose when and where they feel ready to say their goodbyes to their loved ones. Some family members leave shortly after brain stem tests have been performed, other may stay until they go to theatre. This is managed on an individual basis and intense support and compassion is offered by the intensive care and organ transplant team to held family members through this time.

Transplant recipient

Organ transplantation is the treatment of choice for end stage organ failure. Transplant recipients that may benefit from organ transplantation fall into the following categories:

- heart – cardiomyopathy, ischaemic heart disease
- lung
- heart and lung – cystic fibrosis
- liver – primary biliary cirrhosis, chronic active hepatitis
- kidney – polycystic kidney disease, glomerulonephritis.

Allocation of organs and retrieval

Prior to retrieval, the organ must have been accepted by a transplant centre for a suitable waiting list patient. All organs are primarily offered to the local zonal centre. If they do not have any suitable recipients, the organ will then be offered to each of the country's other transplant centres. If none of the UK centres accepts the organ; it is then offered to a European Centre. This is a reciprocal agreement and is important to note that the UK imports more organs than it exports. In the event that the organ cannot be placed to a potential organ recipient, then the organ will not be retrieved.

All potential organ donors will be required to have a virology screen to exclude HIV, hepatitis B and C. Furthermore, the organ transplant coordinator is required to ask family members about the patient's social behaviour so that they have a detailed history of the patient's past. Once again, this information will be documented within the patient's medical notes.

What to do after the patient has died

- Family should be able to spend as much time with their loved one as they want; this should not exclude children
- Doctor will be called to certify the death
- Date and time of death are recorded in the patient's notes.

Grieving process

- Grieving the loss of a child is a profoundly difficult experience for parents and families. Grief is suffered by bereaved parents more acutely than any other relationship, and has the ability to inspire prolonged emotional disturbances, post-traumatic stress reactions and an increased risk of suicide (Raphael 2006).
- Some parents and mothers in particular feel that they cannot continue to live if their child dies because of their intense and prolonged emotional investment in their child's dying trajectory.
- Clinicians caring for dying children and their families should aim to recognize signs of the above described experiences so that appropriate therapeutic interventions can be offered (Raphael 2006).

Cost of caring for the nurse

- Working closely with dying children can cause emotional distress for the nurse and can be very painful. Nurses caring for need adequate support systems in both their professional and personal lives. It is imperative that all staff members realize their needs following death of a patient.

- Need for continuous up-dating and training on breaking bad news and a shared professional goal with reflections, discussions and feedback about the caring aspect of critical care work.
- Need for a support group for staff.
- Death education is important, a topic which is difficult to teach but issues need to be explored.
- Training should include knowledge about death, grief and bereavement, communication skills either at breaking bad news or to deal with discomfort felt by staff when they

were dealing with relatives showing extreme emotions.

The children's nurse needs to recognize internal signs of stress and develop strategies for coping:

- Spacing for holidays and time off is important to recharge lost energy.
- Continuous training and education about bereavement and palliative care.
- Take time to debrief with colleagues and time out to share stories.
- Concise written recording can be therapeutic and assist in the letting go of particularly stressful situation.
- Keep a reflective diary.
- Being honest and sharing vulnerabilities will help a team relate and work well together.

Section 6

Drug administration

6.1 Pharmacokinetics and pharmacodynamics

This is about the basic principles of drugs following its administration (see Neal 2002, Galbraith et al 1999). Why are certain drugs given specific routes of administration? Patients are reliant on all nurses to ensure medicines are administered appropriately. It is vital for nurses to have a sound understanding of the two classes of pharmacology: pharmacokinetics, the way the body affects the drug with time (absorption, distribution, metabolism and excretion of drugs) and pharmacodynamics, which is the effects of the drug on the body.

Pharmacokinetic processes

Pharmacokinetics considers the passage of a drug through the body, and is concerned with absorption, distribution, metabolism and excretion.

Absorption

Drugs must be absorbed across a cell membrane (with the exception of IV drugs). Before entering the systemic circulation a drug must traverse the GIT layers before the drug reaches the bloodstream and cell membranes. Oral drugs are absorbed in the upper small bowel because of its large surface area (Neal 2002), which is determined by the chemical nature of the drug. Absorption occurs by simple diffusion, determined by molecular size:

- Drugs absorbed from the GIT enter the portal circulation and some are extensively metabolized as they pass through the liver.
- Drugs that are lipid soluble are readily absorbed orally and rapidly distributed throughout the body.
- Many drugs are bound to albumin and equilibrium forms between the bound and free drug in the plasma. The drug that is bound to albumin does not exert a pharmacological action.
- Bioavailability is the fraction of the administered dose that reaches the systemic circulation – 100% in drugs administered IV.

Drugs administered orally have to overcome the physical barrier of the gut wall. The absorption process is affected by many factors:

- formulation
- stability to acid and enzymes
- motility of gut
- food in the stomach
- degree of first pass metabolism (discussed later)
- lipid solubility.

Distribution

Distribution around the body occurs when the drug reaches the circulation. It must then penetrate tissues to act. Factors that affect drug distribution are:

- plasma protein binding sites albumin – competition
- specific drug receptor sites in tissues

- regional blood flow
- lipid solubility
- blood–brain barrier
- GIT membrane
- highly water-soluble drugs, e.g. gentamicin
- disease
- liver disease – low plasma protein levels
- renal disease – high blood levels.

Metabolism

Metabolism of drugs occurs in the liver and involves a group of enzymes that transform drugs into products that are more water soluble and easier to excrete. The majority of drug metabolism occurs in the liver and involves two general types of reactions:

1. Phase 1 reaction – the biotransformation of the drug – oxidations are the most common reactions and these are catalysed by mixed function oxidases.
2. Phase II reactions – drugs from phase I cannot be excreted efficiently by the kidneys and are made more hydrophilic by conjugation with compounds in the liver.

Metabolism also occurs in the gut lining, kidney and lungs. The majority of drugs that are metabolized are:

- inactivated (propranolol)
- activated (enalapril)
- remain unchanged (atenolol)
- the products of metabolism (metabolites) are longer acting than the original drug (diazepam).

Concomitant drug administration may influence metabolism, for example:

- phenytoin can induce liver enzymes by increasing the metabolism of other drugs
- cimetidine can inhibit liver enzymes by reducing metabolism.

These can have serious consequences if the patient is already on other drug therapies.

Other factors can affect drug metabolism:

- age (including infants/children)
- alcohol consumption
- immaturity of drug-metabolizing enzymes in neonates and infants
- disease (impaired liver function, dose reduction may be necessary for drugs metabolized in the liver), e.g. chlormethiazole
- smoking.

The first pass metabolism

Drugs absorbed from GIT pass into the bloodstream and are immediately transported to the liver. Some drugs are inactivated the first time they pass through the liver; this affects drug dose and route of administration (e.g. propranolol):

- if given IV the dose is 1 mg
- if give orally the dose is 40 mg
- affects possible routes of administration, e.g. GTN cannot be given orally except by by-passing the liver such as sublingually.

Excretion

The main route of excretion is the kidney in the urine. Excretion of drugs can occur in the faeces. The drug is circulated in blood to the liver then passes into the bile into the GIT. If renal or liver impairment is present a reduced dose may be required, for example with digoxin or gentamicin. Drug can be reabsorbed and re-enter the liver. Metabolism can be reversed (by enzymes present in the gut or by gut microflora), converting the drug so that it can be reabsorbed. This can lead to a cycle known as the enterohepatic recirculation and accounts for the prolonged effect of some drugs. Excretion varies with age and can lead to discoloration of the urine or faeces.

Frequent blood samples may be required for some drugs; in order for them to be effective a certain blood level has to be obtained. Drugs are generally poisonous and at higher blood level concentrations can lead to serious consequences, even death. To avoid drug toxicity in infants (<1 year) lower doses are prescribed or their administration intervals widened. For all drugs there is also a minimum effective concentration, below which there will be not any therapeutic effect.

Factors affecting excretion:

■ renal failure
■ blood flow to the kidneys
■ GFR
■ Urine flow rate and pH, which indirectly alters:
  – passive reabsorption
  – active tubular secretion.

Pharmacodynamics

This is the study of effects of drugs on the body or the biological processes. It is concerned with the pharmacological effect of drugs at its site(s) of action and considers mechanisms of action for both therapeutic and adverse effects of the drug.

■ Pharmacological responses are initiated by the molecular interactions of drugs with cells, tissues or other body constituents.

■ Drug molecules must exert some chemical influence on one or more cellular constituents to produce a pharmacological response.

■ To affect functioning of cellular molecules, the drug must approach the molecules closely.

■ Another requirement is that the drug must have some sort of non-uniform distribution within the body or the chance of interaction if the drug molecules are distributed at random would be negligible. This means that a drug must bind in some way to constituents of the cell to produce an effect.

■ For most drugs the site of action is at a specific biological molecule – the receptor. A receptor is the primary site of action of a drug.

■ Various types of receptor exist, and each responds to a different chemical or hormone, e.g. histamine, acetylcholine, epinephrine (adrenaline) and dopamine.

■ Many endogenous hormones, neurotransmitters and other mediators exert their effects as a result of high affinity binding or specific macromolecular protein or glycoprotein receptors in plasma membranes or cell cytoplasm.

■ When these receptors are bound to a certain chemical, this directs a change to occur in the cell, which then alters an activity of the cell.

The commonest ways in which drugs produce their effects

Not all drugs work via receptors for endogenous mediators and many drugs exert their effect by combining with other regulatory proteins and interfering with their function:

- Ion channels – physical blocking of channel by the drug molecule – sodium channel blocking by local anaesthetics or by binding to accessory sites to facilitate opening of channels.

- Enzymes – many drugs are targeted in this way:
  - substrate analogues and act as competitive inhibitors, either reversible inhibitors (neostigmine on acetylcholinesterase) or irreversible inhibitors (aspirin on cyclo-oxygenase).
  - many act as a false substrate – fluorouracil replaces uracil and blocks DNA synthesis.
  - some drugs are pro-drugs and need enzymic degradation to convert them to the active form, e.g. diamorphine to morphine.

- Transport proteins – drugs may interfere with the uptake of ions or small molecules across the cell membrane:
  - cocaine interferes with the re-uptake of noradrenaline (norepinephrine)
  - digoxin interferes with the sodium/potassium pump.

- Other cellular macromolecules – these do not involve regulatory proteins:
  - chemical action, e.g. antacids (magnesium hydroxide)
  - drugs that act by physical action – osmotic diuretics (mannitol)
  - drugs that act by a physicochemical action – inhaled anaesthetics, which act by altering the protein of cell membranes.

Most drugs produce their effects by acting on specific protein molecules usually located in the cell membrane. These proteins are called receptors and normally respond to endogenous chemicals in the body. A chemical that binds to a receptor is known as a ligand, many drugs cause their effects by combining with these receptors and are of the following types:

- Agonists – these interact with a receptor mimicking the effect of a natural mediator. Epinephrine (adrenaline) is a beta-receptor agonist, which stimulates the cardiac beta-receptors and increases heart rate.

- Partial agonists – the maximal response falls short of the full response block access of the natural agonist, e.g. pindolol, oxprenolol beta blockers, which are partial agonists.

- Antagonists block a receptor to prevent such an effect. Atenolol is a beta-receptor antagonist that slows heart rate by blocking the cardiac beta-receptors and reducing physiological stimulation. They are selective but not specific (they act on more than one receptor and produce side effects). Amitriptyline (tricyclic antidepressant) blocks cholinergic and histamine receptors, which leads to dry mouth, blurred vision, constipation and drowsiness.

Potency of drugs

The interaction between a drug and the binding site of the receptor depends on the 'fit' of the two molecules.

The closer the fit and the greater number of bonds the stronger will be the attractive forces between them:

- If a drug is potent it produces effects at low concentration.
- If a drug has a high potency it is a consequence of high affinity for a specific receptor.
- Affinity is the tendency to bind to receptors.
- Efficacy is the ability once bound, to initiate changes, which lead to effects.
- If a drug is specific small changes in drug structure lead to profound changes in potency or causes a change from agonist to antagonist:
  - selectivity is the phenomenon that allows drugs to be useful; a drug must act selectively on particular cells and tissues
  - specificity is reciprocal – individual classes of drug bind only to certain targets, and individual targets only recognize certain classes of drug
  - no drug acts with complete specificity – will only produce one effect.
- Potency is independent of efficacy and efficacy is usually more important than potency when selecting a drug for clinical use.
- The lower the potency of a drug and the higher the dose needed, the more likely that sites of action other than the primary one will assume significance:
  - this is often associated with the appearance of unwanted side effects, of which no drug is free – varies from trivial to fatal
  - pharmaceutical companies try hard to manufacture drugs that are more selective and thus less dangerous to other tissues.

Mode of action

If the basic mode of action of a drug is via a receptor then it is likely that:

- it will be potent
- it will have biological specificity and may produce opposite effects on apparently similar tissue type
- it will have chemical specificity and changes in the chemical structure of a drug molecule may have a large or small effect on its pharmacological activity
- specific antagonists will abolish the effects of the drug on the tissue
- if plasma concentration of the drug is too high (outside the therapeutic range) toxicity will occur
- if plasma concentration is too low treatment will fail
- the aim of treatment is to keep the plasma concentration within the therapeutic range via blood levels.

Drug interactions

Drugs are chemicals and may interact with one another. When this happens, a drug's action may be:

- suppressed
- rendered completely inactive
- increased.

The therapeutic action of one drug can interfere with the therapeutic action of another.

Combinations of drugs must be carefully considered to avoid drug interactions.

As the number of medications prescribed for a patient increases (polypharmacy) so does the potential for drug interactions. With so many drugs given at the same time and so many drugs available, it is impossible to predict the interactions that can occur. Any adverse reaction needs to be reported to the appropriate authorities. The British National Formulary (BNF) and the BNF for children website (www.bnf.org/bnf/) contain lists of known interactions, and these should always be consulted before drug mixtures are administered. Some produce minor problems, others can be fatal. The types of drug interactions that occur are:

- outside the body – generally due to storage conditions, too much light, oxygen or moisture, interactions with containers whereby the chemicals contained within the drug are prone to degradation
- in the GIT – some food chemicals may react with drugs
- after absorption – where the most known interactions take place, usually when more than one drug is administered concurrently.

Pharmacogenetics

After taking all of the issues related to pharmacokinetics and pharmacodynamics, and the age, level of nutrition, occupation, state of health into consideration, there are still individual differences in drug metabolism. This is described in terms of a person's genetic make-up. How some patients metabolize or inactivate drugs and facilitate their excretion is to a large extent determined by inheritable traits. In addition, different ethnic groups show different pharmacokinetic profiles for a number of drugs.

There are many issues to consider administering individual patient therapy. A good understanding of the fundamental principles of drug therapy should help nurses to optimize patient care. An increase in nurses' contribution to multidisciplinary care in relation to drug administration/therapy is currently being explored.

Drug calculations

In children there are cardiac support and other drugs, which require careful and meticulous calculations to ensure the correct dose is given to patients. Included here are some of the common drug formulas and other useful information.

IV and oral therapy are common administration routes for drugs. It is in your interest to use some of your time to observe and learn about some of the drugs that patients are prescribed. In addition to this, in your role as a nurse you will be expected to check a drug and later to ensure correct calculation, draw up and calculate drug dosages.

The following are some of the drug calculation formulae that may help you in this role:

1000 µg in 1 mg
1000 mg in 1 g

Ampicillin 500 mg in diluted in 10 ml, you require 200 mg

$$\frac{\text{What you want}}{\text{What you have got}} \times \text{What it is in}$$

$$\frac{200}{500} \times 10 = 4\,\text{ml}$$

Epinephrine comes in strengths of 1:1000 (1 mg/ml) and 1:10 000 (10 mg/ml)

(i) If you require 1.6 mg of 1:1000 strength epinephrine, use the formula

$$\frac{\text{What you want}}{\text{What you have got}} \times \text{What it is in}$$

$$\frac{1.6}{1} \times 1 = 1.6\,\text{ml}$$

(ii) If you require 2.5 mg of 1:10 000 strength epinephrine, use the formula

$$\frac{\text{What you want}}{\text{What you have got}} \times \text{What it is in}$$

$$\frac{2.5}{1} \times 10 = 25\,\text{ml}$$

Lidocaine comes in either a 1% solution or a 2% solution; this means that:

A 1% solution is equal to	1 gram	in	100 ml
	1000 mg	in	100 ml
	10 mg	per	ml
A 2% solution is equal to	2 g	in	100 ml
	2000 mg	in	100 ml
	20 mg	per	ml

There are other drugs used for infusion such as dopamine, epinephrine (adrenaline), dobutamine, noradrenaline (norepinephrine), which require to be calculated in μg/kg/min.
First calculate μg/ml
  For these drugs use the formula.
This is a different calculation to the %

concentrations / dosages that adrenaline comes in:

$$\frac{\text{μg required} \times \text{kg} \times \text{min}}{\text{Concentration in μg}}$$

Nurse prescribing

Nursing is moving into the reality of nurse prescribing (Jones 2004, Beckwith and Franklin 2007). Any children's nurse who is interested in the extension of nurse prescribing rights will appreciate the significance of the Crown Report, which proposed a new framework for prescribing, supply and administration of medicines inside and outside the NHS and made three main recommendations:

1. The majority of patients continue to receive medicine on an individual patient basis.
2. The current prescribing authority of doctors, dentists, and certain nurses (in respect of a limited list of medicines) continues.
3. New groups of professionals would be able to apply for authority to prescribe in specific clinical areas, where this would improve patient care and patient safety could be assured.

  It is the third recommendation, that a 'new group of professionals' who currently do not have prescribing rights might apply for this authority to be extended to them and this can happen in two ways:

1. Independent prescribing

    This is identified as someone who is responsible for assessment of patients with undiagnosed conditions and for decisions about the clinical management required, including prescribing (DH 1999 p 39).
    Children's nurses who are currently prescribing from the Children's Nurse

Formulary can continue to do so. However, nurses not currently able to prescribe, who are in a position to undertake the assessment of patients with undiagnosed conditions (e.g. hypokalaemia) and make a prescribing decision (e.g. potassium added to fluids can become newly legally authorized independent prescribers). This will entail a childrens' nurse to undertake a relevant nurse prescribing course. There is a larger space definition in the page above.

2. Dependent prescribing

Crown defines the dependent prescriber as someone who does not have the diagnostic and assessment ability to make a decision about an initial prescription, but will have sufficient knowledge to determine whether that prescription should be continued, or whether to alter the dosage. Furthermore, a dependent prescriber may still be able to prescribe a drug for the first time, but this would be within the parameters of clinical guidelines for a given condition, and the care plan of a patient. This is about protocol arrangement.

There is no reason in the area of children's nursing whereby practitioners would consider themselves working at specialist level could, by undertaking a recognized accredited nurse prescriber course, become an independent or dependent prescriber.

6.2 Medicines management

Safe use of medicines

This includes the clinical, cost effective and safe use of medicines to ensure patients get

the maximum benefit from the medicines they need, while at the same time minimizing potential harm or side effects of the drug (www.mhra.gov.uk).

Healthcare professionals must adhere to the five 'rights' medication administration (NMC 2008). These are:

Right medication – check the name of medication against the prescription.
Right patient – check the name against the prescription and verify with parent/carer.
Right dose – check that the dose is correct for the age of the child.
Right route – check that the route is correct for the child and that the correct medication has been prescribed.
Right time and frequency – check that time and frequency of the drug is correct for the child.

The key contributors to the management of medicines are:

- The primary care trust
- social services, care workers, home help
- primary care pharmacist
- care home staff
- GPs and practice staff
- families and carers
- voluntary organizations
- hospital and all staff
- community pharmacy
- community nurses.

This list shows the complexity of the number of people and organizations involved in the delivery of safe and effective medicines management.

The nurses' role in medicines management:

- interpretation of prescription
- assessing the child

- administering the drug prescribed
- communicating with the child and family, other health care professionals, e.g. doctors and pharmacists
- providing information about the drug to the family, e.g. action and side effects, when to take it
- teaching and support for the patient, e.g. being a patient advocate
- anticipate any potential side effects
- monitor the drug for effectiveness, the patient's response to the medication
- evaluate and review the response to the drug treatment e.g. blood pressure, nausea
- record the administration of the drug
- report any changes in the child after administration of the drug
- this may involve:
  - diagnosis
  - solving any problems
  - prioritization
  - analysis of the child's condition.

Most nurses see medicine management as just their involvement in the task of its administration. Yet nurses do more than this; they facilitate the engagement of patients and their families, so enabling them to make what they see as best use of their prescribed medicines.

The key priorities influencing and directing medicines management are:

- National standards framework (NSF) – these are national standards for key conditions and diseases, which are central to improving quality of services to patients.

- Management of medicines – a resource to support implementation of the wider aspects of medicines management for the NSFs for diabetes, renal services and long-term conditions.

- National Institute for Clinical Excellence (NICE) – provides patients, health professionals and public with guidance on best practice for some medicines and treatments

- The expert patient programme – NHS-based training initiative that provides people with new skills to manage their condition.

- The medicines partnership programme, which supports patients and professionals to enable patients to be more involved in decisions about their medicines.

These priorities are proposed to give patients informed choice and control over care, allowing medicines management to be more personalized and encourages patients, health professionals to work together.

Polypharmacy

There is no widely accepted definition, but in the UK when four or more medicines are prescribed for an individual this is considered as polypharmacy (DH 2001). A child with multiple diseases and complicated medicine regimes may affect a child and their family's ability to manage their own medication regime.

The reasons for polypharmacy are:

- multiple pathologies – a child may have more than one condition
- multiple prescribers – patients may see several doctors and nurses each of whom may prescribe
- self medication – some children may take over-the-counter, herbal and homeopathic medicines given by their parents or carers

- misuse – there may be confusion following discharge and patients may continue to take their previous regime as well as the new regime

- expectations – many patients (parents) expect to leave a consultation with a prescription in their hand.

There needs to be improvement in this area of medicines management:

- non-compliance with prescribed medications

- large quantities of unused medicines returned to pharmacies

- increase in admissions attributed to adverse drug reactions

- poor control of chronic conditions despite effective medicines being available

- unmet patient and carer needs for information concerning treatment

- poor review of treatment

- patients not tolerating side effects that affect their quality of life.

The nurses' role in improving medicines management:

- Ensuring treatment is evidence based – using the NICE guidelines to ensure consistence of care, involvement of a nurse specialist or nurse prescriber.

- When treatments are stopped – the nurse needs to co-ordinate care to ensure unwanted medicines are not continued to be prescribed.

- Identify where under treatment is occurring – children may benefit from additional medicines and identify where under treatment is occurring

- Managing the introduction of new drugs – nurses need to be involved in decisions regarding new treatments, this will involve examining the evidence of effectiveness, the clinical significance of benefit, advantages over existing treatment and cost-effectiveness.

- Monitoring medicine taking – conducting a medication review, encouraging discussion between the health care professional and the child and parent and offer the an opportunity to ask questions such as:
  – are medicines being taken?
  – are they being taken correctly?
  – does the child or parent understand how to take their medication?
  – will a change in dose affect the child's lifestyle in any way?

- Treatment review – some people have reported not being asked about their medicines by their doctor or other health care professional.

Concordance

Concordance advocates a partnership approach to medicine prescribing and taking, and suggests:

- Negotiation between equals.

- It must be recognized that children and parents can make their own decisions about whether or not to take a prescribed treatment.

- That it must be acknowledged that well-informed children and parents may decline treatment after learning about the relative benefits and risks.

- That a child/parents' beliefs about their medicines are likely to be the most important consideration in whether to take their medications or not.

- More involvement of the child and parents.

Concordance means:

- Children and parents should have enough knowledge to participate as partners:
  - children and parents are helped to access information about their condition
  - the relevant medication which is based on their needs, clear, accurate and in sufficient detail
  - children and parents need information about:
    • what the medication is for and what it does
    • how to use it
    • the dos and don'ts
    • side effects and what to do about them
    • how to tell if the medicine is working
    • information about the disease or condition
    • this information will need to be tailored to individuals
- Prescribing consultations involve the child and their parents as partners:
  - children and parents are involved in treatment decisions
    • children and parents are invited to talk about their diagnosis and to express any concerns
    • professionals explain the agreed treatment fully
    • children and parents are invited to talk about their understanding of and ability to follow treatments.
  - children and parents are supported in taking medication:
    • all opportunities are used to discuss medicines and medicine taking
    • children and parents are asked for their views on how their treatment is progressing
    • information is effectively shared between professionals

- medicines are reviewed regularly with child and parents
- practical issues in taking medicines are addressed.

Compliance

Compliance describes the patients' medicine taking in relation to the prescribers' instructions. The reasons for non-compliance (BNF 2008) can be complex but involves the following:

- difficulty in taking the medication
- child or parents forgets
- child and parents make a conscious decision not to take the medicine
- treatment regime is complicated, instructions and purpose of medication unclear
- unpleasant taste, side effects are perceived to be risky
- child and parents are having difficulty coming to terms with the diagnosis
- complicated lifestyle
- certain health beliefs of the family
- a child and families support network
- the cost of the medicines
- breakdown in communication between services e.g. hospital and home
- poor knowledge levels.

6.3 Classification of drugs used in children

The classification of drugs (Table 6.1) is massive and is thus too huge to do it all justice. The classes of drugs outlined in

Table 6.1 Classes of drugs

Class of drug	Action of drug class
Anti-emetic	Nausea, vomiting
Anti-coagulant	Prevent or reduce clotting of the blood in blood vessels, e.g. heparin or warfarin
Antiplatelet	Decrease platelet aggregation – aspirin and dipyridamole
Antihypertensive	Used to reduce blood pressure – examples are beta-adrenergic antagonists (beta blockers) such as atenolol, ACE inhibitors such as captopril, calcium channel blockers, e.g. nifedipine and diuretics such as bendrofluazide
Analgesic	Relieves pain
Hypnotic	Induces sleep – dependency producing, e.g. triazolam.
Anxiolytic	Relieves anxiety – used to alleviate acute and severe anxiety states, e.g. diazepam
Anaesthetic	Insensible stimuli – loss of sensation Local anaesthesia – sensory nerve impulses are blocked and the patient remains alert General anaesthesia – loss of consciousness and patient is unaware of and unresponsive to painful stimulation, can be maintained by inhalation of anaesthetic gases
Antibiotic	Anti-bacterial: length of treatment depends on the nature of the infection and the response to treatment, e.g. penicillin, ampicillin, erythromycin, metronidazole and vancomycin
Antacids	Neutralize the acidity of the gastric juice, given in dyspepsia, gastritis, peptic ulcer and oesophageal reflux
Anti-arrhythmic	Given to prevent or reduce cardiac irregularities of rhythm, e.g. digoxin, amiodarone
Antihistamine	Blocks the release of histamine – released in an allergic reaction, used for insect bites and stings to reduce irritation and inflammation
Antispasmodics	Relax smooth muscle as found in the gut – useful in abdominal colic and distension as in irritable bowel disorder
Antidepressant	Relieves depression – these may be tricyclics such as amitriptyline and imipramine or mono-amine oxidase inhibitors
Antipyretic	Reduces temperature – such as aspirin, paracetamol

(Continued)

Table 6.1 Classes of drugs—cont'd

Class of drug	Action of drug class
Antiepileptic	Epilepsy control – to prevent the occurrence of seizures, only one drug and combinations is to be avoided e.g. phenytoin, sodium valproate, carbamazepine
Bronchodilator	Dilates airways – relax the bronchial smooth muscle and cause dilatation of the air passages, e.g. salbutamol, Atrovent
Cytotoxic	Used in the treatment of cancer, e.g. methotrexate and vincristine
Corticosteroid	Synthetic steroid hormones synthesized by the adrenal cortex – anti-inflammatory and suppress the immune system
Diuretic	Increases urine output – best given in the morning, e.g. furosemide, bendrofluazide, reduce the circulating volume in heart failure and hypertension
Fibroinolytic	Digest fibrin in blood clots – used to dissolve the blood clot and restore circulation to the heart following myocardial infarction, e.g. streptokinase
Immunosuppressive	Suppress the immune system and are used in autoimmune disorders or following transplantation to reduce rejection of the donor organ, e.g. azathioprine
Inotrope	Affect the contraction of the heart muscle, e.g. digoxin.
Laxative	Promote a softer or bulkier stool or to encourage a bowel action, given for constipation, e.g. lactulose
Miotic	Constrict the pupil of the eye – used in glaucoma to open up drainage channels, e.g. pilocarpine.
Muscle relaxant	In conjunction with general anaesthetics to produce complete muscle relaxation, prevent muscles from contracting, stop respiration for ventilation, e.g. atracurium and vecuronium.
Neuroleptic	Acts on nervous system, antipsychotic
Vasodilator	Dilates blood vessels to reduce BP
Hypoglycaemic agent	Glucagon to treat hypoglycaemic states
Hyperglycaemic agents	Insulin for intravenous and subcutaneous use in type I diabetes
	Oral drugs for the use in type II diabetes

this section are brief. However, there are many texts (Neal 2004, Galbraith et al 2007, BNF for children updated twice per year) that go into much more detail regarding the drugs used in children. For further information it is recommended that you use these and/or others for more in-depth information.

Poisoning/overdose

This may be encountered in children of any age, but the causes differ.

Neonatal poisoning

- Usually as a result of therapeutic doses of drugs or self-poisoning in the late stages of labour. Could be due to the miscalculation of doses.

Children

- Accidental poisoning is commonest between the ages of 1 and 5 years when children like to explore the environment with their mouths as well as their eyes and fingers!

Older children

- Usually as a result of a mishap at school or at work, e.g. inhalation of gases or fumes from organic solvents or ingestion whilst pipetting.

Deliberate self-poisoning

- This is the commonest form of poisoning in adults, but it is not uncommon below the age of 15.

Diagnosis

Unlike adults children are not always able to tell us what they have taken but the presence of signs and symptoms may help to see how severe the poisoning is:

- The time to diagnosis is imperative limiting the period from ingestion to supportive treatment is important.
- Always consider the level of consciousness and neurological signs.
- Consult with parents, relatives, friends, general practitioners and pharmacists who may provide valuable information.
- Check:
  - haemodynamic status
  - body temperature
  - body surface – head or body injury, venepuncture marks
- Investigations:
  - urinalysis
  - chest X-ray
  - electrolytes and creatinine
  - ABC analysis.
- Drug levels, e.g. paracetamol and paraquat.

Removal and lavage

- Gastric lavage is rarely required and the benefits outweigh the risks to the child and only considered if a large amount of the drug can be life threatening and only if ingested within the preceding hour.
- Bowel irrigation – it is unclear if this procedure improves outcome and advice should be sought.

- Administration of laxatives alone has no role in the management of the poisoned child and is not recommended as a method of gut decontamination (BNF 2005).

Prevention of absorption

- Activated charcoal given by mouth can reduce the effects of many poisons in the gastrointestinal system reducing their absorption. The earlier this is given the more effective it is. It may still be effective up to one hour after ingestion of the poison.

- A second dose may be necessary if blood levels of the drug continue to increase. For specific drugs and their antidotes see Table 6.2.

Toxbase is the primary clinical toxicology database of the National Poisons Information service and is available on the internet to registered users only (www.spib.axl.co.uk). This service provides information about routine diagnosis, treatments and management of children exposed to drugs, household products and industrial and agricultural chemicals.

Central nervous system drugs

Anxiolytics and hypnotics

These groups of drugs are used for sleep disorders (anxiolytics) and acute anxiety states (hypnotics), dominated by the benzodiazepines, which:

- induce sleep when given in high doses

- provide sedation and reduce anxiety when given in low, divided doses during the day.

The role of drug therapy is the management of anxiety disorders in children and adolescents is uncertain and administered only by specialists.

Benzodiazepines have been used but adverse effects may be problematic in children and so are not used for children.

Hypnotics and anxiolytics may impair judgement and increase reaction time, and so affect ability to drive or

Table 6.2 Administration of specific overdose and antidote

Drug	Antidote
Paracetamol	Acetylcysteine, methionine (Parvolex)
Anticholinesterase	Atropine
Narcotic	Naloxone (Narcan)
Benzodiazepine	Flumazenil (Anexate)
Heparin	Protamine sulphate
Digoxin	Antidigoxin antibodies (Digibind), atropine, phenytoin (Epanutin)
Warfarin	Vitamin K

perform skilled tasks and may impair performance during the day when taken at night.

Hypnotic drugs

- Chloral hydrate – for night sedation, sedation for painful procedures, long-term sedation.

Anxiolytics

- Diazepam – night terrors, status epilepticus, febrile convulsions, muscle spasm, perioperative.

Antipsychotic drugs

This group of drugs relieves psychotic symptoms such as thought disorder, hallucinations and delusions and can prevent relapse:

- Clozapine is used when other antipsychotics are ineffective or not tolerated.

- Chlorpromazine is still widely used, despite the side effects, but is useful in treating violent children. Used in:
  - childhood schizophrenia and other psychoses
  - relief of acute symptoms of psychoses but with caution
  - induction of hypothermia
  - neonatal abstinence syndrome.

- Haloperidol may be preferable for rapid control of hyperactive psychotic states:
  - motor tics (including Gilles de la Tourette syndrome)
  - schizophrenia and other psychoses
  - mania
  - short-term adjunctive management of psychomotor agitation, excitement and violent or dangerously impulsive behaviour.

Antimanic drugs

These drugs are used in mania, both to control acute attacks and also to prevent their recurrence:

- Benzodiazepines may be useful in the early stages of treatment until lithium achieves its full effect.

- Antipsychotic are drugs used in an acute attack.

- Lithium salts are used in the:
  - prophylaxis and treatment of mania,
  - prophylaxis of bipolar disorder (manic-depressive disorder)
  - prophylaxis of recurrent depression (unipolar illness or unipolar depression) and only under specialist advice in children.

- Advise children should maintain adequate fluid intake and avoid dietary changes that reduce or increase sodium intake.

Antidepressants

Used in children with depression and anxiety and the major classes and should take into consideration existing therapy, suicide risk and previous response to antidepressant therapy:

- Tricyclic antidepressants (such as amitriptyline hydrochloride) are used in depression and nocturnal enuresis.

- Selective serotonin re-uptake inhibitors (such as fluoxetine) are effective in depressive illness in children. Many other drugs in this group, e.g. citalopram, escitalopram, paroxetine and sertraline have failed to show benefits and have an increase in harmful outcomes.

Table 6.3 Centrally acting analgesic receptor sites

Endogenous opioid	Receptor type	Major locations	Effects of binding
Not known	Delta	Limbic system – emotions	Behavioural changes Hallucinations
Enkephalin	Epsilon	Hippocampus Amygdala	Dysphoria Psychotic effects
Dynorphin	Kappa	Hypothalamus	Hypothermia Miosis Sedation Analgesia
Endorphin	Mu	Dorsal horn of spinal cord Thalamus	Analgesia Respiratory depression Euphoria

- Other drugs used for attention deficit hyperactivity disorder:
  - atomoxetine for attention deficit hyperactivity disorder should only be prescribed by a specialist managing the condition
  - methylphenidate for attention deficit hyperactivity disorder is initiated by a specialist
  - dexamphetamine sulphate for hyperkinesias is initiated by a specialist.

Analgesic drugs

A child with many medical or surgical conditions, wounds, palliative care all stimulate pain receptors and can lead to severe/moderate/mild pain. The children's nurse in this situation (if applicable) has to assess the level of pain using the appropriate pain assessment tool and administer prescribed medication. However, when there is severe pain together with other changes observed narcotic analgesics may be prescribed. These drugs mimic endogenous opioids by causing prolonged activation of the opiate receptors. The body produces endogenous opioids, which suppress centrally controlled pain mechanisms:

- endorphins
- enkephalins
- dynorphins.

Centrally acting analgesics all act upon receptors within the CNS; there are at least four different receptors for these compounds (Table 6.3). This produces analgesia, respiratory depression, euphoria and sedation. Assessment tools and patient controlled analgesia may be added as soon as the initial emergency is over.

Morphine

Morphine can be used for severe pain following trauma or cancer. Morphine does not only relieve pain, but also relieves the anxieties related to it and gives a sense of euphoria. The analgesic effects start within 20 minutes when given by subcutaneous injection and within 10 minutes of intravenous infusion. The vasodilation produced by morphine may result in hypotension, particularly if administered as a bolus dose. Discontinuation of morphine can cause withdrawal effects such as: sweating, pupillary dilation, lacrimation, rhinorrhoea, tachycardia, tachypnoea, pyrexia, hypertension, vomiting, abdominal pain, diarrhoea, yawning, muscle pains, joint pains, restlessness, irritability, and anxiety.

- Morphine has a short half-life of about 4 hours; therefore frequent dosing is required; this is shortened to 2 hours when given as single doses of 0.1 mg per kg. Morphine can be administered by either continuous infusion or repeated intermittent doses.

- Infants younger than 6 months in the postoperative period should receive continuous morphine infusions starting at 0.01 mg/kg per hour (BNF for children 2008).

- Children as well as infants older than 6 months of age who require opioids during the postoperative period should receive continuous morphine infusions starting at 0.025–0.04 mg/kg per hour (Wood et al 2002).

- As with rectal administration, the oral use of morphine poses setbacks due to variations in bioavailability and initial onset.

- Side effects include: itching, nausea, vomiting, urinary retention, constipation and respiratory depression.

- Respiratory depression warrants the most concern, but severe forms are rarely reported and can be avoided through careful dosage regimens and observation.

Codeine

Codeine is related to morphine but is less potent. Codeine is partly converted into morphine in the liver. Approximately 10% of the population is lacking the enzyme responsible for this conversion (Galbraith et al 1999), which explains why some patients gain little pain relief from high doses of codeine. Thus, codeine is not commonly used on its own, but it is prescribed as an antidiarrhoeal and enhances the analgesic activity of paracetamol and aspirin and is often combined with them.

Diamorphine

Depresses the exaggerated respiratory effort, reduces the child's distress and helps redistribute some of the increased cerebral blood volume to the peripheries. Diamorphine is generally given intravenously for a rapid effect, as orally it is less effective as it is almost completely converted into morphine. Diamorphine is the choice for severe pain when reduced respiratory functioning can lead to severe complications. It can be administered by subcutaneous syringe driver if oral morphine sulphate (MST) can no longer be tolerated.

Pethidine

The analgesic effect of pethidine is not as strong as morphine, but it is widely used for moderate to severe pain, as it causes less respiratory depression. It is useful in labour as it does not suppress uterine contractions, but fetal respiratory rate can be affected. Pethidine is not recommended for long-term use due to its metabolite norpethidine, which can lead to serious convulsions.

Fentanyl

Fentanyl is commonly used as a neuroleptoanalgesic due to its short duration of therapeutic action, which allows patients to recover quickly from its effects and it is popular in the use of maintenance of ventilation.
Its characteristics are:

- synthetic opioid with approximately 100 times the analgesic potency of morphine

- relatively short half-life of 30–60 minutes

- highly soluble lipid so rapid onset of action

- a reduced incidence of hypotension

- clearance is affected by hepatic blood flow

- in neonates the duration of action is prolonged as the central nervous system is more sensitive to its effects.

Entonox (nitrous oxide)

- Homogeneous gas containing 50% nitrous oxide and 50% oxygen

- Anaesthetic gas so should be administered in theatre

- Effective analgesia for short-term relief for children undergoing painful procedures

- Potent analgesic

- Very soluble so fast acting.

Naloxone

Naloxone is a pure antagonist at the opioid receptors and can be used to reverse narcotic analgesia in the case of overdose. The result can be quite dramatic, but the drug only has a half life of 1 hour, and therefore in cases of overdose the patient

needs to remain under observation for a considerable time.

Other narcotic analgesics

- Methadone – used as a morphine or heroin substitute as it produces fewer withdrawal symptoms.

Nonsteroidal anti-inflammatory drugs (NSAIDs) and paracetamol

This group of drugs has in various degrees analgesic, anti-inflammatory and antipyretic actions. NSAIDs have the ability to inhibit cyclo-oxygenase (COX) and the resulting inhibition of prostaglandin synthesis, which is an enzyme critical for the stimulation of the inflammatory responsible and responsible for their therapeutic effects.

- Diclofenac – oral, suppository and can be given by injection safely. Very appropriate as pre-emptive analgesics. Prostaglandin inhibitors and reduce the local tissue response to injury.

- It should be noted that NSAIDs have a ceiling effect and their long-term use may lead to gastrointestinal bleeding and irritation, renal dysfunction, platelet inhibition and bone marrow suppression.

- Mild analgesics – ibuprofen, aspirin and paracetamol.

- Moderate analgesics – diclofenac and naproxen.

- Strong analgesic – change to indomethacin equal to or superior to naproxen.

Other analgesic drugs available

- Paracetamol – no anti-inflammatory action, usually tried first. In overdose give acetylcysteine and protects the liver if given within 24 hours of ingestion, most effective within 8 hours.

- Codeine and dihydrocodeine – stronger than paracetamol but more side effects.

- Paracetamol + codeine phosphate (co-codamol).

- MST for acute pain over short periods (modified release formulation) of morphine, not suitable for acute pain (12 hourly).

Topical anaesthetics

- EMLA/Ametop cream applied for 1 hour under occlusive dressing.

- Lidocaine gel, ointment or spray may be used to provide analgesia after circumcision.

- Tetracaine (amethocaine) used for cornea, skin and oropharynx.

Other anaesthetics

- Wound instillation – Marcain (bupivacaine) solution.

- Peripheral nerve block: Marcain (bupivacaine) solution – 8 hours action

- Regional block: larger areas can be anaesthetized by blocking nerve plexuses, e.g. brachial plexus and spinal blocks.

- Intradural (spinal) – local anaesthetic deposited into the cerebrospinal fluid at lumbar puncture affects the spinal cord and nerve roots directly.

- Extradural (epidural) – solution is placed in the space surrounding the dura at thoracic, lumbar or sacral (caudal) levels.

Antiepileptic drugs

Epilepsy is a chronic disease in which seizures result from the abnormal discharge of cerebral neurones. The seizures are classified empirically and the correct classification is important as it determines the choice of drug treatment (see Section 4).

The aim of treatment is to control the seizures with one drug, but sometimes combination therapies are required only when single therapy with several alternative drugs has proved ineffective:

- carbamazepine and oxcarbazepine will control tonic–clonic and partial seizures, neuropathic pain and some movement disorders

- ethosuximide for absence seizures, myoclonic seizures

- phenytoin can be used for all types of epilepsy with the exception of absence seizures

- valproate is similar to phenytoin but should not be used in children under 2 years old

- vigabatrin can be given in combination with other antiepileptic treatment or the sole treatment of infantile spasms.

- the benzodiazepines, e.g. clonazepam – can also be used but have a sedative effect.

Drugs used in status epilepticus

- Diazepam – also used in febrile convulsions, convulsions caused by poisoning.

- Lorazepam – this is the initial treatment, diazepam can be used, but lorazepam has a longer duration of antiepileptic action.

- Phenytoin can be given slowly intravenously with ECG monitoring. Alternatively fosphenytoin can be given more rapidly but still requires ECG monitoring.

- Paraldehyde also remains useful, as it can be given rectally and when resuscitation facilities are poor.

Endocrine drugs

Hypoglycaemic agents

Prompt treatment is required in children from any cause:

- Initially glucose 10–20 g is given by mouth.

- Hypoglycaemia that causes unconsciousness or fitting is an emergency and glucagon (a polypeptide hormone produced by the alpha cells of the islets of Langerhans in the pancreas), increases plasma-glucose concentration by mobilizing glycogen stored in the liver. It can be given by injection. It is used to treat drug-induced hypoglycaemic states where intravenous glucose cannot be administered. Nausea is a principal side effect, and the preparation needs to be protected from light.

- Chronic hypoglycaemia is useful in management of children with chronic hypoglycaemia from excess insulin secretion from an islet cell tumour or hyperplasia, e.g. diazoxide.

Hyperglycaemic agents

There are two different types – parenteral and oral:

1. Parenteral – insulin administered IV or subcutaneously – used in type I diabetes:
   - The greater the concentration of zinc or the presence of protamine in the insulin preparation, the more prolonged the duration and delayed the action of the insulin itself.
   - Sources of insulin – bovine (ox), porcine (pig) and human (genetically modified for commercial use).
   - Types:
     • soluble insulin (short acting):
       • bovine or porcine neutral – Hypurin
       • human - Actrapid, Velosulin, Humulin S, Insuman
     • intermediate and long-acting insulin
       • isophane insulin for twice daily insulin injections and may be mixed with soluble insulin
       • insulin zinc suspension (crystalline) has a more prolonged duration of action
       • protamine zinc insulin given once daily, but now rarely used
       • insulin detemir (once or twice daily) and insulin glargine (once daily)
     • biphasic insulin – premixed insulin preparations containing various combinations of short-acting (soluble) and rapid-acting (analogue) insulin and an intermediate acting insulin:
       • biphasic insulin aspart intermediate acting insulin, e.g. NovoMix

- biphasic insulin lispro intermediate acting insulin, e.g. Humalog
- biphasic isophane insulin intermediate acting insulin, Mixtard.

2. Oral hypoglycaemic agents are used in type II diabetes mellitus, and should only be prescribed to a child if they fail to respond adequately to restriction of energy and carbohydrate intake and an increase in physical activity. However, type II diabetes mellitus does not usually occur until adolescence and so treatment using anti-diabetic drugs in children is limited:
   - Sulphonylureas are not the first choice and are used when metformin is contraindicated or not tolerated:
     - stimulate the release of insulin from the pancreas
     - inhibit the process of gluconeogenesis (forming glucose from amino acids and fatty acids) in the liver
     - increase the number of insulin receptors on target cells
     - adverse effects – hypoglycaemia overdose, allergy, depression of bone marrow and gastrointestinal disturbances
     - available – tolbutamide.
   - Biguanide (metformin)
     - acts by promoting glucose uptake into cells through enhanced insulin-receptor binding
     - slows absorption of glucose from the gut
     - inhibits glucagon secretion and stimulates tissue glycolysis
     - adverse effects – drug tolerance and acidosis.

Thyroid and antithyroid drugs

Thyroid hormones are used in hypothyroidism (juvenile myxoedema) and in non-toxic goitre, congenital or neonatal hypothyroidism and Hashimoto's thyroiditis (lymphadenoid goitre):

- levothyroxine sodium – drug of choice for maintenance therapy
- liothyronine sodium – similar to levothyroxine but is more rapidly metabolized.

Antithyroid drugs are used for hyperthyroidism either to prepare children for thyroidectomy or for long-term management. However, treatment must be undertaken by a specialist:

- Carbimazole is the most commonly used drug; can lead to bone marrow suppression and if there are any signs of neutropenia treatment needs to stop immediately.
- Propylthiouracil may be used when the child suffers sensitivity reactions to carbimazole.
- Iodine is used as an adjunct before partial thyroidectomy; radioactive sodium iodide is used increasingly for the treatment of thyrotoxicosis at all ages.
- Propranolol is useful for rapid relief of thyrotoxic symptoms and used in conjunction with antithyroid drugs or to radioactive iodine.
- Thyrotoxic crisis is an emergency needing intravenous fluids, propranolol and hydrocortisone as sodium succinate, as well as oral iodine solution and carbimazole or propylthiouracil, which may need to be administered via nasogastric tube.

Posterior pituitary hormones and antagonists

Diabetes insipidus is caused by a deficiency of antidiuretic hormone (ADH, vasopressin) secretion (cranial, neurogenic or pituitary diabetes insipidus) or failure of the renal tubules to react to secreted ADH (nephrogenic diabetes insipidus).

- Vasopressin is used in the treatment of pituitary diabetes insipidus, dosage is to produce a regular diuresis every 24 hours. Treatment may be required permanently or for a limited time such as in diabetes insipidus following trauma or pituitary surgery. In addition it can be used in acute massive haemorrhage of the gastrointestinal tract or oesophageal varices.

- Desmopressin is more potent and longer lasting than vasopressin. It can also be used as a test for suspected diabetes insipidus.

Respiratory drugs

Bronchodilators

Selective beta$_2$ adrenoceptor agonists used in asthma act on beta$_2$ receptors in the lungs; stimulation of these causes:

- bronchodilation to help breathing
- increased skeletal muscle excitability
- vasodilation of blood vessels to the brain, heart, kidneys and skeletal muscle
- stabilization of the membrane of the mast cells preventing the release of inflammatory mediators
- beta$_2$-agonists are usually given by inhalation

- adverse effects include fine tremor, nervous tension and tachycardia, but this is usually a problem when the drug is given by inhalation

- drugs include:
  - salbutamol (Ventalin)
  - terbutaline
  - formoterol – used for long-term regular bronchodilator therapy.

Beta$_2$ antagonist bronchodilators such as ipratropium (Atrovent) by nebulizer may be added to the treatment of asthma when standard therapy fails to improve a child's condition. However, beta$_2$ agonists act more quickly.

Theophylline is a bronchodilator used for chronic asthma. When added in conjunction with small doses of beta$_2$ agonists the combination may lead to an increased risk of side effects such as hypokalaemia. Theophylline is generally given by slow intravenous infusion, and the theophylline level needs to be kept constant to prevent complications.

Glucocorticoids

These effectively increase the airway calibre in asthma. Steroids act by reducing bronchial mucosal inflammatory reactions (e.g. oedema, mucus hypersecretion) and by modifying the allergic reactions of asthma and anaphylaxis. These include:

- betamethasone – local treatment of short-term inflammation
- hydrocortisone acetate – can be given orally, more common use intravenously (shock, status asthmaticus), topically (eczema)
- prednisolone – orally for inflammatory and allergic diseases
- dexamethasone – used in inflammatory and allergic disorders.

They have many adverse effects:

- metabolic effects such as redistribution of fat to the face and trunk, tendency to bruise easily, disturbed carbohydrate metabolism may lead to hyperglycaemia and occasionally diabetes, wasting and weakness, osteoporosis
- fluid retention
- adrenal suppression
- infections due to immunosuppressive effects of glucocorticoids
- peptic ulceration.

Antihistamines

The term antihistamine is usually reserved for use when describing the H_1 blockers or antagonists (Table 6.4). They are used in the treatment of:

- allergies
- nausea
- symptoms of the common cold
- influenza
- skin allergies or insect bites and are used topically.

A common side effect of these drugs is they can lead to drowsiness so patients should be advised not to drive or operate hazardous machinery:

- cetirizine and loratadine are less likely to cross the blood–brain barrier and lead to drowsiness
- promethazine is good at promoting drowsiness – it is commonly used as a sedative.

Antituberculous drugs

Tuberculosis is treated in two phases

1. Initial phase using at least three drugs used to reduce the bacterial population as rapidly as possible and prevent drug-resistant bacteria and can be required for longer than 2 months. The drugs of choice are:
   - isoniazid
   - rifampicin
   - pyrazinamide.
2. Continuation phase using two drugs. This is continued for a further 4 months with:
   - isoniazid
   - rifampicin.

Table 6.4 Antihistamine receptors

Receptor	Receptor abb.	Major locations	Effects of binding
Histamine	H_1	Smooth muscle and exocrine glands and respiratory tract	Used in the treatment of allergies and prevent release of histamine from mast cells, acid production
	H_2	Parietal cells of the stomach	Prevents the release of acid from the stomach H_2 antagonist

Treatment should be under supervision by a specialist paediatrician especially in families in whom concordance may be problematic. Compliance with therapy is a major determinant of its success and incorrect prescribing by physicians. Urine examination (rifampicin gives an orange-red coloration) and may be an indicator of compliance with treatment.

> ⚠ Tuberculosis involves resistant organisms and may affect non-respiratory organs.

Cardiovascular drugs

Sympathomimetics (adrenergic receptor stimulation/agonist)

These drugs are within the domain of sympathetic nervous system function. The properties vary according to whether they act on alpha or beta adrenergic receptor sites and can vary considerably in children. It is important to titrate the dose to the desired effect and closely monitor the child.

Inotropic sympathomimetics

- Epinephrine (adrenaline) acts on both alpha and beta adrenergic receptors; others include, dopamine hydrochloride, dobutamine (Table 6.5). They:
  - increase rate and force of contraction of the heart, increase cardiac output and exact positive chronotropic and inotropic effects
  - increase level of lipid concentration in blood
  - depress digestion and gastrointestinal motility.
- Dopamine is a naturally occurring neurotransmitter, acting on B_1 receptors in cardiac muscle:
  - it increases cardiac contractility of heart with little effect on heart rate
  - a low dose acts on dopamine receptors in the kidneys and increases renal perfusion

Table 6.5 Dose of IM epinephrine from anaphylactic shock

Age	Dose	Volume injection 1 in 1000 (1mg/ml)
Under 6 years	150 micrograms	0.15 ml
6–12 years	300 micrograms	0.3 ml
12–18 years	500 micrograms	0.5 ml

Repeat every 5 minutes if necessary

- increased doses cause vasoconstriction and exacerbate heart failure
- it increases systolic pressure
- it is titrated to blood pressure
- dosage is calculated in μg/kg/min
- the drugs should be changed if results are not satisfactory.

■ Dopexamine – artificial, primarily effective on beta-receptors, improves renal blood flow, increases mean arterial blood pressure and cardiac output.

■ Dobutamine – artificially formulated, B_1 agonist. Has an inotropic effect without increase in heart rate and making heart work faster; has a more inotropic effect than chronotropic effect, sometimes used in cardiogenic shock.

■ Isoprenaline – increases heart rate and contractility, used for short-term treatment of heart block and bradycardia.

Epinephrine (adrenaline)

Anaphylaxis is a systemic immediate hypersensitivity reaction caused by an immunoglobulin (Ig) E-mediated immunological release of mediators of mast cells and basophils, and with potentially life-threatening consequences. For epinephrine (adrenaline) doses in children see Table 6.5. The focus here is on medicines and epinephrine (adrenaline) provides physiological reversal of the immediate symptoms (BNF for children 2005):

■ Adrenaline – increases systolic blood pressure, heart rate, force of contraction. Also used in acute anaphylactic reactions –intramuscular adrenaline is effective as an emergency measure.

■ There has been an increasing use of medicines and antibacterials leading to an increase in medicine induced anaphylaxis and anaphylactoid reactions.

■ Other causative agents are NSAIDs, anaesthetics, muscle relaxants, latex and radio contrast media.

Anaphylaxis is often unpredictable and so we need to focus on how to decrease risks. Strategies:

■ Ensure a detailed patient history and full physical examination is done,

■ Consider the route of the medicine and the rate of the medicine and/or fluid flow.

■ Identification of patients with known causes of anaphylaxis.

■ Sound knowledge of the medicine, as some cross react and also are contraindicated if there is a known history of anaphylaxis.

■ The greater number of years since the last administration of the offending agent, the less the chance of a recurrence.

■ The parenteral route increases the severity and frequency of a reaction, so review the choice of the medicine and route, and if the patient still needs IV route, they remain under medical supervision for 20–30 minutes after medicine administration.

Recommendations:

Immediate actions following anaphylaxis depends on the severity of the reaction and these can range from a mild skin reaction to cardiovascular collapse.

■ discontinue suspected medicine

■ get help, resuscitation call (MET/ outreach/resuscitation team)

- administration of epinephrine (adrenaline):
  - IM route – has a rapid onset of action quicker than if given subcutaneously (dosages of epinephrine (adrenaline) IM are given in Table 6.5)
  - IV route – reserved for extreme emergency when doubt about adequacy of circulation and absorption from the intramuscular site.
- administer oxygen and IV fluids
- start ABCDE
- start CPR if no pulse
- monitor patient; oxygen saturation, vital signs, ECG
- if conscious, will be very anxious, and so nurses' role would be to provide reassurance and adequate information and communication
- at least 2 hours' observation if mild and in severe cases at least 24 hours monitoring of the patient
- ensure prompt and appropriate reporting and recording in the patient case records and consideration of the Yellow Card Reporting scheme, which advocates the reporting of adverse medicine reactions
- the patient will require advice for the future and this might include: the use of a Medic-Alert (e.g. bracelet) ID system and an Epinephrine kit.

Vasoconstrictor sympathomimetics

- Act directly on beta$_1$ adrenoreceptors. Indirect action by causing a release of norepinephrine (noradrenaline) from the stores at nerve endings (amphetamines):
  - preventing reuptake of norepinephrine (tricyclic antidepressants – amitriptyline)
  - preventing destruction of norepinephrine – monoamine oxidase inhibitors
  - preventing the release of norepinephrine – guanethidine
  - causing nerve endings to synthesize a false transmitter – methyldopa.
- Raise blood pressure by acting on alpha$_1$ receptors in the peripheral blood vessels and is used when other emergency methods of raising blood pressure has failed (BNF for children 2005). If infusions of high doses are required to raise blood pressure this can be at the expense of the perfusion of other vital organs (e.g. the kidneys). Drugs include:
- norephinephrine (noradrenaline)
- ephedrine hydrochloride
- metaraminol
- phenylephrine hydrochloride.

Adrenoreceptor (adrenergic receptor blocking/antagonists)

The uses of adrenoreceptor antagonists in children is limited to only a few. Beta receptor antagonists:

- Block the beta receptors in the heart, peripheral vasculature, bronchi, pancreas and liver.
- Have little effect on heart rate, cardiac output or arterial pressure at rest; they reduce the effect of excitement or exercise on these.

- Reduce coronary blood flow, but less oxygen consumption, oxygenation is improved.
- Reduce the force of cardiac contraction and slow the heart rate; they can precipitate heart failure in patients with weak contractility.
- Have an anti-hypertensive effect – produce a gradual fall in blood pressure over a period of several days.
- Increase airways resistance – dangerous in children with asthma and can produce severe asthma attacks, should be avoided.

These drugs act selectively on either alpha or beta receptors, they do not usually act on both. They slow the heart and can depress the myocardium and can be used for:

- hypertension – labetalol
- arrhythmias – esmolol, sotalol
- heart failure – carvedilol
- thyrotoxicosis – propranolol
- tetralogy of Fallot – esmolol or propranolol.

Parasympathomimetic drugs

- Action similar to those of the parasympathetic nervous system and act on cholinergic receptors:
  - carbachol – used in urinary retention, causes contraction of the bladder muscle.
  - anticholinesterases potentiate the transmission of anticholinesterase at the neuromuscular junction
  - physostigmine prevents the breakdown of acetylcholine by inhibiting the enzyme cholinesterase, causes constriction of the pupil, used in glaucoma, use replaced in myasthenia gravis by neostigmine
  - neostigmine – synthetic substance, direct effect on the neuromuscular junction of voluntary muscle and less effect on the eye
  - muscarinic antagonists – weak central stimulant but at high doses causes a tachycardia – atropine.

Other inotropes

The positive inotropic effect of these drugs is to increase the contractility of the cardiac muscle and so improve cardiac function and increase cardiac output.

- The only inotrope used in cardiac failure is digoxin, which is also an anti-arrhythmic drug:
  - increases the force of cardiac contraction in the failing heart
  - particularly effective in heart failure caused by atrial fibrillation.
  - can lead to drug toxicity.

Antihypertensive drugs

Angiotensin-converting enzyme (ACE) inhibitors

- These drugs act by inhibiting the renin–angiotensin system by preventing the conversion of angiotensin I to angiotensin II by ACE therefore preventing the formation of angiotensin II. This process is overactive in heart failure:
  - captopril
  - enalapril
  - cilazapril
  - lisinopril
  - perindopril
  - quinapril
  - ramipril.

- They reduce aldosterone and so increase sodium loss and thus water loss.
- They also vasodilate, which reduces the strain on the failing heart by reducing the preload and the afterload.
- Proven to be beneficial in heart failure:
  - dyspnoea reduced
  - exercise tolerance increased
  - hospital care reduced
  - life expectancy in increased in moderate to severe heart failure.
- Other potential value:
  - may improve coronary blood flow at the same time as decreasing oxygen demand.

Adverse effects:

- hypotension
- renal damage – regular monitoring is essential
- cough – dry productive worse at night
- skin rash
- aplastic anaemia – rarely.

Vasodilator drugs

These drugs act directly on the smooth muscle of the blood vessels or block the calcium channels in the muscle membrane.

Calcium antagonists

These have actions on the heart by increasing the refractory period of the heart, lengthening the period of time calcium remains in the cardiac cell during depolarization. They relieve angina, mainly by causing peripheral arteriolar dilatation and afterload reduction. Increasingly they are replacing hydralazine in the use of hypertension. The drugs include:

- nifedipine in patients who have a related bronchospasm or left ventricular failure
- diltiazem only a slight negative inotropic effect less potent than nifedipine
- verapamil used in SVT.

Can lead to flushing, dizziness, headaches and oedema of the ankles.

Nitrates

Their main effect is to cause peripheral vasodilation, especially in the veins, by a direct action on the vascular smooth muscle.

Glyceryl trinitrate (GTN) is generally short acting and lasts for about 30 minutes:

- a rapid acting drug that causes coronary vasodilatation and ventilation promoting more oxygen rich blood to move towards the heart
- acts by dilating both veins and arteries reduces the filling pressure of the heart as well as the resistance against which the heart has to pump
- consequently, myocardial work and oxygen demand is reduced
- suffers from first pass effect when given orally and is thus given by other routes:
  - sublingually
  - transdermally
  - intravenously
- it has a very short duration of action, but onset of action is rapid – within 2 minutes.
- there are longer-acting nitrates whose onset of action is later (30 minutes):
  - isosorbide mononitrate
  - isosorbide dinitrate

Adverse effects – the vasodilator effect, can produce a headache and flushing, these can be severe, palpitations and hypotension.

Nitropresside

This is used for severe hypertension crisis, acts by direct action vasodilatation of smooth muscle, quick acting, reduces systemic vascular resistance of both veins and arteries.

Diuretics

Diuretics cause an increased secretion of urine in the kidneys. They all produce their effect by decreasing the reabsorption of water and electrolytes by the renal tubules and thus allowing more to be excreted. The kidney filters about 100 litres of fluid per day, but only 1500 ml is lost as urine.

They are useful in the following conditions:

- heart failure
- hypertension
- nephrotic syndrome
- cirrhosis of the liver
- acute pulmonary oedema
- oedema formation from heart disease and cirrhosis
- hypercalcaemia and occasionally in hyperkalaemia.

Types of diuretics

- Ingestion of water – fails to work in heart failure.
- Osmotic diuretics – mannitol increases osmotic pressure in filtrate and causes more water to be excreted, used in:
  – forced diuresis in drug overdose
  – cerebral oedema
  – maintain diuresis during surgery.

- Xanthines – theophylline, caffeine, a weak diuretic action.
- Thiazide diuretics – relatively weak diuretics, inhibit sodium/chloride reabsorption in the early segment of the distal tubule, chlorothiazide, hydrochlorothiazide, bendrofluazide. May lead to hypokalaemia, increased uric acid and cholesterol levels.
- Loop diuretics – most powerful of all diuretics – capable of causing 15–25% of the sodium filtrate to be excreted. Action similar to thiazide, but sodium/chloride reabsorption takes place in the ascending loop of Henle, a very rapid onset of action but of fairly short duration, powerful and can cause electrolyte imbalance, dehydration and hypovolaemia, e.g. furosamide, bumetanide, ethacrynic acid.
- Potassium-sparing diuretics – weak when used alone, but cause potassium retention, often given with a thiazide or loop diuretic to prevent hypokalaemia:
  – triamterene, amiloride – work on the distal tubule and the collecting ducts.
  – frumil is a combination of frusamide and amiloride.
  – spironolactone – an aldosterone antagonist.

Antiarrhythmic drugs

The rhythm of the heart is generally determined by the pacemaker cells in the sinoatrial node, but it can be disturbed in many ways leading to discomfort to heart failure or even death (Neal 2004):

- Serious arrhythmias, e.g. ventricular tachycardia are associated with heart disease.

- Supraventricular arrhythmias arise in the atrial myocardium or atrioventricular node.
- Ventricular arrhythmias may be caused by ectopic focus, which starts firing at a higher rate than the normal pacemaker.
- Re-entry mechanisms can occur, where action potentials are delayed for some pathological reason, re-invade nearby muscle fibres leading to a loop of depolarization.

Many antiarrhythmic drugs are generally local anaesthetics or calcium antagonists, but they are generally classified into those which are effective in:

- supraventricular arrhythmias:
  – adenosine
  – digoxin
  – verapamil
- ventricular arrhythmias
- lidocaine, both types
  – disopyramide quinidine
  – flecainide amiodarone.

Antiplatelet drugs

In the situation where there is some type of clotting disorder, it is possible to use drugs that interfere with blood coagulation processes and thus reduce or prevent further thrombus formation.

Aspirin

- Used to reduce platelet aggregation, thus reducing the chances of increasing or causing clots in patients at risk of stroke.
- Works by inhibiting the production of thromboxane produced by the platelets from prostaglandin precursors, which is a powerful inducer of both aggregation of platelets and vasoconstriction.

Fibrinolytic agents

These drugs are used in children to dissolve intravascular thrombi and unblock occluded shunts and catheters. Treatment should be started immediately. The safety and efficacy of treatment remains uncertain especially in neonates. The three drugs used are alteplase, streptokinase and urokinase.

Streptokinase

- Streptokinase is an exotoxin from β-haemolytic streptococci and a potent plasminogen activator, and when given in large doses as a short infusion it accelerates the conversion of plasminogen to plasmin.
- This breaks down fibrin within the clot forming soluble fibrin degradation products (FDP), leading to the dispersal of the thrombus.
- The treatment must preferably be performed as soon as possible after the onset and can re-establish blood flow in approximately 3 minutes.
- It is administered via intravenous infusion over a period of one hour. Streptokinase has a half-life of approximately 20 minutes.
- Patients may have antibodies to streptokinase, from a streptococcal infection or if they have received streptokinase previously.
- There is a general agreement that streptokinase should not be administered again within 2 years.
- In 1–2% of patients, signs of an allergic reaction may develop, such as urticaria, wheezing or even hypotension and anaphylaxis.
- Streptokinase is contraindicated in patients with severe hypertension and in those with a history of blood

disorders or stroke and children who have had streptococcal infection in the last 12 months.

- The main risk factor with treatment is the risk of bleeding as fibrinolysis is increased.

Alteplase (t-PA)

- Alteplase is an endogenous enzyme found in vascular endothelium.
- Alteplase activates plasminogen and is used to dissolve clots, and hinder new thrombosis formation to help reduce mortality.
- The plasma half-life is 5–8 minutes and unlike streptokinase repeated dose is possible.
- Alteplase is the agent of choice for patients who have previously received streptokinase.

Anticoagulants

Parenteral anticoagulants

Heparin works fast because it binds to plasma anti-thrombin III, which is a natural anticoagulant in the blood. In so doing it inactivates thrombin, plasmin and other serine proteases of coagulation. The amount of heparin required to produce anticoagulant effect depends on each individual and their activated partial thromboplastin time (APPT).

- The normal APPT is 40 seconds.
- The concentration of heparin will prolong APTT from 2–2.5 times over the control value, this should be maintained and measured 6 hourly.
- Can suffer from haemorrhage, cot apnoea and hypertensive reactions; patients require regular measure of BP and heart rate.

- Urine and stools are closely monitored for any signs of blood.
- If overcoagulation of heparin occurs, the effect may be rapidly reversed by administration of protamine sulphate.

Low molecular weight heparins (LMWH)

These include Dalteparin, enoxaparin and tinzaparin can be used as a prophylaxis. It has been identified that the advantage of LMWH is that they do not need close monitoring of blood coagulation tests in older children and minimal monitoring is required in younger children and neonates. It has a longer life therefore requiring once a day dosage.

Oral anticoagulants

Warfarin is prescribed while heparin is running because it takes about 8–12 hours to deplete clotting factors. This highlights the need for warfarin to be started in conjunction with heparin in order to initiate the start of the effect of warfarin in the system before taking the patient off of heparin.

Patients on warfarin need to be warned about bleeding disorders that may occur, especially bleeding of the gums when brushing teeth, excessive or easy skin bruising and unexplained nose bleeds due to the reduced effect of platelets and coagulation factors. Occurrence of any of the above factors would mean a withdrawal from the drug, which restores normal clotting factors.

The vital signs the nurse has to look for include when a patient appears to be in shock or having difficulty in breathing and pain

- Warfarin is measured as a ratio compared with a standard PTT. A standard level represents 25% of the normal rate and this should be maintained for a longer-term therapy.

- Warfarin should be omitted if normal activity is less than 20% until activity rises to above 20%. The international normalized ratio (INR) represents the target levels of 2.5–3.5 to be recommended.

- Blood tests need to be taken regularly to determine the maintenance dose prescribed.

- A recommendation of INR was to be measured once monthly, as it is the recommendation for long-term patients. Once a patient has suffered a PE, the risk of recurrence is high.

- Warfarin given after heparin therapy should continue for at least 6 months as recurrent multiple emboli may require lifelong therapy.

> For warfarin poisoning vitamin K is given slowly intravenously as an antidote. This reverse may take several hours' therefore, in urgent cases fresh frozen plasma is given.

Renal drugs

Urinary incontinence

Involuntary detrusor muscle contractions cause urgency and urge incontinence, usually with frequency of micturition and nocturia. Antimuscarinic drugs may reduce these contractions and increase bladder capacity. Use of these drugs should be reviewed every 3 months:

- Oxybutynin has a direct relaxant effect on urinary smooth muscle and should be considered first for children under 12 years. However, side effects limit the use of oxybutynin, but can be reduced by starting with a low dose and titrating it upwards

- Tolterodine is effective in urinary incontinence and may be considered for children over 12 years or if younger children have failed to respond to oxybutynin.

Nocturnal enuresis

This is a common occurrence in young children but may persist in as many as 5% by 10 years of age. Treatment is not appropriate in children under 5 years and not needed in those aged under 7, however, children over 10 usually require prompt treatment:

- Desmopressin is an analogue of vasopressin and can be used for nocturnal enuresis; it can be given intranasally or by mouth. Desmopressin should not be continued for longer than 3 months without stopping for a full assessment.

Gastrointestinal tract drugs

Antiemetic

- Metoclopramide is a dopamine antagonist that stimulates gastric emptying; it is used to treat nausea and vomiting.

■ Prochlorperazine is a phenothiazine that is widely used as an antiemetic; it is less sedative than chlorpromazine.

Antacids

These usually contain aluminium or magnesium compounds, are all weak bases and rapidly combine with hydrochloric acid and neutralize it. They give short-term relief of symptoms of ulcer dyspepsia and non-erosive gastro-oesphageal reflux in children. Antacids raise the gastric luminal pH, provide effective but short relief of dyspepsia and symptomatic relief in peptic ulcer, gastritis and oesophageal reflux and heartburn. These are usually basic compounds of:

■ aluminium hydroxide

■ magnesium trisilicate

■ aluminium–magnesium complexes, e.g. hydrotalcite

■ compound alginate antacids thicken in the stomach and float on the surface of the contents to reduce reflux and protect the oesophageal mucosa, used in the management of mild gastro-oesphageal reflux (e.g. Gaviscon, Rennies).

Sucralfate

Sucralfate has minimal antacid properties and is a combination of sugar sucrose and aluminium, which only acts in the presence of acid. Once ingested it forms a thick paste like substance, which adheres to the gastric mucosa protecting it from acid. It is not licensed for children but may be used to prevent ulceration in children in intensive care.

Antispasmodics

These include antimuscarinics and alter gut motility, used to be termed anticholinergics. Can be used in the management of irritable bowel syndrome but response varies. They have other uses, for example for asthma, motion sickness, premedication or palliative care. When used for gastrointestinal smooth muscle spasm these include:

■ dicycloverine hydrochloride

■ propantheline bromide

■ hyoscine butylbromide – Buscopan.

Histamine H$_2$ receptor antagonists

These work by reducing gastric acid output as a result of histamine H$_2$-receptor blockade, they can relieve dyspepsia and gastro-oesophageal reflux.

■ Histamine H$_2$-receptor antagonists (cimetidine and ranitidine) block the action of histamine on the parietal cells and reduce acid secretion.

■ Cimetidine has been found to slow down metabolism of many other drugs, resulting in enhancement of their effects.

Antidiarrhoeal drugs

Antimotility drugs relieve symptoms of acute diarrhoea, not recommended in children under 12 years old. They are generally used in uncomplicated acute diarrhoea.

Infectious diarrhoea is a common cause of illness or a complication of some interventions, such as antibiotics, enteral feeding. Antimotility drugs are used to provide symptomatic relief:

- loperamide or Imodium are generally used
- codeine phosphate also reduces bowel motility.

Laxatives

Laxatives are used to increase motility of the gut and encourage defecation. They should be discouraged unless prescribed by a doctor:

- Bulk laxatives – increase the volume of intestinal contents stimulating peristalsis e.g. ispaghula husk, methylcellulose.
- Stimulant laxatives – increase motility by acting on mucosa or nerve plexuses, which can cause damage in prolonged use, e.g. bisacodyl, Dahntron, glycerol, senna
- Lubricants – promote defecation by softening and/or lubricating faeces and assisting evacuation, e.g. arachis oil, liquid paraffin.
- Osmotic laxatives – increase the amount of water in the large bowel, either by drawing fluid from the body into the bowel or by retaining the fluid they were administered with, e.g. lactulose, macrogols, magnesium salts, phosphates (rectal), sodium citrate (rectal).

Anaesthetics

General anaesthetics

These drugs lead to the absence of sensation associated with a reversible loss of consciousness. Anaesthesia depresses all excitable tissues including central neurones, cardiac muscle, smooth and striatal muscle. However, it is possible to administer anaesthetic agents at concentrations that produce unconsciousness without unduly depressing the cardiovascular and respiratory centres of the myocardium:

- Intravenous anaesthetics are thiopental and propofol – unconsciousness occurs within seconds and is maintained by the administration of an inhalation anaesthetic such as halothane.
- Inhaled anaesthetics include halothane – unconsciousness maintained by this inhalation anaesthetic, replaced by less toxic agents such as desflurane and isoflurane
- Nitrous oxide is used in the maintenance of anaesthesia with concentrations of 50–70% in oxygen is a widely used anaesthetic agent in combination with other drugs – causes sedation and analgesia but not sufficient alone to maintain anaesthesia.

Muscle relaxants

Anaesthetists in theatre and in intensive care use muscle relaxants to relax skeletal muscles during surgical operations and to prevent movement and breathing during mechanical ventilation. These drugs are given intravenously and distributed in the extracellular fluid.

Neuromuscular blocking agents compete with acetylcholine for muscle receptors but do not initiate ion channel opening, these include:

- Pancuronium – has a long duration of action, an atropine like action on the heart and can lead to a tachycardia.

- Vecuronium – it depends on hepatic inactivation and recovery takes 20–30 minutes so it is popular for short procedures.
- Atracurium – has a duration action of 15–30 minutes, it is only stable when kept cold and at low pH. At body pH and temperature it decomposes spontaneously in plasma and does not depend on renal or hepatic function for its elimination; good for patients with renal or hepatic disease.

Depolarizing blockers act on acetylcholine receptors, but trigger the opening of ion channels and are not reversed by anticholinesterases. The only drug of this type used is:

- suxamethonium – rapid onset and very short duration of action (3–7 minutes).

Sedative and analgesic perioperative drugs

- For sedation for clinical procedures and include diazepam, lorazepam, midazolam and temazepam
- Non-opioid analgesics such as the NSAIDs diclofenic or ibuprofen
- Opioid analgesics such as alfentanil or fentanyl.

Immune system drugs and vaccines

These are used to prevent tissue rejection after organ transplantation and to treat autoimmune diseases:

- prednisolone is used in combination with azathioprine.

- mycophenolate mofetil, ciclosporin and tacrolimus are potent immunosuppressants that are used with prednisolone.

These drugs have serious adverse effects and like cytotoxic drugs increase a patient's vulnerability to infection.

Infections

Antibacterial drugs

Antibiotics work in three different ways:

1. Inhibit nucleic acid synthesis.
   - Sulphonamides – their use has decreased as a result of increasing bacterial resistance and are being replaced by antibacterials, which are generally more active and less toxic, e.g. co-trimoxazole, trimethoprim.
2. Inhibit cell wall synthesis.
   - Penicillin
     • benzylpenicillin, most staphylococci are resistant to benzylpenicillin; flucloxacillin remains active and can be given orally or by injection
     • broad-spectrum penicillin – amoxicillin, ampicillin
     • antipseudomonal penicillins – piperacillin, ticarcillin
     • metronidazole is an antimicrobial drug and works against anaerobic bacteria and protozoa – an alternative when patients are allergic to penicillin.
   - Cephalosporins – cefadroxil (for urinary tract infections), cefuroxime (as a prophylactic in surgery), ceftazidime and ceftriaxone.

- Vancomycin – septicaemia or endocarditis can cause renal failure and hearing loss.
3. Inhibit protein synthesis
   - Aminoglycosides – gentamicin, amikacin, netilmicin, tobramycin streptomycin.
   - Tetracyclines – tetracycline, minocycline, doxycycline, oxytetracycline
   - Macrolides – erythromycin and clarithromycin
   - Chloramphenicol – broad-spectrum antibiotic associated with serious haematological side-effects and is reserved for life-threatening infections caused by *Haemophilus influenzae* and typhoid fever. Eye drops are available.

Antifungal and antiviral drugs

Fungal infections may be superficial or systemic; the later occurring in immunocompromised patients such as those with acquired immune deficiency syndrome (AIDS).

- Amphotericin is highly toxic.
- Nystatin is too toxic for parenteral use; it is mainly used in the treatment of thrush and applied to mucous membranes as a cream or ointment or suspension in the mouth or pessaries in the vagina.
- Flucytosine.
- Imidazoles.
- Triazoles – fluconazole.

Viruses are intracellular and are small and lack independent metabolism. They can replicate only within living host cells. Vaccines are generally the major method for controlling viral infections (poliomyelitis, rabies, measles, mumps, rubella). Some effective antiviral drugs have been developed and act in two different ways:

1. Stop the virus entering or leaving the host cell:
   - amantadine
   - zanamivir.
2. Inhibit nucleic acid synthesis:
   - acyclovir – selectively antiviral
   - antiretroviral drugs – used to suppress the replication of human immunodeficiency virus in patients with AIDS

References

ACT, 2003. A guide to the development of children's palliative care services. Association for Children with Life-threatening or Terminal Conditions and their families (ACT). Bristol, UK.

Advanced Life Support Group, 2005. Advanced paediatric life support: the practical approach (4th Edition). Blakwell Publishing, London.

Allen, D., Gillen, E., Rixson, L., 2009. Systematic review of the effectiveness of integrated care pathways: what works, for whom, in which circumstances? International Journal of Evidence Based Healthcare 7 (2), 61–74.

Allen, H.D., Driscoll, D.J., Shaddy, R.E., Feltes, T.F., 2008. Moss and Adams' heart disease in infants, children and adolescents, including fetus and young adults (7th Edition). Lippincott; Williams and Wilkins, Philadelphia.

Ambuel, B., Hamlett, K.W., Marx, C.M., Blumer, J.L., 1992. Assessing distress in the pediatric intensive care environments: the COMFORT scale. J. Pediatr. Psychol. 17, 95–109.

American Thoracic Society, 2000. Care of the child with a chronic tracheostomy. Am. J. Respir. Crit. Care Med. 161, 297–308.

Ashwal, S., 2004. Pediatric vegetative state: Epidemiological and clinical issues. NeuroRehabilitation 19, 349–360.

Asmussen, K., 2010. Key facts about child maltreatment. National Society for the Prevention of Cruelty to Children, London.

Baines, P., 2008. Medical ethics for children: applying the four principles to paediatrics. J. Med. Ethics 34 (3), 141–145.

Barker, P., 2004. Basic child psychiatry, seventh ed. Blackwell Publishing, Oxford.

Bear, L.A., Ward-Smith, P., 2006. Interrater reliability of the COMFORT Scale. Pediatr. Nurs. 32, 427–434.

Beckwith, S., Franklin, P., 2007. Oxford handbook of nurse prescribing. Open University Press, Oxford.

Bee, H.L., Boyd, D., 2009. The developing child. Allyn & Bacon, New York.

Birchley, G., 2010. What limits, if any, should be placed on a parent's right to consent and/or refuse to consent to medical treatment for their child? Nurs. Philos. 11 (4), 280–285.

Blew, H., Kenny, G., 2006. Attention deficit hyperactivity disorder: the current debate and neglected dimensions. J. Child Health Care 10, 251–263.

Boud, D., Keogh, R., Walker, D. (Eds.), 1985. Reflection: turning experiences into learning. Kogan Page, London.

Bowlby, J., 1952. Maternal child care and mental health. World Health Organization, Geneva.

Bowlby, J., 1980. Attachment and Loss, vol. 3. Penguin, London.

Bowlby, J., Ainsworth, M., Boston, M., Rosenbluth, D., 1956. The effects of mother–child separation: A follow-up study. Br. J. Med. Psychol. 29, 211–247.

Breen, M., 2010. Parents of children who died from their brain tumours share common challenges during the neurological deterioration of their child, including balancing competing responsibilities and talking to their child about death. Evid. Based Nurs. 14, 7–8.

Brewer, S., Gleditsch, S.L., Syblik, D., Tietjens, M.E., Vacik, H.W., 2006. Pediatric anxiety: Child life intervention in day surgery. J. Pediatr. Nurs. 12 (1), 13–22.

British Thoracic Society, 2008. Guidelines for emergency oxygen use in adult patients. Thorax 63 (Suppl. V1), vi1–vi73.

British National Formulary, 2008. BNF for children. BMJ Publishing Group, London.

Butler, V., 2005. Non-invasive ventilation (NIV) an adult audit across the north central London critical care network (NCLCCN). Intensive Crit. Care Nurs. 21 (4), 243–256.

Cancer Research UK, 2010a. CancerStats key facts: childhood cancer. Cancer Research UK, London.

Cancer Research UK, 2010b. Childhood cancer – Great Britain & UK. Cancer Research UK, London.

Carnevale, F.A., Razack, S., 2002. An item analysis of the COMFORT scale in a pediatric intensive care unit. Pediatr. Crit. Care Med. 3, 177–180.

Carpenter, K.D., 1991. Oxygen transport in the blood. Crit. Care Nurse 11 (9), 20–31.

Casey, D., 2007. Nurses' perceptions, understanding and experiences of health promotion. J. Clin. Nurs. 16 (6), 1039–1049.

Cassidy, J., Shaver, P.R., 2008. Handbook of attachment: theory, research, and clinical applications. Guilford Press, New York.

Chambliss, C.R., Heggen, J., Copelan, D.N., Pettignano, R., 2002. The assessment and management of chronic pain in children. Pediatric Drugs 4, 737–746.

Chesson, R.A., Chisholm, D., Zaw, W., 2004. Counseling children with chronic physical illness. Patient Educ. Couns. 55, 331–338.

Children's Cancer and Leukaemia Group, 2010. Childhood cancer: Fact Sheet for general practitioners. Children's Cancer and Leukaemia Group, Leicester.

Cho, H.H., O'Connell, J.P., Cooney, M.F., Inchiosa, M.A., 2007. Minimizing tolerance and withdrawal to prolonged pediatric sedation: case report and review of the literature. J. Intensive Care Med. 22, 173–179.

Children's Workforce Development Council, CWDC, 2010. The children and young people's workforce: Refreshing the common core of skills and knowledge. CWDC, Leeds.

Clarke, D.J., Holt, J., 2001. Philosophy: a key to open the door to critical thinking. Nurse Educ. Today 21, 71–78.

Cochrane, H., Liyanage, S., Nantambi, R., 2007. Palliative care statistics for children and young adults. Department of Health, London.

Collishaw, S., Maughan, B., Natarajan, L., Pickles, A., 2010. Trends in adolescent emotional problems in England: a comparison of two national cohorts twenty years apart. J. Child Psychol. Psychiatry 51, 885–894.

Coyne, I.T., 2006. Children's experiences of hospitalisation. J. Child Health Care 10 (4), 326–336.

Craig, F., Abu-Saad Huijer, H., Benini, F., et al., 2008. Impact: Standards of paediatric palliative care in Europe. European Journal of Palliative Care 14 (3), 109–114.

Critchley, L.A., Oh, T.E., 1997. Electrical safety and injuries. In: Oh, T.E. (Ed.), Intensive care manual, fourth ed. Butterworth Heinemann, Oxford.

Dacie, J.V., Lewis, S.M., 1997. Practical haematology (8th Edition). Churchill Livingstone, Edinburgh.

Darke, J., Bushby, K., Le Couteur, A., McConachie, H., 2006. Survey of behaviour problems in children with neuromuscular diseases. Eur. J. Paediatr. Neurol. 10, 129–134.

Davies, R., 2005. Mothers' stories of loss: their need to be with their dying child and their child's body after death. J. Child Health Care 9 (4), 288–300.

De Jonghe, B., Cook, D., Appere-De-Vecchi, C., et al., 2000. Using and understanding sedation scoring systems: a systematic review. Intensive Care Med. 26L, 275–285.

Department of Health, 1999. Working together to safeguard children. HMSO, London.

Department of Health, 2001. The expert patient: a new approach to chronic disease management for the 21 Century. HMSO, London.

Department for Health and Children, DC, 2004. Ready, Steady, Play, National Play Policy. Department for Health and Children, DOHandC, Dublin.

Department of Health and Children, DOH, 2000a. Report of the Public Consultation for the National Children's Strategy. Department of Health and Children, Dublin.

Department of Health and Children, DOH, 2000b. The National Children's Strategy: our children – their lives. Department of Health and Children, Dublin.

Department of Health, DOH, 2003. Getting the right start: The National Service Framework for Children, Young People and Maternity Services – Standards for Hospital Services. Stationery Office, London.

Department of Health, DOH, 2004. Il child standard, National service framework for children, young people and maternity services. Department for Education and Skills, London.

Department of Health, DOH, 2008. Better Care Better Lives: Improving Outcomes and Experiences for Children, Young People and Their Families Living with Life-Limiting and Life-Threatening Conditions. Department of Health, London.

Department of Health, Department for Education and Skills, DfES, 2009. Healthy lives, brighter futures: The strategy for children and young people's health. DOH, London.

Diagnostic and Statistical Manual of Mental Disorders, fourth ed. 1999. American Psychiatric Association, Washington DC.

Dick, M.C., 2008. Standards for the management of sickle cell disease in children. Archives of Disease in Childhood – Education and Practice 93, 169–176.

Dick, M., Anie, K., Darbyshire, P., et al., 2006. Sickle cell disease in childhood. NHS Sickle Cell and Thalassaemia Screening Programme, London.

Doocey, A., Reddy, W., 2010. Integrated care pathways – the touchstone of an integrated service delivery model for Ireland. International Journal of Care Pathways 14 (1), 27–29.

Eaton, N., 2000. Children's community nursing services: models of care delivery. A review of the United Kingdom literature. J. Adv. Nurs. 32, 49–56.

Edgtton-Winn, M., Wright, K., 2005. Tracheostomy: A guide to nursing care. Aust. Nurs. J. 13, 17–20.

Edwards, S.L., 1998a. Hypovolaemia: pathophysiology and management options. Nurs. Crit. Care 3 (2), 73–82.

Edwards, S.L., 1998b. High temperature. Prof. Nurse 13 (8), 523–526.

Edwards, S.L., 1999. Hypothermia. Prof. Nurse 14 (4), 253–258.

Edwards, S.L., 2000. Fluid overload and monitoring indices. Prof. Nurse 15 (9), 568–572.

Edwards, S.L., 2001a. Regulation of water, sodium and potassium: implications for practice. Nurs. Stand. 15 (22), 36–42.

Edwards, S.L., 2001b. Shock: types, classifications and exploration of their physiological effects. Emerg. Nurse 9 (2), 29–38.

Edwards, S.L., 2002a. Myocardial infarction: nursing responsibilities in the first hour. Br. J. Nurs. 11 (7), 454–468.

Edwards, S.L., 2002b. Physiological insult/injury: pathophysiology and consequences. Br. J. Nurs. 11 (4), 263–274.

Edwards, S.L., 2003a. Cellular patho-physiology. Part 1: changes following tissue injury. Prof. Nurse 18 (10), 562–565.

Edwards, S.L., 2003b. Temperature regulation (Chapter 5). In: Brooker, C., Nicol, M. (Eds.), Nursing Adults: the practice of caring. Mosby, Edinburgh.

Edwards, S.L., 2003c. The formation of oedema. Part 1: pathophysiology, causes and types. Prof. Nurse 19 (1), 29–31.

Edwards, S.L., 2004. Compartment syndrome. Emerg. Nurse 12 (3), 32–38.

Edwards, S.L., 2005a. Pathophysiological mechanisms of shock (Chapter 13). In: O'Shea, R.A. (Ed.), Principles and practice of trauma nursing. Elsevier, Edinburgh.

Edwards, S.L., 2005b. Maintaining calcium balance: physiology and implications. Nurs. Times 101 (19), 58–61.

Edwards, S.L., 2006. Tissue viability: understanding the mechanisms of injury and repair. Nurs. Stand. 21 (13), 48–56.

Edwards, S.L., 2007. Critical thinking: a two-phase framework. Nurse Education in Practice 7, 303–314.

Edwards, S.L., 2008. Pathophysiology of acid base balance: the theory practice relationship. Intensive Crit. Care Nurs. 24, 28–40.

Edwards, S.L., Manley, K., 1998. Care of adults in hospital (Chapter 25). In: Hinchliff, S., Norman, S., Schober, J. (Eds.), Nursing practice & Health Care: a foundation text, third ed. Arnold, London.

Edwards, S.L., Sabato, M., 2009. A nurses' survival guide to critical care. Elsevier, Edinburgh.

References

Eiser, C., Eiser, J.R., Stride, C.B., 2005. Quality of life in children newly diagnosed with cancer and their mothers. Health Qual. Life Outcomes 3, 1–5.

Ellerton, M., Merriam, C., 1994. Preparing children and families psychologically for day surgery: An evaluation. J. Adv. Nurs. 19, 1057–1062.

Emerson, E., Hatton, C., 2007. Mental health and children and adolescents with intellectual disabilities in Britain. Br. J. Psychiatry 191, 493–499.

Endean, P., 2006. Unconscious patients. Nurs. Stand. 20, 67.

Finn, L., 1997. Nurses' documentation of infection control precautions: 2. British Journal of Nursing 6 (12), 678–684.

Fletcher, S., Dhrampal, A., 2003. Acid–base balance and arterial blood gas analysis. Surgery 21 (3), 61–65.

Frankenburg, W.K., Dodds, J.B., 1967. The Denver Developmental Screening Test. J. Pediatr. 71, 181–183.

Freebairn, R.C., Oh, T.E., 1997. Burns. In: Oh, T.E. (Ed.), Intensive care manual, fourth ed, Butterworth Heinemann, Oxford, pp. 622–630.

Freeman, N., Gazendam, J., Levan, L., Pack, A., Schwab, R., 2000. Abnormal sleep/wake cycles and the effect of environment noise on sleep disruption in the intensive care unit. American Journal of Respiratory and Critical Care Medicine 163, 451–457.

Friebert, S., 2009. Pain management for children with cancer at the end of life: beginning steps toward a standard of care. Pediatr. Blood Cancer 52 (7), 749–750.

Gailbraith, A., Bullock, S., Manias, E., Hunt, B., Richards, A., 1999. Fundamentals of pharmacology: a text for nurses and health professionals. Addison Wesley Longman Limited, London.

Gailbraith, A., Bullock, S., Manias, E., Hunt, B., Richards, A., 2007. Fundamentals of pharmacology: a text for nurses and health professionals (2nd Edition). Addison Wesley Longman Limited, London.

Galbraith, A., Bullock, S., Manias, E., Bunt, B., Richards, A., 2008. Fundamentals of pharmacology: an applied approach for nursing and health, second ed. Pearson Education, Edinburgh.

Gehlbach, B.K., Hall, J., 2007. Overview of mechanical ventilation. Merck Manual Online. Available from http://www.merck.com/mmpe/sec06/ch065/ch065b.html (accessed 20.02.12).

Giles-Corti, B., Salmon, J., 2007. Encouraging children and adolescents to be more active. Br. Med. J. 335 (10), 677–678.

Gillick v West Norfolk and Wisbech Area Health Authority 1985 3 All ER 402, 1985. Gillick v West Norfolk and Wisbech Area Health Authority.

Goldman, A., 2007. An overview of paediatric palliative care. Med. Princ. Pract. 16 (1), 46–47.

Grindstaff, R.J., Tobias, J.D., 2004. Applications of bispectral index monitoring in the pediatric intensive care unit. J. Intensive Care Med. 19, 111–116.

Guyton, A., Hall, J., 2000. Textbook of medical physiology, tenth ed. WB Saunders, Philadelphia PA.

Haggerty, L.A., Grace, P., 2008. Clinical wisdom: the essential foundation of 'good' nursing care. J. Prof. Nurs. 24 (4), 235–240.

Hain, R., Wallace, A., 2008. Progress in palliative care for children in the UK. J. Paediatr. Child Health 18 (3), 141–146.

Hanneman, S.K., 2004. Weaning from short-term mechanical ventilation. Crit. Care Nurse 24 (1), 70–73.

Harpin, V.A., 2005. The effect of ADHD on the life of an individual, their family, and community from preschool to adult life. Arch. Dis. Child. 90, i2–i7.

Harris, K.M., 2010. An integrative approach to health. Demography 47 (1), 1–22.

Hazinski, M., 1992. Nursing care of the critically ill child (4th Edition). Mosby, St Louis.

Hockenberry, M.J., Barrers, P., 2007. Communication and physical and developmental assessment of a child. In: M.J. Hockenberry and D. Wilson (Editors), Wong's nursing care of infants and children. Mosby Elsevier, Missouri.

Hooker, L., Milburn, M., 2000. Taking practice forward in paediatric oncology: the impact of a newly developed education programme for nurses working in shared-care hospitals. Eur. J. Oncol. Nurs. 4, 48–54.

Howard, R.F., 2003. Current status of pain management in children. J. Am. Med. Assoc. 290, 2464–2469.

Holm-Knudsen, R.J., Rasmussen, L.S., 2009. Paediatric airway management: basic aspects. Acta Anaesthesiol. Scand. 53 (1), 1–9.

Holmes, O., 1993. Human acid–base physiology: a student text. Chapman & Hall Medical, London.

Horgan, M.F., Glenn, S., Choonara, I., 2002. Infant distress scale. Journal of Child Health Care 6 (2), 96–106.

Holtzclaw, B.J., 1993. Monitoring body temperature. AACN 4 (1), 44–55.

Hulst, J., Joosten, K., Zimmermann, L., et al., 2003. Malnutrition in critically ill children: from admission to 6 months after discharge. Clin. Nutr. 23, 223–232.

Infection control nurses association, 1984. Report of an infection control nurses association working party. ICNA, London.

International Classification of Diseases, tenth ed. 1992. World Health Organization, Geneva.

International Council of Nurses, 2005. The ICN Code of Ethics for Nurses. International Council of Nurses, Geneva.

International Neonatal Network, 1993. The CRIB (clinical risk index for babies) score: a tool for assessing initial neonatal risk and comparing performance of neonatal intensive care units. Lancet 342, 193–198.

Ista, E., de Hoog, M., Tibboel, D., van Dijk, M., 2009. Implementation of standard sedation management in paediatric intensive care: effective and feasible? J. Clin. Nurs. 18, 2511–2520.

Jasper, E.V.P., 2008. Specimen collection. In: J. Kelsey and G. McEwing (Editors), Clinical skills for child health practice. Churchill Livingstone, London.

Jones, M. (Ed.), 2004. Nurse prescribing: politics to practice. Balliere Tindall, Edinburgh.

Jones, S.C., McVie, D., Noble, G., 2008. You are what your children eat: using projective techniques to investigate parents' perceptions of the food choices parents make for their children. The Open Communication Journal 2 (March), 23–28.

Justus, R., Wyles, D., Wilson, J., et al., 2006. Preparing children and families for surgery: Mount Sinai's multidisciplinary perspective. Pediatr. Nurs. 32, 35–43.

Kain, Z.N., Caldwell-Andrews, A.A., Mayes, L.C., et al., 2007. Family-centered preparation for surgery improves perioperative outcomes in children. Anesthesiology 106, 65–74.

Kaminski, M., Pellino, T., Wish, J., 2002. Play and pets: The physical and emotional impact of child-life and pet therapy on hospitalised children. Child. Health Care 31 (4), 321–335.

Keogh, S., 2004. Weaning ventilated children safely. Aust. Nurs. J. 11 (11), 39.

Kirk, S., 2001. Negotiating lay and professional roles in the care of children with complex health care needs. J. Adv. Nurs. 34, 593–602.

Kirk, S., Glendinning, 2002. Supporting 'expert' parents – professional support and families caring for a child with complex health care needs in the community. Int. J. Nurs. Stud. 39, 625–663.

Kirkham, F.J., Newton, C.R., Whitehouse, W., 2008. Paediatric coma scales. Development Medicine and Child Neurology 50 (4), 267–274.

Knight, K.M., McGowan, L., Dickens, C., Bundy, C., 2006. A systematic review of motivational interviewing in physical health care settings. Br. J. Health Psychol. 11, 319–332.

Krauss, B., Green, S.M., 2006. Procedural sedation and analgesia in children. Lancet 367, 766–780.

Limbers, C.A., Turner, E.A., Varni, J.W., 2008. Promoting healthy lifestyles: behavior modification and motivational interviewing in the treatment of childhood obesity. Journal of Clinical Lipidology 2 (3), 169–178.

Lindsay, G., Dockrell, J.E., Strand, S., 2007. Longitudinal patterns of behaviour problems in children with specific speech and language difficulties: child and contextual factors. Br. J. Educ. Psychol. 77, 811–828.

London Safeguarding Children Board, 2010. London Child Protection Procedures. London Safeguarding Children Board, London.

Longden, J.V., Mayer, A.T., 2007. Family involvement in end-of-life care in a paediatric intensive care unit. Nurs. Crit. Care 12 (4), 181–187.

Lundqvist, A., Nilstun, T., 2007. Human dignity in paediatrics: the effects of health care. Nurs. Ethics 14 (2), 215–228.

Lutman, D., Mok, Q., 2006. Airway management and chest drains. Great Ormond Street Hospital, London.

Lykkeslet, E., Gjengedal, E., 2006. How can everyday practical knowledge be understood with inspiration from philosophy? Nurs. Philos. 7 (2), 79–89.

Marieb, E., 2004. Human anatomy and physiology. Benjamin/Cumming, San Francisco.

Marieb, E., 2006. Essentials of human anatomy & physiology, eighth ed. Addison Wesley Longman, San Francisco.

McCulloch, R., Comac, M., Craig, F., 2008. Paediatric palliative care: coming of age in oncology? Eur. J. Cancer 44 (8), 1139–1145.

McCurry, M.K., Revell, S.M.H., Roy, C., 2009. Knowledge for the good of the individual and society: linking philosophy, disciplinary goals, theory, and practice. Nurs. Philos. 11 (1), 42–52.

Mesiano, G., Davis, M., 2008. Ventilatory strategies in the neonatal and paediatric intensive care units. Paediatr. Respir. Rev. 9, 281–289.

Middleton, S., Barnett, J., Reeves, D., 2001. What is an integrated care pathway? Evid. Based Med. 3 (3), 1–8.

Midson, R., Carter, B., 2010. Addressing end of life care issues in a tertiary treatment centre: lessons learned from surveying parents' experiences. J. Child Health Care 14 (1), 52–66.

Miller, J.F., 2006. Opportunities and obstacles for good work in nursing. Nurs. Ethics 13 (5), 471–487.

Milner, Q.J., Gunning, K.E., 2000. Sedation in the intensive care unit. British Journal of Intensive Care 10 (1), 12–17.

Monaghan, A., 2005. Detecting and managing deterioration in children. Paediatric Nursing 17 (1) 32–35.

Morgan, S., 1990. A comparison of three methods of managing fever in the neurologic patient. J. Neurosci. Nurs. 22 (1), 19–24.

National Institute of Clinical Excellence, 2007. Head injury: triage, assessment, investigation and early management of head injury in infants, children and adults. NICE clinical guideline 56, NICE, London

National Society for the Prevention of Cruelty to Children, 2010. Child protection factsheet: The child protection system in the UK, National Society for the Prevention of Cruelty to Children, London.

Navalesi, P., Fanfulla, F., Frigerio, P., Gregoretti, C., Nava, S., 2000. Physiologic evaluation of noninvasive mechanical ventilation delivered with three types of masks in patients with chronic hypercapnic respiratory failure. Crit. Care Med. 28 (6), 1785–1790.

National Institute for Health and Clinical Excellence, 2006. Methylphenidate, atomoxetine and dexamfetamine for attention deficit hyperactivity disorder (ADHD) in children and adolescents. National Health Service, Department of Health, London.

National Institute for Health and Clinical Excellence, 2008. Attention deficit hyperactivity disorder. National Health Service, Department of Health, London.

Neal, M., 2002. Medical pharmacology at a glance (4th Edition). Blackwell Sciences, Oxford.

Neal, M., 2004. Medical pharmacology at a glance (4th Edition). Blackwell Sciences, Oxford.

Nursing and Midwifery Council, 2004. Standards of proficiency for pre-registration nursing education. Nursing and Midwifery Council, London.

Nursing and Midwifery Council, 2007. Introduction of essential skills clusters for pre-registration nursing programmes. NMC Circular 07/2007. NMC, London.

Nursing and Midwifery Council, 2008. The code: Standards of conduct, performance and ethics for nurses and midwives. Nursing and Midwifery Council, London.

NMC, 2008. Standards for medicine management. NMC, London.

O'Brien, J.E., Birnkrant, D.J., Dumas, H.M., et al., 2006. Weaning children from mechanical ventilation in a post-acute care setting. Pediatr. Rehabil. 9 (4), 365–372.

Office for National Statistics, 2008. News release: Childhood stress link to emotional disorders. Office for National Statistics, Newport.

Paediatric Formulary Committee, 2005. British National Formulary for children. Pharmaceutical Press, London.

Palmer, A., Burns, S., Bulman, C., 1994. Reflective practice in nursing: the growth of the professional practitioner. Blackwell Scientific Publications, Oxford.

Panella, M., Vanhaecht, K., Sermeus, W., 2009. Care pathways: from clinical pathways to care innovation. International Journal of Care Pathways 13 (2), 49–50.

Parekh, S.A., 2006. Child consent and the law: an insight and discussion into the law relating to consent and competence. Child Care Health Dev. 33 (1), 78–82.

Parentline Plus, 2009. You can't say go and sit on the naughty step because they turn round and say make me'. Aggressive behaviour in children: parents' experiences and needs. Parentline, London.

Parker, L., 2000. Applying the principles of infection control to wound care. Br. J. Nurs. 9, 394–404.

Patel, D., Meakin, G.H., 2000. Paediatric airway management. Current Anaesthesia and Critical Care 11 (5), 262–268.

Peate, I., McGrory, C., 2009. Caring for the unconscious person. British Journal of Healthcare Assistants 3, 190–193.

Playfor, S., Jenkins, I., Boyles, C., et al., 2006. Consensus guidelines on sedation and analgesia in critically ill children. Intensive Care Med. 32, 1125–1136.

Pollack, M.M., Ruttiman, U., Getson, P.R., 1988. Pediatric risk of mortality (PRISM) score. Crit. Care Med. 16, 1110–1116.

Purvis, Y., Edwards, S., 2005. Initial needs of bereaved relatives following sudden and unexpected death. Emerg. Nurse 13 (7), 26–34.

Randolph, A.G., Wypij, D., Venkataraman, S.T., et al., 2002. Effect of mechanical ventilator weaning protocols on respiratory outcomes in infants and children: a randomized controlled trial. J. Am. Med. Assoc. 288 (20), 2561–2568.

Raphael, B., 2006. Grieving the death of a child. Br. Med. J. 332, 620–621.

Robinson, M., Cottrell, D., 2005. Health professionals in multi-disciplinary and multi-agency teams: changing professional practice. J. Interprof. Care 19 (6), 547–560.

Richards, A., Edwards, S., 2008. A nurse's survival guide to the ward, second ed. Churchill Livingstone, Edinburgh.

Richardson, P., 1996. Report of the WHO/ISFC task force on the definition and classification of cardiomyopathy. Circulation 93, 341–342.

Ridling, D.A., Martin, D.A., Bratton, S.L., 2003. Endotracheal suctioning with or without installation of isotonic sodium chloride in critically ill children. Am. J. Critical Care 12, 212–219.

Rossen, B.E., McKeever, P.D., 1996. The behavior of preschoolers during and after brief hospitalizations. Issues Compr. Pediatr. Nurs. 19, 121–133.

Royal College of Nursing, 2003. Standards for Infusion Therapy. RCN, London.

Royal College of Paediatrics and Child Health, RCPCH, Ethics Advisory Committee, 2000. Guidelines for the ethical conduct of medical research involving children. Arch Dis. Child. 82 (2), 117–182.

Ruland, C.M., Hamilton, G.A., Schjødt-Osmo, B., 2009. The complexity of symptoms and problems experienced in children with cancer: a review of the literature. J. Pain Symptom Manage. 37, 403–418.

Schon, D., 1983. The reflective practitioner: how professionals think in action. Guildford, Arena, New York.

Sellman, D., 2010. Mind the gap: philosophy, theory, and practice. Nurs. Philos. 11 (2), 85–87.

Simon, K., Lobo, M.L., Jackson, S., 1999. Current knowledge in the management of children and adolescents with sickle cell disease: part 1, physiological issues. J. Pediatr. Nurs. 14, 281–295.

Smith, L., Daughtrey, H., 2000. Weaving the seamless web of care: an analysis of parents' perceptions of their needs following discharge of their child from hospital. J. Adv. Nurs. 31, 812–820.

The Status Epilepticus Working Party, 2000. The treatment of convulsive status epilepticus in children. Arch. Dis. Child. 83, 415–419.

Steer, C.R., 2005. Managing attention deficit/hyperactivity disorder: unmet needs and future directions. Arch. Dis. Child. 90, i19–i25.

Streetly, A., Latinovic, R., Henthorn, J., 2010. Positive screening and carrier results for the England-wide universal newborn sickle cell screening programme by ethnicity and area for 2005–07. J. Clin. Pathol. 63, 626–629.

Suarez, M., Mullins, S., 2008. Motivational interviewing and pediatric health behavior interventions. J. Dev. Behav. Pediatr. 29, 417–428.

Taylor, L.K., Miller, M., Joffe, T., et al., 2010. Palliative care in Yorkshire, UK 1987–2008: survival and mortality in a hospice. Arch. Dis. Child. 95 (2), 89–93.

Telfer, P., Coen, P., Chakravorty, S., et al., 2007. Clinical outcomes in children with sickle cell disease living in England: a neonatal cohort in East London. Haematologica 92, 905–912.

Theunissen, N.C.M., Tates, K., Visser, A., 2004. Educating and counseling children about physical health. Patient Educ. Couns. 55, 313–315.

Thoburn, J., 2009. Effective interventions for complex families where there are concerns about, or evidence of, a child suffering significant harm. The Centre for Excellence and Outcomes in Children and Young People's Services (C4EO), London.

Thompson, W.R., 1990. Severe head injuries. In: Oh, T.E. (Ed.), Intensive care manual, third ed. Butterworths, Sydney.

Tingberg, B., Bredlöv, B., Ygge, B.M., 2008. Nurses' experiences in clinical encounters with children experiencing abuse and their parents. J. Clin. Nurs. 17 (20), 2718–2724.

United Nations, 1989. Convention on the Rights of the Child. United Nations, Geneva.

Vasey, J., 2009. Consent and refusal: selective respect for a young person's autonomy. Journal of Community Nursing 23 (4), 32–34.

Vincent, S., 2008. Child protection statistics: A UK comparison. University of Edinburgh/NSPCC Centre for UK-wide Learning in Child Protection, Edinburgh.

Watson, A.T., Visram, A.A., 2003. Children's preoperative anxiety and postoperative behavior. Paediatr. Anaesth. 13, 188–204.

Whitehead, D., 2009. Reconciling the differences between health promotion in nursing and 'general' health promotion. Int. J. Nurs. Stud. 46 (6), 23–28.

Whiting, L., Miller, S., 2009. Traditional, alternative and innovative approaches to health promotion for children and young people. Paediatr. Nurs. 21 (2), 45–51.

Wikstrom, B.M., 2005. Communicating via expressive arts: The natural medium of self-expression for hospitalised children. Pediatr. Nurs. 31 (6), 480–485.

Willis, D.G., Grace, P.J., Roy, C., 2008. A central unifying focus for the discipline: facilitating humanization, meaning, choice, quality of life, and healing in living and dying. Advances in Nursing Science 31 (1), E28–E40.

Wilne, S., Collier, J., Kennedy, C., et al., 2007. Presentation of childhood CNS tumours: a systematic review and meta-analysis. Lancet Oncol. 8, 685–695.

Wilson, M., 2005. Paediatric tracheostomy. Paediatr. Nurs. 17 (3), 38–44.

Woodnorth, G.H., 2004. Assessing and managing medically fragile children: Tracheostomy and ventilatory support. Lang. Speech Hear. Serv. Sch. 35, 363–372.

Woodrow, P., 2004. Arterial blood gas analysis. Nurs. Stand. 18 (21), 45–52.

Woodward, S., 2008. What do unconscious patients understand? British Journal of Neuroscience Nursing 4, 205.

Wong, M., Elliott, M., 2009. The use of medial orders in acute care oxygen therapy. Br. J. Nurs. 18 (8), 3–5.

Yucha, C., 2004. Renal regulation of acid-base balance. Nephrol. Nurs. J. 31 (2), 201–206.

Zelcer, S., Cataudella, D., Cairney, A.E.L., Bannister, S.L., 2010. Palliative care of children with brain tumors. Arch. Pediatr. Adolesc. Med. 164 (3), 225–230.

Appendix 1
Normal vital signs

Normal values of heart rate, blood pressure and respiratory rate				
Age of baby/ child	**Heart rate (beats/min)**	**Blood pressure (mmHg)**	**Blood pressure (mmHg)**	**Respiratory rate (breaths/ min)**
		Systolic	*Diastolic*	
Newborn (3 kg)	100–180	50–70	25–45	30–60
Infant	100–160	85–105	55–65	30–60
Toddler	80–110	95–105	55–65	24–40
Preschool	70–110	95–110	55–65	22–34
Adolescent	65–110	95–110	55–70	18–30
Young person	60–90	110–120	65–80	12–16

Source: adapted from Hazinski 1992.

Normal vital signs

Full blood count for normal infants and children

	Units	Age			
		Newborn Full-term	Up to 6 months	2–6 years	6–12 years
Red blood cells (RBC)	$\times 10^{12}$/l	6.0–6 1.0	3.8–0.8	4.6–0.7	4.6–0.6
Haemoglobin (Hb) g/dl		16.5–3.0	11.5–2.0	12.5–1.5	13.5–2.0
Packed cell volume (PCV)	l/l	0.54–0.10	0.35–0.07	0.37–0.03	0.40–0.05
Mean corpuscular volume (MCV)	fl	110–10	91–17	81–6	86–8
Mean corpuscular haemoglobin (MCH)	pg	34–3	30–5	27–3	29–4
Platelets	$\times 10^9$/l	150–400	150–400	150–400	150–400
White blood count (WBC)	$\times 10^9$/l	18–8	12–6	10–5	9–4
Neutrophils	$\times 10^9$/l	5.0–13.0	1.5–9.0	1.5–8.0	2.0–8.0
Lymphocytes	$\times 10^9$/l	3.0–10.0	4.0–10.0	6.0–9.0	1.0–5.0
Monocytes	$\times 10^9$/l	0.7–1.5	0.1–1.0	0.1–1.0	0.1–1.0
Eosinophils	$\times 10^9$/l	0.2–1.0	0.2–1.0	0.2–1.0	0.1–1.0
Reticulocytes	$\times 10^9$/l	200–500	40–100	20–200	20–200

Source: from Dacie and Lewis 1997.

Urea and electrolytes		
	Value	**Standard units**
Sodium	135–145	mmol/l
Potassium	3.5–5.0	mmol/l
Chloride	98–107	mmol/l
Bicarbonate	22–32	mmol/l
Anion gap	7–17	mmol/l
Urea	2.5–7.5	mmol/l
Creatinine	40–90	µmol/l
Calcium	2.19–2.51	mmol/l
Alb. corrected calcium	2.19–2.51	mmol/l
Magnesium	0.65–0.95	mmol/l
Phosphate	1.2–1.8	mmol/l
Total protein	62–81	g/l
Albumin	37–56	g/l
Alkaline phosphatase	145–320	U/l
Total bilirubin	0–22	µmol/l
Alanine transaminase	0–55	U/l
Aspartate transaminase	0–35	U/l
Gamma glutamyl transpeptidase	8–78	U/l
C reactive protein	7	mg/l

Appendix 2

Units of measurement

Units (SI), the metric system and conversions

The International System of Units (SI) or Système International d'Unités is the measurement system used for scientific, medical and technical purposes in most countries. In the United Kingdom SI units have replaced those of the Imperial System, e.g. the kilogram is used for mass instead of the pound (in everyday situations, both mass and weight are measured in kilograms although weight, which varies with gravity, is really a measure of force).

The SI comprises seven base units with several derived units. Each unit has its own symbol and is expressed as a decimal multiple or submultiple of the base unit by using the appropriate prefix, e.g. millimetre is one thousandth of a metre.

Base units

Quantity	Base unit and symbol
Length	Metre (m)
Mass	Kilogram (kg)
Time	Second (s)
Amount of substance	Mole (mol)
Electric current	Ampere (a)
Thermodynamic temperature	Kelvin (K)
Luminous intensity	Candela (cd)

Derived units

Derived units for measuring different quantities are reached by multiplying or dividing two or more base units.

Quantity	Derived unit and symbol
Work, energy, quantity of heat	Joule (J)
Pressure	Pascal (Pa)
Force	Newton (N)
Frequency	Hertz (Hz)
Power	Watt (W)
Electrical potential, electromotive force, Potential difference	Volt (V)
Absorbed dose of radiation	Gray (Gy)
Radioactivity	Becquerel (Bq)
Dose equivalent	Sievert (Sv)

Factor, decimal multiples and submultiples of SI units

Multiplication factor	Prefix	Symbol
10^{12}	tera	T
10^{9}	giga	G
10^{6}	mega	M
10^{3}	kilo	k
10^{2}	hecto	h
10^{1}	deca	da
10^{-1}	deci	d
10^{-2}	centi	c
10^{-3}	milli	m
10^{-6}	micro	μ
10^{-9}	nano	n
10^{-12}	pico	p
10^{-15}	femto	f
10^{-18}	atto	a

Rules for using units and writing large numbers and decimals

- The symbol for a unit is unaltered in the plural and should not be followed by a full stop except at the end of a sentence: 5 cm not 5 cm. or 5cms.
- Large numbers are written in three-digit groups (working from right to left) with spaces not commas (in some countries the comma is used to indicate a decimal point): fifty thousand is written as 50 000; five hundred thousand is written as 500 000.

- Numbers with four digits are written without the space, e.g. four thousand is written as 4000.

- The decimal sign between digits is indicated by a full stop positioned near the line, e.g. 50.25. If the numerical value of the decimal is less than 1, a zero should appear before the decimal sign: 0.125 not .125.

- Decimals with more than four digits are also written in three-digit groups but this time working from left to right, e.g. 0.000 25.

- 'Squared' and 'cubed' are expressed as numerical powers and not by abbreviation: square centimetre is cm^2 not sq. cm.

Commonly used measurements requiring further explanation

- Temperature – although the SI base unit for temperature is the kelvin, by international convention temperature is measured in degrees Celsius (°C).

- Energy – the energy of food or individual requirements for energy are measured in kilojoules (kJ); the SI unit is the joule (J). In practice many people still use the kilocalorie (kcal), a non-SI unit, for these purposes.

- 1 calorie = 4.2 J

- 1 kilocalorie (large calorie) = 4.2 kJ

- Volume – volume is calculated by multiplying length, width and depth. Using the SI unit for length, the metre (m), means ending up with a cubic metre (m^3), which is a huge volume and is certainly not appropriate for most purposes. In clinical practice the litre (L or l) is used. A litre is based on the volume of a cube measuring 10 cm × 10 cm × 10 cm. Smaller units still, e.g. millilitre (ml) or one thousandth of a litre, are commonly used in clinical practice.

- Time – the SI base unit for time is the second (s), but it is acceptable to use minute (min), hour (h) or day (d). In clinical practice it is preferable to use 'per 24 hours' for the excretion of substances in urine and faeces: g/24 h.

- Amount of substance – the SI base unit for amount of substance is the mole (mol). The concentration of many substances is expressed in moles per litre (mol/l) or millimoles per litre (mmol/l) which replaces milliequivalents per litre (mEq/l). Some exceptions exist and include haemoglobin and plasma proteins in grams per litre (g/l); and enzyme activity in International Units (IU, U or iu).

- Pressure – the SI unit of pressure is the pascal (Pa) and the kilopascal (kPa) replaces the old non-SI unit of millimetres of mercury pressure (mmHg) for blood pressure and blood gases. However, mmHg is still widely used for measuring blood pressure. Other anomalies include cerebrospinal fluid, which is measured in millimetres of water (mmH_2O), and central venous pressure, which is measured in centimetres of water (cmH_2O).

Measurements, equivalents and conversions (SI or metric and imperial)

Length

1 kilometre (km)	= 1000 metres (m)
1 metre (m)	= 100 centimetres (cm) or 1000 millimetres (mm)
1 centimetre (cm)	= 10 millimetres (mm)
1 millimetre (mm)	= 1000 micrometres (μm)
1 micrometre (μm)	= 1000 nanometres (nm)

Conversions

1 metre (m)	= 39.370 inches (in)
1 centimetre (cm)	= 0.3937 inches (in)
30.48 centimetres (cm)	= 1 foot (ft)
2.54 centimetres (cm)	= 1 inch (in)

Volume

1 litre (l)	= 1000 millilitres (ml)
1 millilitre (ml)	= 1000 microlitres (μl)

NB The millilitre (mL) and the cubic centimetre (cm^3) are usually treated as being the same.

Conversions

1 litre (L)	= 1.76 pints (pt)
568.25 millilitres (ml)	= 1 pint (pt)
28.4 millilitres (ml)	= 1 fluid ounce (fl oz)

Weight or mass

1 kilogram (kg)	= 1000 grams (g)
1 gram (g)	= 1000 milligrams (mg)
1 milligram (mg)	= 1000 micrograms (μg)
1 microgram (μg)	= 1000 nanograms (ng)

NB To avoid any confusion with milligram (mg) the word microgram (μg) should be written in full on prescriptions.

Conversions

1 kilogram (kg)	= 2.204 pounds (lb)
1 gram (g)	= 0.0353 ounce (oz)
453.59 grams (g)	= 1 pound (lb)
28.34 grams (g)	= 1 ounce (oz)

Temperature conversions

To convert Celsius to Fahrenheit:

multiply by 9, divide by 5, and add 32 to the result:
e.g. 36°C to Fahrenheit:

$36 \times 9 = 324 \div 5 = 64.8 + 32 = 96.8°F$
therefore $36°C = 96.8°F$

To convert Fahrenheit to Celsius:

subtract 32, multiply by 5, and divide by 9:
e.g. 104°F to Celsius:

$104 - 32 = 72 \times 5 = 360 \div 9 = 40°C$
therefore $104°F = 40°C$

Temperature comparison

°**Celsius**	°**Fahrenheit**
100	212
95	203
90	194
85	185
80	176
75	167
70	158
65	149
60	140
55	131
50	122
45	113
44	112.2
43	109.4
42	107.6
41	105.8

(Continued)

Temperature comparison – (cont'd.)

°Celsius	°Fahrenheit
40	104
39.5	103.1
39	102.2
38.5	101.3
38	100.4
37.5	99.5
37	98.6
36.5	97.7
36	96.8
35.5	95.9
35	95
34	93.2
33	91.4
32	89.6
31	87.8
30	86
25	77
20	68
15	59
10	50
5	41
0	32
−5	23
−10	14

NB Boiling point $= 100°C = 212°F$
Freezing point $= 0°C = 32°F$

Appendix 3

Drug measurement and calculations

The International System of Units (SI) is used for drug doses and concentrations and patient data (including weight and body surface area), drug levels in the body and other measurements (see Appendix 1 for more information).

Weight

Grams (g) and milligrams (mg) are the units most often encountered in drug dosages. Doses of less than 1 g should be expressed in milligrams, e.g. 250 mg rather than 0.25 g. Similarly, doses less than 1 mg should be expressed in micrograms, e.g. 200 micrograms rather than 0.2 mg. Whenever drugs are prescribed in microgram dosages, the units should be written in full, e.g. digoxin 250 micrograms, as the use of the contracted terms μg or mcg may in practice be mistaken for mg and, as this dose is one thousand times greater, disastrous consequences may follow.

Drug dosages are often described in terms of unit dose per kg of body weight, i.e. mg/kg, μg/kg, etc. This method of dosage is frequently used for children and allows dosages to be tailored to the individual patient's size.

Volume

Litres (L or l) and millilitres (mL or ml) account for almost all measurements expressed in unit volume for the prescription and administration of drugs.

Concentration

When expressing concentration of dosages of a medicine in liquid form, several methods are available.

- Unit weight per unit volume – describes the unit of weight of a drug contained in unit volume, e.g. 1 mg in 1 ml, 40 mg in 2 ml. Examples of drugs in common use expressed in these terms: pethidine injection 100 mg in 2 ml; chloral hydrate mixture 1 g in 10 ml; phenoxymethylpenicillin oral solution 250 mg in 5 ml.

- Percentage (weight in volume) – describes the weight of a drug expressed in grams (g) which is contained in 100 ml of solution, e.g. calcium gluconate injection 10% which contains 10 g in each 100 ml of solution, or 1 g in each 10 ml or 100 mg (0.1 g) in each 1 ml.

- Percentage (weight in weight) – describes the weight of a drug expressed in grams (g) which is contained in 100 g of a solid or semisolid medicament, such as ointments and creams, e.g. fusidic acid ointment 2% which contains 2 g of fusidic acid in each 100 g of ointment.

- Volume containing '1 part' – a few liquids and to a lesser extent gases, particularly those containing drugs in very low concentrations, are often described as containing 1 part per 'x' units of volume. For liquids, 'parts' are equivalent to grams and volume to millimetres, e.g. epinephrine (adrenaline) injection 1 in 1000 which contains 1 g in 1000 ml or expressed as a percentage (w/v) – 0.1%.

- Molar concentration – only very occasionally are drugs in liquid form expressed in molar concentration. The mole is the molecular weight of a drug expressed in grams and a one molar (1 M) solution contains this weight dissolved in each litre. More often the millimole (mmol) is used to describe a medicinal product, e.g. potassium chloride solution 15 mmol in 10 ml indicates a solution containing the molecular weight of potassium chloride in milligrams × 15 dissolved in 10 ml of solution.

Body height and surface area

Drug doses may be expressed in terms of microgram, milligram or gram per unit of body surface area. This is frequently the case where precise dosages tailored to individual patients' needs are required. Typical examples may be seen in cytotoxic chemotherapy or in drugs given to children. Body surface area is expressed as square metres or m^2 and drug dosages as units per square metre or units/m^2, e.g. cytarabine injection 100 mg/m^2.

Formulae for calculation of drug doses and drip rates

Oral drugs (solids, liquids)

$$\text{Amount required} = \left\{ \frac{\text{Strength required} \times \text{Volume of stock strength}}{\text{Stock strength}} \right\}$$

Parenteral drugs

(a) Solutions (IM, IV injections)

$$\text{Volume required} = \left\{ \frac{\text{Strength required} \times \text{Volume of stock strength}}{\text{Stock strength}} \right\}$$

(b) Powders

It is essential to follow the manufacturer's directions for dilution, then use the appropriate formula.

(c) IV infusions

$$\text{Rate (drops/min)} = \left\{ \frac{\text{Volume of solution (ml)} \times \text{Number of drops per ml}}{\text{Time (min)}} \right\}$$

Macrodrip (20 drops/ml) – clear fluids

1. $\text{Rate (drops/min)} = \left\{ \dfrac{\text{Volume of solution (ml)} \times 20}{\text{Time (min)}} \right\}$

2. Macrodrip (15 drops/ml) – blood

$$\text{Rate (drops/min)} = \left\{ \frac{\text{Volume of solution (ml)} \times 15}{\text{Time (min)}} \right\}$$

(d) Infusion pumps

$\text{Rate (ml/h)} = \text{Volume (ml)} \div \text{Time (h)}$

(e) IV infusions with drugs

$$\text{Rate (ml/h)} = \left\{ \frac{\text{Amount of drug required (mg/h)} \times \text{Volume of solution (ml)}}{\text{Total amount of drug (mg)}} \right\}$$

NB After selecting the appropriate formula, ensure that all strengths are in the same units, otherwise convert.
1% solution contains 1 g of solute dissolved in 100 ml of solution.
1:1000 means 1 g in 1000 ml of solution, therefore 1 g in 1000 ml is equivalent to 1 mg in 1 ml.

Other useful formulae

Children's dose (Clarke's Body Weight Rule)

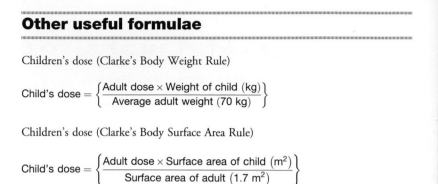

$$\text{Child's dose} = \left\{ \frac{\text{Adult dose} \times \text{Weight of child (kg)}}{\text{Average adult weight (70 kg)}} \right\}$$

Children's dose (Clarke's Body Surface Area Rule)

$$\text{Child's dose} = \left\{ \frac{\text{Adult dose} \times \text{Surface area of child } (m^2)}{\text{Surface area of adult } (1.7 \ m^2)} \right\}$$

Acknowledgements

The measurement section was adapted from Henney C R et al 1995 Drugs in Nursing Practice, 5th edn. Churchill Livingstone, Edinburgh, with permission; and the formulae from Havard M 1994 A Nursing Guide to Drugs, 4th edn. Churchill Livingstone, Edinburgh, with permission.

Useful websites

UK children's charities: health and medicine

British Institute for Brain Injured Children: Offers training, information and support to families and professionals caring for children with conditions affecting the brain (e.g. autism, cerebral palsy, Down's syndrome, traumatic or acquired brain injury, etc.). http://www.bibic.org.uk/

Cardiac Risk in the Young: Provides information, counselling and bereavement support to families affected by sudden cardiac death in young people. http://www.c-r-y.org.uk/index.htm

Children with Cancer: Supports the parents and families of children with leukaemia through welfare projects and programmes within local communities. http://www.childrenwithcancer.org.uk/

Great Ormond Street Hospital Children's Charity: Provides accommodation and support to seriously ill children and their families.
http://www.gosh.org/gen/why-we-need-your-help/our-mission/

Rainbow Trust: Provides counselling, bereavement support and home care services to the parents and families of seriously ill children.
http://www.rainbowtrust.org.uk/

Teenage Cancer Trust: Funds healthcare services and provides educational resources for young people living with cancer. http://www.teenagecancertrust.org/

The Children's Trust: Offers rehabilitative, nursing and medical services to children with acquired brain injury, multiple disabilities and other complex health conditions. http://www.thechildrenstrust.org.uk/

Well Child: Provides financial support and medical care to children with serious illnesses and complex health conditions. http://www.wellchild.org.uk/

UK children's charities: mental health and emotional wellbeing

Action for Sick Children: Supports vulnerable and neglected children through youth programmes, parenting initiatives and advocacy work. http://actionforsickchildren.org/

Bullying UK: Provides resources, counselling and social support to children dealing with bullying in their schools and communities. http://www.bullying.co.uk/

ChildLine: Offers online information and help lines to children dealing with social and emotional problems, such as anxiety, depression, family problems, substance abuse, eating disorders and bullying. http://www.childline.org.uk/explore/Pages/Explore.aspx

KidScape: Works to prevent bullying and develop children's self-confidence through workshops, support groups and educational resources. http://www.kidscape.org.uk/

PAPYRUS: Works to prevent suicide in young people through help line support, education and training. http://www.papyrus-uk.org/

The Beat – Young People: Provides online resources and help line support to young people struggling with eating disorders. http://www.b-eat.co.uk/

The Lucy Faithfull Foundation: Safeguards children and young people from sexual abuse through professional training, counselling and advocacy work. http://lucyfaithfull.org/

Young Minds: Supports young people's mental health and emotional wellbeing by providing advice, information and training to young people, parents and professionals. http://www.youngminds.org.uk/

UK children's charities: social, community and housing support

Depaul UK: Helps homeless young people find emergency accommodation and safe, affordable housing. http://www.depauluk.org/

Family Lives: Provides educational resources and help line support to parents and families dealing with a range of topics, including parenting, bereavement, divorce, abuse, housing, education and childcare. http://familylives.org.uk/

National Children's Bureau: Promotes the social, emotional and physical wellbeing of children through advocacy work, education and support. http://www.ncb.org.uk/

National Deaf Children's Society: Provides information and advice to deaf children, their families and professionals working with deaf children. http://www.ndcs.org.uk/

National Society for the Prevention of Cruelty to Children (NSPCC): Works to prevent child abuse through research, education and the provision of professional and family support services. http://www.nspcc.org.uk/what-we-do/what-we-do-hub_wdh71749.html

Shelter: Gives advice, information and support to young people, families and professionals dealing with homelessness. http://england.shelter.org.uk/about_us

St. Basil's: Provides emergency accommodation, housing services and help lines to young people facing homelessness. http://www.stbasils.org.uk/

Children's support services in the UK

Children and Family Court Advisory and Support Service (CAFCASS): CAFCASS is a public body within the Department for Education which advocates for the best interests of children who are being represented in the family courts. CAFCASS gives a voice to children undergoing family proceedings for adoption, divorce, care supervision and other legal matters. http://www.cafcass.gov.uk/default.aspx

Child Support Agency: The Child Support Agency operates within the Child Maintenance and Enforcement Commission to ensure that parents living away from their child continue to pay child maintenance. http://www.csa.gov.uk/

Secure Accommodation Network: The Secure Accommodation Network (SAN) promotes and develops the children's homes and emergency shelters of 19 local authorities in England and Wales. A directory of homes and a bed availability service is offered to children and professionals who visit their website. http://www.secureaccommodation.org.uk

Children's Legal Centre: The centre provides legal advice information and representation to young people and professionals working on their behalf. Have a particular focus on protecting the rights of migrant and asylum seeking children, and offer free phone support for issues affecting the rights and wellbeing of children.

Glossary of Terms and Abbreviations

A

Accountability
responsibility for your actions

Actrapid infusion
Actrapid is an artificial insulin; an infusion is given in uncontrolled diabetes

Acute
describes illness or condition of rapid onset and of brief duration, e.g. appendicitis

Acidosis
abnormally high acidity of the blood and tissues

Acute epiglottitis
inflammation of the structures above the glottis caused by bacterial infection

Acute compartment syndrome
raised pressure within a closed fascial space

Advocacy
helping to represent a person's interest or viewpoint

Agglutination
clumping of blood cells

Alveoli
air sacs in the lung

Amputation
surgical removal of a limb (arm, leg) or finger or toe

Anaesthetist
a specialist doctor who oversees respiratory function during an operation.

Anaemia
a condition in which the number of red blood cells in the blood is low

Analgesia
broad term given to the group of drugs that relieve pain

Anaphylaxis
occurs when a sensitized child is exposed to an antigen, to which s/he is allergic

Anion
an ion that carries a negative charge

Anticoagulant
drug that prevents clotting of the blood

Antibody
specialized immune protein produced in reaction to an antigen

ADH
antidiuretic hormone

Apnoea
absence of breathing

Arterial blood gases (ABG)
determined from arterial blood
to measure a patient's acid–base
status and so determine severity of
a particular medical condition, e.g.
asthma, diabetes

Arrhythmia
an abnormality of electrical conduction
through the heart

Anencephaly
a neural tube defect (NTD) that occurs
when the cephalic (head) end of the
neural tube fails to close, usually between
the 23rd and 26th days of pregnancy,
resulting in the absence of a major
portion of the brain, skull, and scalp.

Anxiety disorder
a chronic condition characterized by an
excessive and persistent sense of
apprehension with physical symptoms
such as sweating, palpitations, and
feelings of stress. Anxiety disorders have
biological and environmental causes.

Aseptic technique
sterile technique to prevent infection

Asthma
narrowing and inflammation of
the bronchial airways leading to
difficulty in breathing and wheezing,
precipitated by exposure to a wide
range of stimuli.

Assessment
identifying and documenting the child's
physical, psychological and social needs

Asystole
absence of electrical activity in the heart

Attachment
emotional bond between a child and
another person

Atelectasis
collapse of the lung

Atrial fibrillation (AF)
fast chaotic irregular heart rhythm

Auscultation
listening with the use of a stethoscope

Autonomy
capacity to think and decide freely

Autoclaving
sterilization of instruments

B

Bacterial tracheitis
diffuse inflammation of the larynx,
trachea and bronchi

Bacteraemia
presence of bacteria in the blood

Beneficence
doing good to others

Bereavement
loss of a person due to death

Bradycardia
low heart rate

BiLevel positive airways pressure (BPAP)
non-invasive ventilation, which requires external mask attachment

Bilirubin
waste product of red blood cell breakdown, 99% excreted in faeces, 1% excreted in the urine as urobilinogen

Blood glucose level (BGL)
measure of glucose (sugar) in blood to determine diabetes (high). Can be an indication of malnutrition or dieting if low

Blood pressure (BP)
the pressure in blood that ensures circulation throughout the body from the right side of the heart to the left

Blood products
administered in hospital or emergency situation via the intravenous route to maintain blood pressure and body circulation

Blood results
blood contains a normal level of many of the body's waste products, electrolytes, proteins, haemoglobin, glucose required for normal body function. These can be measured and contribute to a personal diagnosis

Blood transfusion
the introduction of blood into a blood vessel, replacement of lost or destroyed blood by compatible human blood

BM Stix
a thin stick used to measure blood glucose level

Body mass index (BMI)
a measure using the formula weight/height^2 to determine a patient's propensity towards obesity or under nutrition

Bonding
another term for attachment

Brain stem dead
the brain stem is situated at the top of the spine and at the base of the skull, in serious brain injury if this fails to function the patient is termed brain stem dead

Bradycardia
slow heart rate, resulting in a slow pulse rate

Breathless
having difficulty in breathing in or out depending on cause

British National Formulary (BNF)
a book giving all up-to-date information regarding drugs, e.g. names, doses, side effects

Bronchiolitis
inflammation of the bronchioles of the lungs

Bronchopulmonary dysplasia (BPD)
a chronic lung disease of babies, which most commonly develops in the first 4 weeks after birth and most often affects babies born at least 4 weeks before term

Buccal medication
medication given via the oral cavity

C

Cancer
any malignant tumour that arises from the abnormal and uncontrolled division of cells that then invade and destroy the surrounding tissues

Cannula
tube inserted into the body

Cardiac arrest
a state whereby the person's heart stops beating or fails to supply the rest of the body with blood

Cardiogenic shock
occurs when the heart, due to impaired myocardial performance, cannot produce an adequate cardiac output to sustain the metabolic requirements of body tissues

Cardiomyopathy
congenital disease of the heart not caused by a defect or hypertension, generally degenerative and can lead to serious arrhythmia

Cardiopulmonary resuscitation (CPR)
maintains external cardiac and respiratory function through cardiac massage and artificial breathing

Catheter/catheterization
insertion of thin tube into the bladder to facilitate patients to pass urine or to measure urine output

Catabolism
energy burning aspect of metabolism

Cation
an ion carrying a positive electric charge

Central venous pressure (CVP)
measured by placing a small catheter through a neck vein down into the right atrium of the heart

Chemotherapy
use of chemical agents to prevent the growth and spread of a tumour. Related to the treatment of cancer

Chest X-ray (CXR)
radiographic picture of the lungs

Chest pain
type of severe pain between the ribs that generally radiates down the left arm – sign of a heart attack

Child protection (or child safeguarding)
system of protecting children identified as either experiencing neglect or abuse

Chronic
gradual onset and long duration of an illness or condition

Clotting factors
manufactured by the liver and forms a clot when blood loss is threatened

CMV
cytomegalovirus

Coma
depression of the central nervous and respiratory centre systems

Consent
agreement to a procedure

Colostomy
a surgical operation in which a part of the colon is brought through the abdominal wall and opened in order to drain the intestine; may be temporary or permanent

Computerized tomography scan (CT)
a diagnostic procedure used for examining soft tissue

Confusion
a mental state whereby a patient may not know where or who they are, the time or date or recognize family or friends

Cognitive development
ability to reason, think and understand

Cognition
process of thought

Congenital condition
a condition or disease either genetically acquired or caused by damage while in the mother's womb

Coronary care unit (CCU)
A specialist area of nursing, caring for patients with potential for or after having a heart attack

Cricoid cartilage
a ring of cartilage in the throat that is rigid and not distendable

Cricoid pressure
pressure on the cricoid cartilage of the throat to prevent aspiration during intubation

Critical thinking
to use higher-level thinking and reasoning

Crystalloid
intravenous fluid that contains electrolytes

Cyanosis
bluish discoloration of the skin due to lack of oxygen

Cystic fibrosis
hereditary disease that affects the exocrine glands resulting in thick sticky mucus, which builds up and causes problems in many of the body's organs, especially the lungs and pancreas

Cytokines
produced as a result of the immune response recognizing foreign antigens; they activate T cells to achieve cellular inflammatory responses and drive B cells to produce antibodies in the humoral immune response

D

Deep vein thrombosis (DVT)
a blood clot in the vein in the calf of the leg

Dehydration
fluid loss in the cells and blood

Depression
a condition when feelings of sadness and other symptoms make it hard to get through the day, and when the symptoms last for more than a couple of weeks in a row

Diabetes insipidus

excessive urination and extreme thirst as a result of inadequate output of the pituitary hormone ADH (antidiuretic hormone also called vasopressin) or the lack of the normal response by the kidney to ADH

Diabetes mellitus (DM) types I & II

an inability of the pancreas to release insulin. Type I is generally congenital and requires insulin injections and diet control. Type II is generally of late onset and requires oral drugs and diet control and possibly insulin

Diabetic ketoacidosis

occurs when there is insufficient insulin in the body, and the cells cannot utilize glucose and it accumulates in the blood

Difficulty in breathing

breathlessness, unable to effectively move air into the lungs

Dignity

respect for a person's worth

Disseminated intravascular coagulation (DIC)

clotting and bleeding occurring together throughout the body

Diuretics

increase the amount of urine that the kidneys produce

Dysphagia

disorder of swallowing

Dysphasic/aphasia

disorder of language following brain damage

E

Ecological approach

approach that considers the child's home routine and family environment when encouraging long-term lifestyle change

Electrocardiograph (ECG)

measures the electrical impulses running through the heart at regular intervals. There are generally 12 leads, which look at the heart from all angles

Electroencephalogram (EEG)

non-invasive diagnostic test that records electrical activity of the brain

Embolus

an occlusion or obstruction of a vessel by air, cholesterol or thrombus

Emphysema

a long-term, progressive disease of the lungs that primarily causes shortness of breath due to over-inflation of the alveoli

Endotracheal tube (ETT)

oral or nasal tube passed into the lungs on patients who can no longer maintain their own airway e.g. when unconscious

Epistaxis

nose bleed

Extubated

when a breathing tube is removed from a patient who has been unable to maintain their own airway or breathe for themselves due to major illness

Exogenous

outside the patient's body

Exudate
fluid or cells that have oozed out of blood vessels

Endogenous
inside the patient's body

Evaluation
reviewing how the interventions have worked

F

Fracture
a break in the continuity of a bone

G

Gastroschisis
Condition where the bowel herniates through a defect in the abdominal wall

Gastrostomy
a tube passed from the surface of the skin through the abdominal wall into the stomach; usually for artificial feeding

Gingiva
gum in the mouth

Glasgow coma scale (GCS)
a quick and easy measure to determine mental state of an unconscious patient

Glomerulonephritis
a disease affecting the glomerulus, the tiny ball-shaped structure in the kidney composed of capillary blood vessels that is actively involved in the filtration of the blood to form urine. The main sign of the disease is marked proteinuria (protein in the urine)

Guedel airway
a thick plastic tube passed into the mouth when a patient is unconscious and unable to maintain their own airway

H

Haematology
the study of disorders of the blood

Haemolysis
destruction of red blood cells

Haemodilution
dilution of the blood

Haemodynamic
a state of the body, e.g. stable or unstable; generally refers to cardiovascular status e.g. blood pressure, heart rate, respiratory rate, urinary output and temperature

Haemothorax
collection of blood within the pleural cavity

Health promotion
enables children to meet their full potential and develop into healthy young adults

Heart failure
the heart fails as a pump generally due to an underlying cardiac condition

Heart rate (HR)
the rhythmic beat of the heart. It can be counted at various points around the body where an artery flows over a bone, measured in beats per min (bpm)

Heat moisture exchange (HME)
captures the heat and moisture exhaled by the patient and then circulates it back into the patient's inhaled gas

Heimlich manoeuvre
a series of subdiaphragmatic thrusts with the purpose of forcing air out of the lungs

Hepatomegaly
enlarged liver

High dependency unit (HDU)
a specialist area of nursing where patients are acutely ill and require moderate invasive therapies

Homeostasis
the body's attempts to compensate for a threat, e.g. by increasing heart rate, respiratory rate and blood pressure

Hospital acquired infection (HAI)
an infection acquired while the patient is in hospital

Human immunodeficiency virus (HIV)
a virus carried by humans that if infected leads to acquired immune deficiency syndrome (AIDS)

Humidification
adding moisture

Hydranencephaly
a condition in which the cerebral hemispheres of the brain are absent and replaced by sacs filled with cerebrospinal fluid

Hydrocephalus
a congenital condition determined by an excess of cerebral spinal fluid (CSF) inside the skull due to an obstruction to normal CSF circulation

Hyperglycaemia
a high blood glucose level

Hypoglycaemia
a low blood glucose level

Hypercapnia
excess levels of carbon dioxide in the blood

Hyperpyrexia
very high temperature $> 40\,°C$

Hyperkalaemia
high concentration of potassium

Hypotension
a blood pressure that is below the normal range

Hypothermia
a body temperature below $35.5°C$

Hypoventilation
reduced ventilation of the lungs

Hypovolaemia
condition when a person's blood loss is so great the body's homeostatic mechanisms can no longer maintain blood circulation

Hypoxia
when all cells, or a part of the body, are starved of oxygen, e.g. as in a stroke

I

Implementation
carrying out the interventions planned

Internalization
view that illness may be located within the body

Infection control
a list of general principles that prevent infection from transferring from one patient to another in hospital, e.g. hand washing, use of antiseptic hand gel

Inflammatory immune response (IIR)
the body's normal defence mechanism against infection following injury

Integrated care pathways (ICPs)
documented policies and guidelines for delivering integrated care

Intracranial pressure monitoring (ICP)
measure of the pressure within the brain, generally around 0–15 mmHg

Intramuscular injection
injection into a muscle

Insulin
a pancreatic hormone that regulates glucose in the blood, can be given artificially by injection in diabetes

Intensive therapy unit (ITU)
a specialist area of nursing where patients are critically ill and require high technological invasive therapies

Intravenous (IV) cannula/therapy
a needle is placed into a vein so fluids can be administered to replace loss

Intubated, intubation
An act of passing a tube (ETT) into the trachea to initiate artificial breathing (ventilation), involves the use of an ETT (see above)

Irrigation
flushing with a liquid

Ischaemia
loss or reduced blood supply to an organ of the body

J

Jaundice
associated with liver failure and gall stones, when bile cannot drain out of the liver via the bile duct and excess bile is taken up by the tissues and the patient appears yellow in colour

K

Ketones
when cells are starved of glucose, fat is broken down into fatty acids and these fatty acids are converted to ketones in the liver

L

Laryngoscope
instrument that provides a pathway along which the endotracheal tube can be passed into the airway

Laryngoscopy
visual examination of the vocal tissue and glottis

Laryngospasm
involuntary closure of the larynx, obstructing the flow of oxygen

Laryngectomy
surgical removal of the larynx

Last offices
a procedure that takes place by a nurse for a patient following their death

Level of consciousness
the alertness level of the brain and what it takes to awaken it if damaged

Liver failure
a failure of the liver to function adequately, affecting all other body functions

M

Medical assessment unit (MAU)
an area of accident and emergency that initially assesses patients prior to admission to hospital

Melanoma
a tumour arising from the deep cells in the skin

Metabolic diseases (inborn errors of metabolism)
hereditary (genetic) disorders of biochemistry

Metastasis
the distant spread of disease, especially a malignant tumour from its site of origin

Monitoring
a variety of equipment for continuous measurement of heart rate, blood pressure, temperature, respiratory rate and oxygen saturation

Model
a way of grouping ideas into a framework

Multidisciplinary team (MDT)
all health care professionals involved in patient care, e.g. GP, pharmacist, consultant, nurse, physiotherapist, occupational therapist, specialist nurse (pain, wound)

Multidrug resistant *Staphylococcus aureus* (MRSA)
a strain of bacteria that is resistant to most of the current antibiotic therapies

Multiple myeloma
more than one tumour occurring in bone tissue

Myocardial infarction
heart attack

N

Nasogastric tube
an artificial tube passed through the nose into the stomach, used for artificial feeding

Nebulizers
drugs given through oxygen or air under pressure for certain lung conditions, e.g. asthma, chronic obstructive pulmonary disease

Neoplasm
a tumour or an abnormal growth of tissue. The word neoplasm is not synonymous with cancer. a neoplasm may be benign or malignant

Nephrotic syndrome
disease of the kidneys characterized by high levels of protein in the urine

Neurological assessment
a set of criteria that determines neurological deterioration

Neutropenia
lack of neutrophils, which are a type of white blood cell that help the cell to kill and digest microorganisms

Neurogenic shock
result of a severe brain stem injury at the level of the medulla, an injury to the spinal cord, or spinal anaesthesia

Non-maleficence
avoid causing harm to others

Nursing model
framework for providing nursing care

O

Obesity
accumulation of excess fat on the body and having a body mass index (BMI) of greater than 30. The BMI is a measure of your weight relative to your height

Oedema
the abnormal accumulation of fluid in certain tissues within the body

Opioid
a group of narcotics that relieve strong pain

Osmolality
a concentration of solution expressed as osmoles of solute particles per kilogram of solvent

Overweight
child who weighs more than expected

Oxygen saturation
the measure of the molecules of oxygen attached to haemoglobin in the blood

P

Palliative care
medical or comfort care that reduces the severity of a disease or slows its progress rather than providing a cure

Papilloedema
swollen pupils due to fluid movement into the interstitial space usually due to trauma

Paralysis
complete or incomplete loss of nervous function to a part of the body

Parenteral
entering the body not by the alimentary tract but rather by another means (such as the subcutaneous, the intramuscular, or often the intravenous route)

Participation
taking part

Past medical history (PMH)
enquiring into the medical history of a patient

Patient-controlled analgesia (PCA)
pain relief that is controlled and self administered by the patient

Perinatal
the period immediately before and after birth

Petechiae
small haemorrhagic (bruise like) spots generally found on the skin

Polycystic kidney disease
one of the genetic disorders characterized by the development of innumerable cysts in the kidneys, which are filled with fluid, and replace much of the mass of the kidneys, thus reducing kidney function and leading to kidney failure.

Positive end-expiratory pressure (PEEP)
pressure within alveoli which occurs at the start of a breath

Post-traumatic stress
an anxiety disorder that develops in some individuals who have had major traumatic experiences

Pharmacology
the study of drugs and their effects on the body

Philosophy
viewpoint or set of values

Phlebitis
acute inflammation of a vein directly linked to the presence of any vascular device

Planning
setting goals and outcomes for the care plan

Plasmapheresis
the process of removing autoantibodies from the bloodstream mechanically using a process similar to that used in renal failure treatment

Pleurisy
inflammation of the pleural tissue lining of the lungs

Pneumonia
infection of lung tissue by the *Pneumococcus* bacteria

Pneumothorax
collapsed lung due to collection of air between the pleura of the lungs seen in trauma

Polymyopathy
inflammation of the muscles

Postoperative care
care and management of a patient following surgery

Pulmonary embolism (PE)
a clot occurring in one of the major arteries (blood vessels) of the lungs, which generally occurs following long-haul flights

Pulse oximeter
a monitor that is placed on the finger to measure oxygen saturation of blood

Pupil reaction to light
when a light is shined into the eye the pupil should change size quickly indicating the 3rd cranial nerve is functioning

R

Radiotherapy
the treatment of disease (usually cancer) with ionizing radiation

Reflection
paying attention to significant aspects of an experience in order to make sense of it

Renal failure
failure of kidneys to function

Respiration
act of breathing

Respiratory failure
the lungs fail to work, this may require intubation and artificial ventilation

Respiratory rate
respiratory rate – the rate of breathing, the lungs should expand symmetrically

Resuscitation
a term used to indicate the administration of invasive therapy when a patient's condition is deteriorating

Retinopathy
damage to the retina of the eye

Retropharyngeal abscesses
serious infection of the retropharyngeal space

Rewarming
gradual re-warming of the hypothermic patient

Rh factor
antigen found in red blood cells

Robinson drain
a small tube inserted into a wound following surgery to remove excess fluid that may collect internally

S

SABRE system
serious adverse blood reactions and events system

Safeguarding
process of protecting children from abuse or neglect

Semiconscious
a mental state whereby the person is not fully aware of their surroundings; there are varying degrees of this state

Seizures
caused by abnormal electrical discharges in the brain

Self harm
a form of intentional physical self-damage or self-harm that is not accompanied by suicidal intent or ideation. Examples include cutting, burning, stabbing, or excessive rubbing

Sensorimotor
learning is mainly through the senses and physical activity

Septic shock
caused by an overwhelming infection

Shock
a condition associated with circulatory collapse, when the blood pressure is too low to maintain an adequate supply of blood to the tissues

Sickle cell disease
a hereditary blood disease that mainly affects people of African ancestry. It occurs when the sickle cell gene has been inherited from both parents, characterized by an abnormal production of haemoglobin

Sickle cell crisis
a severe attack that causes pain because blood vessels can become blocked or the defective red blood cells can damage organs in the body

Sinus rhythm (SR)
the normal electrical rhythm of the heart shown on a cardiac monitor

Squamous cell carcinoma
a type of cancer that emerges from squamous cells – a specialist type of body tissue that covers external body surfaces

Systolic pressure
pressure of the blood as a result of contraction of the ventricles

Status asthmaticus
acute exacerbation of asthma that may be unresponsive to initial treatment with bronchodilators; the condition becomes progressively worse

Stoma
artificial opening into the body from the outside created by a surgeon

Stridor
noisy sound on inspiration due to obstruction of airway

Stroke/cerebral vascular accident (CVA)
an area of the brain suffers a period of hypoxia due to a bleed or clot (fat or blood)

Subarachnoid haemorrhage (SAH)
rupture of an artery in the brain leading to a stroke

Suctioning
removal of secretions

Supraventricular tachycardia (SVT)
a very fast heart rate that is regular but with abnormal electrical complexes

Systemic lupus erythematosus (SLE)
an autoimmune process that affects all organs of the body

T

Tachycardia
a fast heart rate above normal for age range. Compensatory mechanism of the body to maintain homeostasis

Tachypnoea
rapid breathing

Tamponade
collection of fluid around the heart that can cause cardiac arrest

TED stockings
white elasticized stockings that create pressure on the outside of the legs to prevent oedema and deep vein thrombosis (DVT) formation

Tension pneumothorax
life-threatening condition where air cannot escape from the chest, leading to a build up in the thorax

Terminally ill
a patient who will not recover and eventually will die

Thrombus
a clot in the cardiovascular system formed from constituents of blood

Thrombocytopenia
a lower platelet count in the blood compared to the normal range

Tidal volume
the amount of air which passes in and out of the lungs in normal quiet breathing.

Tinnitus
ringing sound in the ear

Total parenteral nutrition (TPN)
nutrition is administered intravenously via a central venous line (CVP)

Transdermal
medication given via the skin

Tracheostomy
opening in the neck into the trachea to allow breathing

Tracheal stenosis
narrowing of the trachea

Tracheo-oesphageal fistula
opening due to failure of the trachea to separate from the oesophagus before birth

Tuberculosis (TB)
an infectious disease caused by the bacterium *Mycobacterium tuberculosis*

U

Ultrasound
sound waves of extremely high frequency inaudible to the human ear. Can be used to examine the structure of the inside of the body and can be used to break up stones and cataracts

Unconsciousness
state of unawareness and inability to perceive

Urticaria
raised itchy area of skin due to allergic reaction

V

Vasodilation
dilation of a vessel

Vegetative state (VS)
a condition of sleep–wake cycles in which patients experience wakefulness but lack awareness of their self and their surroundings

Venepuncture
insertion of a needle into a vein to obtain a blood sample

Ventilation
mechanical means of infusing the lungs with air and oxygen

Ventilator
machine that supports breathing

Ventricular tachycardia (VT)
a fast undefined heart rate that is life threatening

Ventricular fibrillation
uncoordinated contractions of the cardiac muscle of the ventricles

Ventilation/perfusion (V/Q scanning)
two different isotopes are used, one inhaled to examine lung ventilation and one injected, to examine lung perfusion, used to detect pulmonary embolism

Vital signs
includes blood pressure (BP), heart rate (HR), respiratory rate (RR) and temperature (temp)

W

Wound care
caring for an opening in the skin either from surgery or trauma, uses aseptic technique and a variety of assessment tools, wound dressings and techniques

Index

NB: Page numbers in *italics* refer to boxes, figures, tables.

Index